Kindly submit five copies of new manuscripts to

Albert J. Solnit, M.D.
Yale Child Study Center
P.O. Box 3333
New Haven, CT 06510

The
Psychoanalytic
Study
of the Child

VOLUME FORTY-FOUR

The Psychoanalytic Study of the Child

VOLUME FORTY-FOUR

Kindly submit five copies of new manuscripts to

Albert J. Solnit, M.D.
Yale Child Study Center
P.O. Box 3333
New Haven, CT 06510

The
Psychoanalytic
Study
of the Child

VOLUME FORTY-FOUR

New Haven and London
Yale University Press
1989

Designed by Sally Harris
and set in Baskerville type.
Printed in the United States of America by
Vail-Ballou Press, Inc., Binghamton, N.Y.

Library of Congress catalog card number: 45–11304
International standard book number: 0–300–04594–8

The paper in this book meets the guidelines for
permanence and durability of the Committee on
Production Guidelines for Book Longevity of the
Council on Library Resources.

2   4   6   8   10   9   7   5   3   1

Contents

PSYCHOANALYTIC THEORY

The Place of the Adolescent Process in the Analysis of the Adult

PETER BLOS, Ph.D.

HAVING BEEN INVITED TO SPEAK ON THIS OCCASION WHICH HONORS SIG-
mund Freud by commemorating his birthday every spring makes me
feel pleased and proud. I delivered the Freud lecture in Vienna two
years ago, so today's occasion gives me a sense of completion. Now I
have expressed my indebtedness—intellectually, professionally, philosophically, and aesthetically—to the founder of psychoanalysis in the
best way I know how. I have done this in the two cities where I learned
the fundamentals of psychoanalysis, where I practiced it, where I came
to realize the boundless complexity of this science, and where my
mounting curiosity for the not yet fully understood had become the
natural way of my clinical attention and of my thinking about the
human mind; where, in short, I had followed, like every student of
psychoanalysis, the lengthy and exhilarating, often painful and disap-
pointing journey which we hope leads every analyst to the state and
practice of the art.

My awareness of psychoanalysis as an awesome system of ideas,
promising a limitless comprehension of the human mind, came to me
first in the course of my fortuitous acquaintance with Anna Freud.
This occurred in 1925, soon after I had arrived in Vienna to continue
my studies in biology at the University of Vienna. Due to this circumstance my first impression of psychoanalysis was focused on childhood.
Subsequently, again by fortuitous circumstances, my focus shifted; this

Life Member, American Psychoanalytic Association; faculty, Columbia University
Center for Psychoanalytic Training and Research.

Freud Anniversary lecture, the New York Psychoanalytic Institute and Society, Acade-
my of Medicine, New York, April 12, 1988.

time to the terminal stage of childhood, namely, to adolescence. This occurred in the course of my affiliation with that legendary man, August Aichhorn, who became my teacher, mentor, and paternal friend. These beginnings or years of apprenticeship date back about 60 years. In retrospect I might say that these two personalities had watched unknowingly and unwittingly, like two good fairies, over my psychoanalytic cradle, introducing me patiently to my professional future. Today after 60 years I am still at work in deciphering the mysteries of adolescence and in laying bare its trifold relatedness: one to early childhood, one to its specific function as a developmental phase, and one to its critical involvement in the life of the adult. This broad schema of the crucially conjunctive or linking position which adolescence occupies in human development grew quite naturally out of my analytic work with children, adolescents, and adults, male and female.

In order to delineate the position from which my clinical observations of the adolescent mind originated, I resort briefly to metaphorical speech. I view my growing attention to adolescence as being a determined approach to the two opposing shores of a river, trekking my way closer from the vast hinterlands of childhood and adulthood to the connecting rushing waters between those two shores, namely, to adolescence. Having arrived at this bridging passageway which joins the two shores, I set up my observation post in the middle of this crowded thoroughfare, watching the endless traffic of people moving back and forth from both sides—some rushing ahead, then stopping and waiting in indecision; some retreating, then suddenly changing direction altogether. Viewing this imaginary landscape of movement and direction, you probably have had no trouble in translating it into the psychoanalytic theory of adolescent development.

My adolescent research and the clinical observations on which it was founded, inclusive of its structural and dynamic extrapolations from normal child and adult development, as well as from the psychopathology of these periods of life, have followed the time-honored model of such investigative enterprises. This is to say that clinical observations become translated into theoretical formulations, which in turn are subjected to the testing of their validity or, pragmatically speaking, of their clinical usefulness. This process may lead to a reasoned deletion or judicious modification of traditionally held propositions because at this point in time and this stage of theory-building they have become incomplete or misleading. As a consequence, the ensuing shift in the comprehension of clinical data introduces a revision of theoretical conceptualizations, which in turn are followed by plausible departures from the prevailing technique of the time.

I intend in what follows to give an account of my studies in adolescent psychology, the consequences of which extend far beyond the confines of this particular developmental stage; in fact, they have led me irrefutably to modifications of some aspects of established psychoanalytic theory. The deepening of our understanding of adolescence has affected not only our grasp of early childhood development but quite unexpectedly that of the adult personality, of the epigenesis of the adult neurosis, and therefore of the analysis of the adult. Such claims require empirical evidence which I intend to present. In order to accomplish this task, I have first to set the stage for its delivery by strengthening the logic of my argument and, in addition, link my propositions to the history and tradition of psychoanalytic thought. As part of this effort I shall later take a brief excursion into some of Freud's writings which are of particular relevance for the issues of my investigation.

The first psychoanalytic conceptualization of adolescence was based on Freud's *Three Essays on the Theory of Sexuality* (1905) or, more precisely, on the third essay, "The Transformations of Puberty." The psychoanalytic concept of adolescence was firmly founded on the two commentaries about infantile sexuality, preoedipal and oedipal. Both constitute the preeminent reference points of development which become reanimated by the biological event of sexual maturation. The psychoanalytic theory of adolescence was essentially determined by a reduction to its genetic and dynamic forerunners, namely, the two comprehensively defined and clinically validated developmental stages of prelatency, and preoedipal and oedipal periods. Due to these facts I called the classic psychoanalytic theory of adolescence a recapitulation theory.

At the time I started to work with adolescents, this theory presented the uncontested baseline from which every therapeutic effort with this age group was launched and from which its therapeutic direction and its rationale were derived. All enlightenment with reference to adolescence was derived from the comprehension of infantile sexuality, its history of the concurrent object relations and their implicit conflicts, as well as the relative states of the ego. The dominant concept in the explanatory schema of adolescence, normal and abnormal, was without doubt the oedipus complex as perceived within the larger context of the loosening and final dissolution of parental dependencies. The adolescent process became ever more clearly identified by its specific function of taking the final and definitive step in the resolution of all those straggling preadult immaturities and inner discordances within the scope of whatever they have come to mean over time to any given

individual. Whether adolescent changes are predominantly determined by progressive or regressive moves, we never fail to recognize in
them selective imprints of original interactions between the young
child and his animate and inanimate surround.

As documented in the history of psychoanalysis, refinements and
innovations in theory derived most markedly and repeatedly from
cases of failure or disappointment in analytic work. I am certainly not
the first who has gathered courage in such distressing moments of
work from a comment by Freud (1918) and as a consequence has taken
a fresh look at what previously seemed to be so well understood.
Freud's comment reads: "Something new can only be gained from
analyses that present special difficulties" (p. 10). I allude here to the
time when I slowly came to question the centrality of the oedipus
complex and whether or not it had been given too monolithic a place in
the psychoanalytic understanding of adolescence. Of course, I was
aware of the shift in the comprehension of adolescent psychic reorganization which the structural theory and the refinements of ego
psychology had introduced. I was equally aware of the gradual shift of
focus in adolescent clinical research from drive-centered conflict to
that of a characterologically adaptive and defensive organization,
which renders the last touches during the waning stage of childhood,
called adolescence, to what we generally refer to as personality consolidation. In spite of these mighty advances in theory, the psychoanalytic
conceptual armamentarium at my disposal had come in some crucial
respects to a decline in its usefulness. This was glaringly evident in
some cases, while in others therapy proceeded well in its classic famil-
iarity. Nevertheless, my work with certain adolescents left me with a
mild but distinctive sense of dissatisfaction and incompleteness, especially as to its theoretical perspicuity.

I repeatedly made an observation in my work with adolescents which
attracted my attention. I am referring to the repeated ineffectualness
of oedipal interpretations concerning actions, thoughts, and fantasies
of a typical oedipal nature. This in itself is nothing new or surprising.
Nevertheless I was puzzled as to why these therapeutic interventions
were responded to with such equanimity and indifference. I suspected
that this kind of stalemate in therapy had something to teach me. Since
at this time I was preoccupied with certain questions and suppositions
regarding the classic recapitulation theory of adolescence, I had to be
careful in keeping a clear distinction between what I saw clinically in
my patients and what I wished to see as supportive evidence of my
theory-building. In essence, I was trying to disentangle preoedipal

psychological content from oedipal phenomenology in adolescence, for example, in the boy's proverbial conflict-proneness to his father or the girl's to her mother. I found myself often confronted with an impasse in the resolution of oedipal problems via interpretations and was faced with the technical challenge: where do I go from here?

As a general precaution I had to avoid taking recourse in the too often and too globally applied expedient of relegating this kind of therapeutic impasse to resistance or to transference complications or to unanalyzability. Being familiar with the role of these typical explications in analytic work with adolescents, I was at the time perplexed in such cases by the ineffectuality of oedipal defense analysis. To my surprise the patients showed no signs of negativism to treatment, quite the contrary. I asked myself, can all this be attributed to and subsumed under the concepts of a positive transference or to transference acting out?

What puzzled me was the simultaneity of the patient's ready and willing acceptance of oedipal interpretations and their coincidental ineffectualness on the patient's psychological status. In fact, the patient's affirmation and seemingly gratifying responsiveness to oedipal interpretations, which normally evoke some emotional turbulence, protest, or hesitancy in acceptance, made me suspicious of a perverse gratification being at play, where one might expect an unsettling, yet also liberating, insight to be evoked.

Was it possible that pathogenic determinants were ignored because the current psychoanalytic theory of adolescence was not cognizant of them? Such a posture not only puts the analyst's narcissism on the line but also tends to goad his countertransference potential into treacherous accommodations, such as overloading his empathy system with active participation in the patient's problems. I have in mind the therapist's tender of guidance, advice, or even theoretical explanations to the patient of his disturbed or disturbing behavior and emotions. Might such involvements counteract the patient's secret plot to abandon therapy? Given the adolescent's proclivity to action, this possibility must always be reckoned with. These and similar impasse situations do legitimize interventions of using so-called rational, commonsense advice, as long as its administration is founded on psychoanalytic thought and not on rationalizations of a therapist in distress. Such crisis digressions from standard technique do not, in my opinion, necessarily put the therapeutic process at risk. These typical adolescent vagaries in treatment have repeatedly called the analyzability of adolescents into question. Such doubts and controversies are often argued unconvincingly in the light of the intrinsic nature of adolescence rather than as a consequence of an incompleteness in the prevailing psychoanalytic theory of this age.

No student of adolescence has ever failed to realize the impact of sexual maturation on behavior, mood, thought, and affect. We recognize this impact in the overpowering need of youth for a social acknowledgment of their functioning as an autonomous self (of having "authenticity," as the present-day saying goes) and for a confirmation of their masculinity or femininity, as manifested in social and sexual expressions, realized in fantasy, self-gratification, or bodily affective interaction with the same or other sex. Beyond that we observe volatile mood changes, increased self-absorption, a disposition toward social isolation, as well as an insatiable and irrepressible gregariousness. A solipsistic posture prevails in its broad spectrum from active to passive in relatedness and separateness, in sharing with others and being shared by them. This familiar panorama can be viewed from a developmental perspective as passing stages of tentative role tryouts of the new pubertal self in all its potential realizations working synergically toward a postchildhood identity. This process brings in its course a decrease of developmental plasticity and a growing rigidity or unpliability of the personality; in other words, we witness the emergence of character. This principle applies dramatically to two hallmark aspects of childhood or, more exactly, of preadult life, namely, playfulness and bisexuality.

I might mention as an aside that society has always provided institutionalized occasions in adult life for the exercise of these preadult pleasurable indulgences. At these times superego interdictions are suspended by social consensus, and all kinds of behavioral licenses are granted as to sensual excesses. The respective festivities are calendrically fixed and restricted in duration. I mention as examples the Saturnalia of ancient Rome or the Carneval of the Christian era. The most conspicuous characteristic of this festivity lies in the playful game of publicly dressing up. By the use of mask and costume one's identity becomes changed as to age, sex, and looks, ranging from the hideous to the beautiful. In modern life there is the carousing behavior at convention times or at reunions, which are observed in celebration of "when we were young." Both preadult pleasure modes of which I speak, playfulness and bisexuality, are paradise lost with the closure of adolescence; both seek a last fling before this happens when either extraversive or introversive excesses make their startling but transient adolescent appearance. Neither of these two aspects of childhood lets itself be easily left behind without the person attempting a rescue by compromise. These cherished but largely lost causes, hung onto for dear life, are rediscovered in the analysis of the adult among the far-flung returns of the repressed and within the comprehensive neurosogenic history of the patient. They represent the residual relics from a derailed or never completely traversed adolescence. At a later point I shall return to this train of thought.

Much of what I have thus far related about adolescence has been known to the Western world ever since Aristotle's eloquent and enlightening essay on Athenian youth.[1] It was left to psychoanalysis to transcribe such observations along with those of other perceptive writers as well as the data of descriptive psychology into a developmentally coherent system of psychological principles and concepts.

In dislocating the role of the oedipus complex from its accustomed place in our grasp of adolescent mental functioning and consequently from its time-honored place in the theory of adolescence, I followed the same timeless process of theory-building to which I have alluded. The oedipus complex defines a constellation of object relations which has to be attained and resolved before adolescence can be declared transcended and childhood be declared passed. Nothing about that or about the two-phasic resolution of the oedipus complex—first in early childhood and then in adolescence—appears to be in question. But it needs reminding that the second phase of the oedipal constellation does not move automatically into the center of the adolescent process just because the sexual maturation of the body has arrived. What obstructs the second and final phase of oedipal conflictuality from occurring as vigorously and irresistibly as physical maturation proceeds—that is the focal issue under discussion. Only slowly did I realize the consequences which such an assertion might exert on the preadult timetable of development and on the plotting of the disparate developmental tracks which the two genders follow into adult life. These revisions forced the question how the reformulation of the theory of adolescence would affect the psychoanalytic theory of the adult neurosis.

As I pursued this thought further, my investigation narrowed down to the male adolescent. The reason for this was not, as usually assumed, because I had seen more male than female adolescent patients, but it had its good reason in the fact that the disturbances of the female adolescent and of women in general had been more extensively and repeatedly studied. I refer here not only to Freud's writings but also to the many investigators, predominantly women, who were Freud's contemporaries, co-workers, and successors. In the 1930s Freud ex-

---

1. This essay appeared in *Aristotle: Selections*, ed. W. D. Ross (1927, pp. 323–325).

pressed the opinion—as quoted by Ruth Brunswick (1940) in her paper on which Freud collaborated—that our knowledge of the early development of the boy urgently needs to be deepened in order to equal the one we possess of the preoedipal girl. In the fulfillment of this largely unheeded Freudian legacy, I have formulated a schema from the vantage point of adolescence which enlightens as well as links male preoedipality with male adolescence.

In broad terms, male adolescence was plausibly understood for too long and too complacently within the schema of the oedipus complex, namely, parricide and the taboo of incest. I came to conclude that a major component of the typical rivalrous or rebellious impulse of the male is not necessarily nor singularly what is meant by a manifestation of the oedipus complex. I suspected that the boy's feelings of jealousy, competition, oppositionalism, and defiance in action and thought toward the father are too exclusively categorized under the concept of oedipal strivings. Clinical experience forced me to comprehend the proverbial and universal emotional dislocations between father and son in adolescence as a normal, age-adequate effort to reach a more complete emotional detachment and distancing—not only from the oedipal father, but also from the early dyadic father. Instead of delegating the adolescent boy's aggressive affect predominantly to oedipal strivings and conflicts, I assigned to it a function of defense against a never sufficiently relinquished dyadic attachment emotion from son to father. This emotion becomes extremely disturbing when it surfaces within the adolescent updrift of infantile object attachments. It needs to be stated with emphasis that this regressive updrift of infantile dyadic affects is eventuated by and necessarily coincides with the sexual maturation of the body. Here we detect the source of the transient homosexual preoccupation which, in one form or another, is never absent from adolescent self-awareness. Usually it is only dimly acknowledged or totally ignored.

Earlier I referred to the frequent ineffectualness of oedipal interpretations in which, summarily speaking, the sexual drive has either the mother or the father as object. When my interpretative focus encompassed more confidently the concept of the oedipal defense against the attachment emotions to the dyadic father, I noticed that the whole spectrum of aggressive and negativistic behavior toward the father and the symbolic father representations in the social sphere, like "law and order," gradually lost some of its intensity and uncontrollable drivenness. I feel justified to state that the adolescent revolt, comprehensively directed against the powerful figures on the stage of family and world, asserts itself with greater recklessness and disregard of reason, the more profoundly repressed the son's dyadic father attachment has remained. I observed that once the infantile dyadic father conflict had been worked through on the adolescent level, the advance to the second oedipal phase was rendered not only conceivable but assured. The ensuing expressions of oedipal or triadic conflictuality are easily identified, once we find ourselves on the familiar territory of the oedipus complex.

What has been said about the adolescent who puts his emotions into action is equally relevant for the expressively inhibited boy whose pathology is so often an impenetrable enigma. As is probably apparent from my discussion, besides the conflictedness of drives, we also have to consider those inner discordances in adolescence which arise from simultaneous dyadic and triadic regressions. Both of these synchronous sources of tension are developmentally normal; to some youths they are invigorating while dispiriting to others.

It follows, therefore, that the function of the boy's heightened aggression or passivity toward his father is not always to be found solely or even mainly in the effort to ward off castration by the oedipal father but mainly to protect himself against the regressive pull to the early preoedipal father. There are good reasons why this regressive pull is synchronized with puberty. At this period of life the relationship to the opposite sex undergoes changes in affect and sensation which have a profound influence on body and mind. Telescoping a complex developmental story, I mention only that normatively the adolescent boy's irresistible attraction to the female whom he is now sexually able to possess never fails to revive the infant boy's wish for and fear of reengulfment by the archaic mother, the primordial image of woman.

When the toddler takes his first steps toward autonomy, along with his exuberance, the anxiety of regression is simultaneously aroused. The intensity of this emotion threatens to throw the infant back into the passive state of merger. The projection of this infantile predicament is condensed in the term of the "reengulfing mother."

At this developmental juncture, the idealized rescuer, the father, forcefully enters the toddler's rapidly expanding life. The dyadic father idealization is now at its peak and mobilizes a developmental line which I have traced from this early and primitive same-gender identification all the way to the most complex and advanced formation of the adult ego ideal (Blos, 1974).

Pubertal maturation and the growing independence of the adolescent revive the longing for the protection of the early father; at the same time this is also anathema to him. In any case, the infantile dyadic attachment is carried forward by the male child until the time for its final dissolution has arrived at adolescence. At this juncture the expectable residues of a father bonding present obstacles to the loosening of the same-gender infantile tie. I speak here of the adolescent boy's father complex which dominates every male adolescent's emotional life to a highly variable degree of intensity and duration. The dyadic passions are essentially different from those of the oedipal modality.

At this point, I think, I hear voices spelling out the reminder that precisely due to the expectable shiftiness of infantile emotions which shuttle from attraction to rejection, from love to hate, toward one or the other parent, the designations of a positive (other-gender) and a negative (same-gender) oedipus complex have been formulated. As a rejoinder, I argue that dyadic and triadic object relations are of an intrinsically heterogeneous and mutually exclusive nature. The preclusive distinctness of dyadic and triadic object relations not only need be acknowledged but also clinically and theoretically defined in their influence on drive and ego development. Both modalities of object relations—dyadic and triadic—can coexist in childhood as relationship modes and clearly do so during the stages of early libido development; however, they cannot fuse or become absorbed in each other without undergoing profound restructuring in adolescence. The immature nature of the dyadic object tie becomes apparent in case it survives beyond its normal timing in the adult's emotional instability, fickleness, and irresistible need of changing the object in face of unpleasure. We observe in these cases a habitual fluctuation between passionate possessiveness and equally intense total indifference regarding the object.

In order to sharpen a pertinent distinction between child and adult, I wish to state as a principle of development that emotional maturation during childhood, adolescence included, does not advance in a linear or sequential order of discrete entities of stages; it moves forward in an ad hoc manner. This is to say that during this period of development, we can observe revocable adaptations and compromises between progression, regression, and also what might be called digression. With this term I refer, for example, to the unduly extended perseveration on a developmental level once reached until the lost momentum of growth gets recaptured and the forward move of development is reset into motion. The ongoing resolutions of maternal or paternal attachments and detachments are experienced by the child and adolescent either as a dependency-euphoria or panic and conversely as an independency-exhilaration or anxiety. Paradoxically, these affective states are experienced simultaneously and recurrently during preadult life. Deciphering adolescent emotions and thoughts has often given me the confusing sense of listening to several texts being read in different languages at the same time. Perhaps this is what Siegfried Bernfeld, the first analyst who dedicated himself intensively to research in adolescence, was referring to when back in the 1920s he said to me half-seriously, half-facetiously in an offhand remark, "Adolescence is a normal psychosis."

I will now change abruptly the focus of my presentation and start on the previously announced excursion into Freud's writings. I preface it by reporting an often repeated experience in my life as analyst. Whenever I credited myself with having made a noteworthy psychoanalytic observation or discovery, I subsequently found somewhere in Freud's writings or letters a reference to that idea, either explicit or by innuendo, by analogy or by a hint to what I had thought to be new. The sobering fact emerged that *der Herr Professor,* as we used to refer to Freud in novice modesty during my Vienna years, had already known something about it. And so it was again with the thesis which I report here. Since the references I have in mind are of particular interest for the history of psychoanalytic theory-building about adolescence, I shall refer verbatim to some of the relevant passages from his 1931 paper.

Freud refers to an observation which repeated itself too often in his analytic work with women to be attributed solely to the uniqueness of the individual neurosis, but it had to be attributed, so Freud argued, to the uniqueness of the neurosis in the female gender. His recurrent observation refers to an impasse which he found typical in the analysis of women, namely, that the oedipal material recedes almost to a vanishing point, before it becomes possible to subject it to analysis, and then often only within limits. "I was struck, above all, by two facts. The first was that where the woman's attachment to her father was particularly intense, analysis showed that it had been preceded by a phase of exclusive attachment to her mother which had been equally intense and passionate" (p. 225). The second fact refers to the greatly underestimated and surprisingly long duration of a woman's attachment to her early, dyadic mother, an attachment which never reaches a degree of decline as poignant as it is observed in the male. As I read these previously quoted passages, it occurred to me that the impassioned attachment of female patients to their father, as observed by Freud, represents an analogue to what I have termed "the oedipal defense," which I have observed and defined in male adolescence. The display of these emotions is often mistakenly identified as oedipal strivings, while in fact they are the reflection of preoedipal fixations. Freud did not use the term "defense" but ascribed his observation to a gender-related, emotional proclivity. He let the issue rest there by saying that his female patients "were able to cling to the very attachment to the father in which they had taken refuge from the early phase that was in question" (p. 226). The employment of this oedipal defense in both genders seems to be a normal aspect of development in both sexes. Before an advance to the second oedipal phase of adolescence is possible, a resolution of the same-gender, dyadic, attachment emotions must have taken place.

As I observe the adolescent boy, this conclusion regarding the resurgence of the preoedipal dyadic father connection imposed itself on my mind by the forcefulness of his all-consuming, impersonally tinged, heterosexual preoccupation, coupled with an irresistible oppositionalism to the father, either directly but more often displaced to other human, symbolic or ideational substitutions. In any event, we come to witness what we expect will arrive, namely, the unmistakable prelude to the final enactment of the Sophoclean family drama of the oedipus complex. As we well know, this drama often enough fails to get off the ground or fades away before the last lines have been spoken. These familiar phenomena which are clinically unmistakable in the adolescent boy but which, against all expectations, frequently remain immune to oedipal interpretations, raise in me disquieting and searching questions. The conclusion which Freud drew from his observation deserves our attention in this discourse because, what I had discovered in the adolescent boy as a regressive conflict with the preoedipal or dyadic father, Freud recognized in his female patients as a common phenomenon which demonstrates the specific role played by the fixation on same-gender, dyadic, attachment emotions in the neurosis of women. This infantilizing fixation is hidden from recognition by a defensive father attachment that lies at the bottom of the neurotic illness in women which Freud discussed in his paper.

Following convergent observations, I postulated that the male preoedipal father complex moves during adolescence into the conflictual center of the adolescent's object relations. Schematically stated, I furthermore concluded that an advance to the second oedipal phase during male adolescence requires that it be preceded or accompanied by a resolution of his same-gender, dyadic, attachment emotions. Should this developmental task of the adolescent process lie beyond the male adolescent's mastery, an aborted adolescence will result.

The residue of this particular crisis will be encountered in any treatment that follows later in life and decidedly so in adult analysis. We might expect that these adolescent-specific residua lie embedded in the core of the adult neurosis. The specific manner in which these anachronistic, dyadic, same-gender complexes surface in adult life, and especially in analysis, must remain the subject for another discussion.

At any rate, Freud noted in the analysis of his female patients the loss of all traces of their passionate oedipal attachment to their father when they approached in their analysis the depth of their preoedipal mother fixation. He was so struck by this fact that he likened his findings and their resulting consequences to an exciting discovery in archaeology, namely, to the discovery of the Minoan-Mycenean civilization which lies behind the civilization of Greece (p. 226). By alluding to the profound influence the discovery of Greek prehistory had on the comprehension of classic Greece, Freud implicitly referred to an equally profound influence of his findings in the analysis of women on the comprehension of the classic ocdipus complex. This he explains in greater detail in the same paper.

I counterpose Freud's comparison with my observation, based on the prehistory of male adolescence, where I recognized a phase of defensive heterosexuality as a normal and transient phase, manifest or latent, when full sexual maturity is on the brink of being attained or has fully established itself. It follows that the typical pubertal potential for phallic sexualization of any kind of sensation, perception, and mentation also engulfs the dyadic, same-gender, infantile, attachment emotions and introduces unfailingly the unsettling emotions of homosexuality to this epoch in the life of both sexes. I postulated that the final resolution of the dyadic father attachment in the boy's life must occur in adolescence. It follows that it is here where neurotic complications are bound to occur, causing permanent derailment in the progression to mature object relations and consequently precluding the structuralization of a competent adult self.

Freud's 1931 paper contains another statement which had a crucial influence on the development of the psychoanalytic theory of adolescence and beyond. The stage of an unchallenged or dominant and never abandoned mother attachment in the analysis of his female patients also perplexed Freud in regard to the genealogy of the neurosis: "Since this phase [i.e., of a prolonged total preoedipal mother attachment] allows room for all the fixations and repressions from which we trace the origin of the neuroses, it would seem as though we must retract the universality of the thesis that the Oedipus complex is the nucleus of the neurosis." Freud hastens to comfort the alarmed analyst who might feel "reluctant about making this correction" by suggesting that "there is no need to do so" because "we can extend the content of the Oedipus complex to include all the child's relations to both parents" (p. 226). By taking this step of integrating all beginnings of object relations, including the most archaic ones, into the so-called complete oedipus complex as a broad etiological backdrop to all neurotic formations, Freud rescued the cornerstone of psychoanalytic theory from losing its distinguished place of centrality and exclusivity in the comprehension and definition of the neurosis.

I think it would have served the understanding of infancy and adolescence better in their specific roles which they play in the cumulative progression of neurotic formations, if a sharper differentiation between dyadic and triadic object ties not only had been preserved but also been more precisely related to the developmental conditions in preadult life. I refer to those conditions which either promote, delay, or enfeeble the subsequent ascendancy of the oedipus complex and the confrontation with its triadic conflictuality. Expanding the boundaries of oedipality by the fiat of definition and subjugating the essentially heterogeneous neurotic potentials of dyadic and of triadic object relations to the distention of a complete oedipus complex, hindered rather than helped the understanding of adolescence and of what follows later. The compromise made in this rescue operation of the oedipus complex as the nucleus of the neurosis introduced and maintained controversies in theory-building which have particularly bridled the comprehension of adolescence in its unique contribution to the formation of the adult neurosis.

I may have given the impression that I attribute to the dyadic component of infantile and adolescent object relations an unwarranted importance in comparison to the role which the oedipus complex commands in the individual evolution of the neurosis. This impression is not without foundation. The reason why I give the dyadic component in adolescent development such emphatic prominence is due to the fact that its role and function have remained almost totally neglected in comparison to the eminence of the triadic configuration of the oedipus complex. Nevertheless, the decisive role and function of the oedipus complex in the formation of the neurosis remain unquestioned. My discussion has intended to focus on the preconditional steps which must be taken before the second and conclusive oedipal stage in adolescence can be transacted.[2] This precondition is fulfilled when the termi-

---

2. The mutually exclusive antagonistic positions of dyadic and triadic fixations fit well into Freud's dynamic model of two factors operative in the etiology of neurotic disturbances which stand in inverse proportion to each other. The model I refer to is known as the complemental series, defined by Freud (1916–17, p. 346 and p. 362).

nal resolution of the residual, same-gender, dyadic attachment emotions is achieved during the adolescent period.

I have focused in this discussion on the fate of the dyadic and the triadic developmental lines separately, even though they undergo maturational changes concurrently during the first two decades of life until most of the developmental plasticity of childhood and adolescence is spent and the process of maturation is brought to a natural decline. In fact, we observe in the adolescent boy and girl during the resolution of the dyadic same-gender as well as the triadic oedipal ties their treacherous navigation toward adulthood. The engagement in this enterprise proceeds either without letup or rather intermittently, either demonstratively or in the silence of the heart, either by rejection and withdrawal or by animosity and confrontation. The aim always remains the same, namely, to reach a sufficient loosening of infantile object ties and to set a decisive forward move into the new world of adult object relations into motion. In this progress Freud's female patients had failed early in life and in adolescence again. Freud (1931) concluded that "we had to reckon with the possibility that a number of women remain arrested in their original attachment to their mother and never achieve a true change-over towards men" (p. 226).

My analytic experience with adult men has convinced me that a parallel fixation on the level of same-gender object relation constitutes a nuclear component of their neurosis, equally laborious to reach and to surmount. This parallel might be aligned to Freud's comment by paraphrasing his sentence to read: "a number of men remain arrested in their original attachment to their father and never achieve a true change-over towards women." I am afraid I might sound redundant if I emphasize that I do not speak here of the oedipal father of the negative oedipus complex.

Taking this proposition one step further, I venture to say that not until adolescence has the developmental moment arrived for the oedipal drama to be completed and the realization of mature object relations to be initiated. This step must be taken in adolescence or it never will, certainly not without circumstantial good fortunes and therapeutic intervention—in any case, not without much suffering which not every human adult is capable to endure. My conclusions which parallel the ones which Freud has drawn from his analytic work with female patients also applies *mutatis mutandis* to the other sex. The respective same-gender pathogenic determinant also has to be identified and recognized as a "core-nucleus" in the neurosis in men as well as in women.

BIBLIOGRAPHY

ARISTOTLE. *Selections,* ed. W. D. Ross. New York: Scribner's, 1927.

BLOS, P. (1974). The genealogy of the ego ideal. *Psychoanal. Study Child,* 29:43–88.

BRUNSWICK, R. M. (1940). The preoedipal phase of libido development. *Psychoanal. Q.,* 9:293–319.

FREUD, S. (1905). Three essays on the theory of sexuality. *S.E.,* 7:125–243.

────── (1916–17). Introductory lectures on psycho-analysis. *S.E.,* 15 & 16.

────── (1918). From the history of an infantile neurosis. *S.E.,* 17:3–123.

────── (1931). Female sexuality. *S.E.,* 21:221–243.

Rapprochement and Other Crises

The Specific and Nonspecific in Analytic Reconstruction

LEO RANGELL, M.D.

PSYCHOANALYSIS HAS ALWAYS HAD AS THE MAIN THRUST OF ITS AIM AND method the casting of light on the past to illuminate and understand the present. The gripping effect exerted by Freud's first psychoanalytic assertions stemmed from the two-pronged result that what he was saying was disturbing, even shocking, while at the same time it was affectively felt to be true. The beam cast by Freud's original insights and formulations penetrated through and beyond the resistances they elicited.

The first nuclei of psychic life pointed to by Freud, which were the nodal subjects of both insight and outrage, were such concepts as childhood sexuality, the oedipus complex, repression, preoedipal wishes, latent perversion behind universal behavior. It is generally not appreciated how early in Freud's writings preoedipality accompanied his original contributions about the oedipus complex. Freud (1905) first chartered the area of developmental phases with his bold chronological mapping of the libidinal zones. The libidinal phases themselves spanned from birth through the preoedipal to the oedipal years.

With increasing clinical experience and theoretical expansion, sub-

---

This paper is an outgrowth and expansion of a presentation to the International Symposium on "Separation-Individuation and the Roots of Internalization and Identification," held in honor of Margaret Mahler, Paris, France, November 3, 1985. It is sad that this symposium turned out to be a memorial meeting for Mahler, who died shortly before she was to attend.

sequent elaborations expanded on traumatogenic events and other formative experiences in early childhood. Gradually these pointed to the very earliest stages of life, the original mother-child relationship and its varieties and vicissitudes. Both the original and the new points of etiologic foci have been continually expanded by a combination of clinical observations and theoretical elaborations. Originally the new points of etiologic foci were approached from the direction of reconstruction, reaching earlier neurosogenic influences from more careful and persistent clinical experiences. These were complemented by the burgeoning field of direct observations of childhood development, including various experimentally controlled situations, and carefully conducted longitudinal studies. Most recently, there has been added a group of psychoanalytic researchers engaged in direct observations of the postnatal state, examining minutely the reactions of the newborn infant, and the reciprocal cues, activities, and interactions between the new mother-infant pair.

Contrary to general opinion, preoedipal issues have from the beginning occupied predominant attention in the psychoanalytic literature of those elaborating on Freud's original contributions. The oedipus complex and its attendant castration anxiety, which many consider to have been overemphasized, have actually been the least elaborated upon or made a new and deeper center of investigation.

Among the studies by direct observations, some representative examples are the clinical and experimental approaches by Spitz (1957, 1959), the combined clinical, research, and therapeutic contributions of Anna Freud (1968), and the current body of work by Brazelton (1984) and Stern (1985) as well as many others too numerous to be referred to here. Added to these studies, which include the biological substrates, are the papers by Greenacre (1971), written from a retrospective adult perspective, on genetic patterns and predispositions.

The emphasis, in most direct observational studies of early development, has been to magnify the mental apparatuses with which the infant and child are endowed from the beginning and the initial behaviors resulting from these. One conclusion resulting from these studies, not in the earliest stages but at some further point as the first wave of development moves on, is that preoedipal does not mean pregenital. Awareness of and anxiety about the anatomical differences between the sexes is routinely present during the second year of life. Prospectively, however, both the pregenital and preoedipal shape the oedipal, and together with the oedipal, continue to exert effects throughout life.

MAHLER

Among the most systematic of the observers has been Margaret Mahler. Describing observational data and drawing theoretical conclusions, she has had a widespread and profound influence on current psychoanalytic thinking. Since Freud's original developmental cartography, no other individual has equaled her superimposition of greater detail and a higher power of observation in that large and useful area of preoedipality. The careful stratification she contributed, seen with a higher direct observational lens, was achieved at approximately the center of the first five years of life described by Freud. The focus was on the phase of separation of the evolving child into an individuated self with its own relatively independent borders.

Mahler took as her central focus the very apex of the preoedipal years, of the span from birth to about 4 or 5, concentrating and enlarging upon the self-individuation process during this phase. The area of Mahler's work was perhaps synchronous with Freud's anal phase, a confluence not generally sufficiently articulated. Ego phases and zones have been added to and fused with the libidinal ones. While Freud described this period mainly from the instinctual side (libidinal and later aggressive), Mahler, in complementary fashion, considered primarily the ego side of this stage of development.

Freud's original libidinal phases, which were significantly and convincingly added to in depth, meaning, and sense of conviction by other pioneers among Freud's early associates have in fact entered a long period of disuse. In spite of their having become out of fashion, however, it is remarkable how much these phases are still applicable and powerful in therapeutic practice and in the theory which guides it. I feel that they have retained their clinical usefulness throughout the entire history of psychoanalysis. The addition and integration of these with complementary and correlative ego phases only increase this power. I have never ceased to use oral, anal, and phallic points of fixation and regression, for example, as illuminating concepts both in the understanding of neurosogenesis and the psychoanalytic treatment of pathological phenomena. These have remained in evidence in descriptions of clinical work even by those who claim to have discarded drives in their theoretical thinking. This is similar to the empirical fact that many who discount metapsychology and the structural view continue to use psychic structures in their descriptions of clinical conditions. These terms and their connotations have become part of our language.

Another related aspect of Mahler's studies takes us back to "the psychological birth of the human infant" (Mahler et al., 1975), a felicitous term differentiating mental birth from the moment of physical birth and separation from the body of the mother. In the wider scope of her work, Mahler takes up and spans in detail from the beginnings of life, from physical birth, through autism and presymbiosis, the symbiotic phase, "the psychological birth of the infant," separation-individuation, as well as indicating the further developmental progression of these psychological stages into the later phallic phase, and beyond that to latency, adolescence, and the future path of the processes she describes.

Following her observations on early psychomotor, including affectomotor, manifestations, Mahler enunciated her well-known stratification into the much-quoted subsidiary subphases of the separation process. Following the earlier autistic and symbiotic stages, the four subphases of separation-individuation consist of differentiation, the practicing period, rapprochement, and the consolidation of object and self constancy. There exists even within the rapprochement subphase the rapprochement crisis, presumably an acute affective awareness of the alternatives of being together and being apart, at approximately 17 to 20 months.

RAPPROCHEMENT REVISITED

With each advance in psychoanalytic understanding, coming from the direction either of observation or treatment, the new locus of interest stands in danger of being lifted out of context with a premature wave of enthusiasm which usually distorts more than it adds.

Rapprochement crisis can by such means easily go the way, for example, of projective identification, the overuse of which has become common and well-known. This complex mechanism, which arose first and was limited to a succinct clinical observation, gradually spread to be used as an explanation for all difficult behavior, and in some geographic regions to all conflictful phenomena. From a specific and rather restricted interpersonal occurrence, projective identification has come to be used to explain indiscriminately almost all interpersonal phenomena, from there to be extended as an explanation of the psychology of a difficult age group, such as adolescence, or of a wide and complex sociologic problem, as prejudice against minorities, racial, gender, economic, and others, or even of conservative political views. By a similar mechanism and trend, the proper role of unresolved rapprochement conflicts has come to be obscured by excessive claims, and used, by reductionism, to explain complex and multidetermined surface behavior.

An example of this was a presentation by Fischer (1985) to the Symposium honoring Margaret Mahler in Paris in 1985. He reported on the detailed 4-year psychoanalytic treatment of a case of anorexia nervosa in a 16-year-old girl. From a series of traumas endured by the patient from birth onward, Fischer extracted, in a sensitive treatment and presentation, what he felt was a specific pathognomonic focus of etiology in the patient's rapprochement subphase of development. Confronted by a discouraging and seemingly interminable therapeutic impasse lasting for about two years, the analyst suddenly felt he understood the chaotic drama between patient and analyst as a derivative of unresolved rapprochement conflicts. Interpretation of this insight led to a loosening of the protracted defense, and an opening of the analysis to a more positive course and successful outcome.

It was in this clinical report that I (Rangell, 1985) was impressed with the much wider base of psychopathology which was present in addition to what Fischer felt he had seen of the threatening and inadequately traversed separation-individuation phase. These included anal and urethral medical manipulations beginning immediately after birth, which led to a complex web of anxieties and traumas, present and feared. There were enemas almost on a daily basis for the first 3 months after birth, a series of cystoscopies and repeated catheterizations at age 2, four or five myringotomies from ages 1 to 3, in addition to blood-taking and the more usual medical bodily invasions. Castration anxiety was amply present, continuous with and superimposed upon the earlier oral, anal, urethral, and aural traumatic experiences, involving a continuous invasion of body orifices. Even the deficiencies and anxieties of the separation-individuation phase itself could not be said to present a traumatic base limited to the rapprochement subphase alone.

Such a focal narrowing of etiologic beginnings is, in my experience, quite a common diagnostic occurrence. Evidence for a specific etiology in the rapprochement crisis must be more convincingly forthcoming and demonstrated. The therapeutic impasse in this case, I suggested, which the analyst thought to be due to a reenactment in the transference of a rapprochement crisis, was instead postulated to be due, not to fear of separation, i.e., of space between the patient and the analyst, but the opposite: that space, symbolic of her body space, would be invaded and violated by the analyst, repeating enemas and cystoscopies of the past. It was not, in my opinion, the analyst's interpretations of rapprochement anxiety, but his noninvasiveness which broke the impasse and resulted in a resumption and forward movement of the therapeutic process. The loosening of the therapeutic course came about as a result of the analyst's successful and patient maintenance of the analytic attitude, effecting a deep feeling of safety which led to the more normal and productive, verbal second half of the analysis.

This view of the clinical material does not devalue or make unnecessary Mahler's theory of rapprochement but is to place it into perspective with the entire gamut of her contributions. In this case, the continuous line of invasive traumas from the beginning of the patient's extrauterine life affected the entire early developmental sequence described by Mahler, from the autistic, through the symbiotic, through *all* of the phases and subphases of the separation-individuation stage, and beyond. The succession of traumas from the start, from "the psychological birth of the infant" on, was the basis for the abnormal push-pull between the patient and the analyst more than the rapprochement crisis itself. All levels, from oral, through anal and urethral to genital, resulting in phallic, oedipal, bisexual, castrative conflicts, are involved. As Mahler noted, the rapprochement crisis coincides with the convergence of the three basic anxieties of early life. The fear of object loss has been replaced by a conspicuous fear of loss of love and definite signs of castration anxiety. The direct observations and experimental work of Galenson and Roiphe (1974) bear this out (see also Roiphe and Galenson, 1981).

Rapprochement, as a specific and widely applicable etiologic focus, has been stressed by developmentalists who, in recent years, have attracted a good deal of attention, although the developmental point of view is not necessarily an original one, or separate from others already in common use. Other clinicians and theoreticians also look to this phase within the wider span of the pregenital years. Socarides (1979, 1987), for example, studying the etiology of perversions in general, and homosexuality in particular, offers a unitary theory of sexual perversions based upon fixation at the rapprochement subphase as the specifically affected area. The pivotal nuclear conflict in the etiology of the range of perverse disorders involves "the urge to regress to a preoedipal fixation in which there is a desire for, and dread of, merging with the mother in order to reinstate the primitive mother-child unity" (1979, p. 166). The Tysons (1982), on the other hand, describing pseudonarcissistic psychopathology, see rapprochement conflicts as part of a wide spectrum of pathological influences, including early intrasystemic superego conflicts and inadequate resolution of the oedipal phase.

The naming of this otherwise transient developmental phase as such a specific etiologic point of psychopathology has exerted a wide appeal for intellectual and affective reasons. Its operation as a continuous universal mechanism registers affectively; it is "felt" to be correct because of its ubiquitous applicability. Aside from its operation in general behavior, however, pointing to it as a specific etiology for a wide spectrum of psychopathology poses theoretical and methodological problems. The excessive attribution of specificity has been a widespread fallacy applied from one new insight to another during the course of expanding psychoanalytic theory. Rapprochement conflicts have merely become in recent years one of the most topical examples.

THE SPECIFIC AND NONSPECIFIC

I return to the problem of specific reconstructions in the pregenital years. In these theoretical considerations guidelines are embedded for the question of specificity versus nonspecificity in the psychoanalytic aim during the therapeutic procedure. Interpretation of rapprochement is but one example, a current one, of a principle which applies equally to many other current explanations. What I believe is nonspecific, and crosses individual lines, is the presence or chronic potential experience of the partial traumatic state, and the anxiety that is always adherent to it. This is universal. Interpretations in any patient of the qualitative existence of this state, coupled with the relevant confirmatory data, can be accurate and focal interpretations in themselves, received and reacted to as such by the patient. The automatic interpretation, however, of the cognitive experiences which initiated and sustain these affective states, is unjustified and can be misleading, without the necessary data either observed or logically and convincingly inferred. It is here that "leaps of inference" are introduced which lead to serious criticism of and questions about the psychoanalytic method.

An interpretation of the general affective state can be received accurately with validity and therapeutic influence. This in itself is specific; there are gradations of specificity. More specific, however, are the historical incidents and their cognitive accompaniments, the individual human experiences of external events, internal perceptions, and the complex object relations which make up human life. An unjustified or premature or insufficiently documented leap from the affective result to specific occurrences as their presumable etiologic triggers is what makes for blind spots and questionable links of distant inferences in the therapeutic course. The unempathic mother, an example that may be leaped to as such an explanation, is a current fashion rather than a finding in a particular analysis. Such interpretations, often as familiar to the patient as they are in current vogue by the analyst, can be accepted by the patient, but by different mechanisms and for different reasons. These can be both with positive or negative effects. In a positive sense, they may serve as inexact but still fruitful insights, leading to the search for more precise origins and explanations. They may, however, also serve defensive purposes as screen insights, blocking the further path to deeper and more warded-off psychic content. The same affective state can result from, and can be used to cover, multiple causative events. The nonspecific covers the specific, and the affective covers and takes precedence over the cognitive. In each case, the broader category of experience is used to obscure the more definitive.

Psychoanalysis is a continuous search for individual experiences grafted upon universal experiences, individual repressed causes of trauma and the repressed unconscious experience of them. Both ideational and affective aspects of psychic trauma are repressed, separately and to different degrees. The affective experience, the suffering of the sensation of helplessness and unpleasure, is the element in common in all incidents of trauma, in all individuals. This unwelcome and unassimilable affective state is itself repressed and needs to be uncovered. Within the context of human life, it is a specific and delineated subjective state, often experienced and repeatedly repressed. But with this, the associated event and cognitive experience also are repressed and defended against. "You felt [a description of the subjective traumatic feeling] because of [the exposure of the causative historical incident]" is the total experience uncovered by psychoanalytic interpretation and insight.

While psychoanalytic understanding converges universal experiences, and even common human causes and conditions, into a unified explanatory theory, the individual variants of these belong to that patient alone. Anatomy tells general facts but not the individual somatic example. The theory of dreams can explain all dreams but not any one dream. Seduction, fantasy, the infantile neurosis, constitutional factors, even a common fear of abandonment, loss of love or castration can be captured in one running summary account. But no one of these overall theoretical condensations applies specifically or can be used with validity and expected therapeutic effect in an individual patient.

So it is with rapprochement, or all deprivation, states or crises, or any widely experienced growth conflict, when we look into an individual life history. The oedipus complex occurs to all, yet no one oedipal constellation applies to any. Psychic trauma takes place in any life, yet the quality, the quantity, and the specifics of the subjective experience can be told only by the particular individual, and even by him only after the common work and exploration between patient and analyst uncovers them from his memory.

Rapprochement, as described by Mahler, takes its place alongside all such universal tools of insight. But its enlistment as a distinct memory, or as a developmental year or few months of specifically experienced anxiety, trauma or depression cannot be automatically pointed to, or taken for granted from universal knowledge, as an individually exposed and remembered event or condition or series of experiences. To do so, as has tempted many, without documenting and pointing to the specific memories, affective and cognitive, is to include it in a long series of psychoanalytic clichés, which historically reach a peak of acceptance as explanatory concepts, only to be discarded after their supposed uniqueness and specificity fail to fulfill their promised roles. As infancy should be seen in perspective to later adult stages of development, rapprochement should similarly be seen in perspective to related issues and events before and after as well as during the same pregenital years. Mahler's writings have always stood together as a whole, and been part of the total mainstream of developing psychoanalytic theory. Psychopathology stands on a base, not a point.

Many authors, including Mahler et al. (1975) and Mahler and McDevitt (1982), have pointed out the lifelong applicability of attachment problems which follow the partial achievement of separation-individuation in early life. These fuse with the contributions of Bowlby (1969–73) on attachment, Freud's (1937) adhesiveness of the libido to objects, Kohut's (1971, 1977) use of the selfobject, and my own work (1954, 1955) on poise, holding-on, "the need to belong," the perioral area, and attachment to ground. A classic paper which I found to be a background to this series of thoughts was the work on clinging by the pioneer Hungarian analyst, Imre Hermann (1935), who died in 1984 in Budapest at the age of 95. Some six months after his death, I (Rangell, 1984b) gave a paper to the Hungarian Society in Budapest in his honor. Here is another connection to Mahler. Margaret, who was born in Hungary, first became interested in psychoanalysis as a young girl when, as a student in the gymnasium, she attended the psychoanalytic salon at the home of Vilma Kovacs, the mother of her school friend Alice Kovacs, later to become Mrs. Alice Balint. Vilma Kovacs was one of the analysts of Hermann, to whose work Mahler refers and relates.[1]

---

1. Browsing, a form of research, turns up unexpected surprises. In searching out what Vilma Kovacs may have written, I found references to only two papers. One was on

The search for the specific goes on in psychoanalysis superimposed upon the general. The cognitive details are added to affective states which they caused. The specific infantile traumas, the developmental series of traumatic experiences before, during, and following separation-individuation, are continually sought and exposed. More than is apparent may stem from castration anxiety, viz., Freud's (1905) classic descriptions of regression to the preoedipal level from higher-level castration anxiety. Moreover, with respect to specificity, castration itself is not monolithic but can also be further stratified. Some patients suffer from the feeling of having been castrated, while others are mainly intent on the future possibility. Yet with all of these, such as I described in a homosexual patient who suffered from "penis inferiority," or in another who had surgical manipulations to infections on the penis and felt that the damage already was done, to all the greatest danger is still the imminence of the potential of further and complete castration.

As another common example of a too-automatic linkage, separation anxiety seen in the transference is not necessarily a repetition of the conflicts of the separation-individuation stage. Periods of absence from the analyst can mean the entire gamut of dangers, castration as well as separation. Separation can also mean a threat of the loss of the mastery acquired during the analysis thus far, i.e., the strengthening of the patient's own analytic ego in dealing with instinctual and superego pressures (Rangell, 1987). The automatic assumption of separation anxiety as a definitive interpretation, on weekends or other such fortuitous separations between patient and analyst, is a widespread reflex conclusion on the part of analysts. Moreover, with regard to the even more specific crisis of rapprochement within separation, both separation and with it an anxiety about returning occur before the more organized rapprochement subphase, and typically in such early phases

---

a case of Gilles de la Tourette's disease (Kovacs, 1925). While the important work on tics by Ferenczi, including "maladie des tics," was incorporated in the bibliography of the joint paper written by Mahler and myself (1943), I do not remember Mahler mentioning to me this paper by Kovacs, also from Hungary. Adjacent to the Kovacs paper in the same issue of the *Zeitschrift,* were other papers on tics by Helene Deutsch (1925) and Melanie Klein (1925). The interest in this subject in Central Europe at that time seemed to rival that in Paris some 40 years earlier. Mahler came to New York prepared when she later began her work there on tics and psychomotor disturbances.

Freud's spontaneous reaction to this syndrome is also of interest. When Ferenczi (1921) discussed the meaning of tics with Freud, Freud "mentioned that apparently there was an organic factor in the question" (p. 142). This position is consonant with Mahler and my original views as well as recent literature on the subject.

as well as in the developmental periods which follow, not as crises but as continuities. Problems of separation, and retrospective testing of the environment just turned from, begin from the time of "hatching," and continue throughout life. Mahler herself, pointing out that the autistic and symbiotic phases are also the initial stages of separation-individuation, expresses caution to see these problems of relatedness and object relations in perspective to other developmental conflicts which precede and follow them. I have pointed to the crucial significance of the age of 17 in preparing the psychological soil for the final definitive separation-individuation which marks the passage into adult life, even though problems of attachment and separation continue for the entire life-span. All stages are to be pointed to when indicated and linked in continuity of associations (Rangell, 1988).

The automatic leap in current interpretations to lack of maternal empathy, or separation anxiety, or mourning, or even in previous years to castration anxiety, is what gives psychoanalysis a dubious look. This can be the case equally in the "here and now" of transference as in reconstruction. What is needed in the analytic method may be not more empathic immersion but greater discipline, a restraint to require more clinical bridges for interpretations.

However, while I have cautioned against the excessive emphasis of the rapprochement subphase and ignored its surrounding behavioral matrix, it would be equally incomplete to leave this out. The individual's unique and characteristic experiences in all their developmental aspects are an integral and indispensable part of the analytic search and procedure. Although premature and automatic interpretations to historically far-distant etiologic nuclei are made with great frequency, rendering the interpretative procedure artificial and toward the wild side rather than a valid experience, the better examples, of appropriate interpretations made on prepared psychological ground and leading to deeply convincing insight, occur with frequency and regularity as well.

Rapprochement, when detected and adequately revealed, in the transference or in its historical antecedents, can be pointed to with confidence and profit to the analysis, as can other specific distant reconstructions. Preoedipal reconstruction has been elegantly demonstrated as possible to the earliest years of life in many papers by Greenacre (1971) in specific syndromes such as fetishism, clearly applicable from there to others. Other careful clinical explorations dedicated to such efforts, e.g., by E. Kris (1956), Bak (1968), Rosen (1955a, 1955b), Blum (1974, 1977), Harley (1978), van Dam (1989), and many other psychoanalytic writers, have similarly succeeded in linking various psychopathological syndromes to specific early pregenital determinants, to the enhancement not only of the clinical reports but of the credibility of the psychoanalytic method. The wheat is retained while the chaff is discarded. In each case, the methodological pitfalls of reductionism or leaps of inference have been avoided. Rapprochement does shine through, in dreams, actions, symptoms, transference, and extra-transference manifestations. But while reconstruction of the rapprochement period was essential, Harley (1978) illustrated the interactions of rapprochement with libidinal and aggressive drive development, and the gamut of succeeding pathological conflicts. In these instances, as in the history of science, "a willingness to explore the new has resulted in a keener eye with which to appreciate the old."

The traumas of early life, revealed through adult observations or in adult analyses, also extend from mild to severe, from general and diffuse to specific and circumscribed. Even without interpretations or specific memories linking these to the past, patients can put appropriate words and ideation to these currently experienced traumatic affects themselves, which lead to self-directed unconscious insights. One patient, recounting his childhood, again and again stated, "I felt terminally unloved," comparing his state then, in its repetitive forms, to the terminal illnesses of a number of people. In a combination of the general and the specific, as these usually exist clinically, psychoanalysis often reconstructs a traumatogenic childhood rather than a circumscribed experience, a condition rather than an event. The patient who saw himself as "terminally unloved" reconstructed a childhood which was a melange of roles toward him played by mother, father, an older brother, and two younger siblings who added their parts to his feelings of deprivation, hostility, and neglect. In a similar fashion, another patient described the childhood behind his acquired homosexuality as diffusely traumatogenic in all aspects. "I never did then or since fit in with the world."

It was this finding of diffuse rather than circumscribed, chronic rather than acute, strain rather than shock trauma which led E. Kris (1956) to question whether one ever really knows "what happened on the staircase." This observation and thought were carried further—too far, in my opinion—by many who, following Spence (1982a, 1982b), feel that there can be only narrative truth, never historical truth. The quest of psychoanalysis becomes mitigated, aiming to reach only the patient's perceptions, not reality. Conditions can be as "real" as events, both of them a combination of the objective filtered through the subjective, idiosyncratic processes of the patient. An atmosphere, ambience, the characteristics of the surround are not without meaning or importance in a psychoanalytic procedure. An unempathic mother or schizophrenogenic parent to a particular patient cannot be regarded entirely as the patient's perceptions. The subjective but also the objective are grist for the analytic mill, and especially the methods, meanings, and reasons for the distortions of one by the other. One cannot interpret distortions without having an actuality as a base. This applies to general conditions as to specific experiences in the evolving life history.

In this regard, psychoanalysis is more adapted to specific, distant, but appropriate reconstructions than is psychotherapy, although such rational and effective therapeutic links are also available in properly conducted and monitored psychoanalytic psychotherapy. Even in a psychoanalytic procedure, transference, usually more exposed and interpreted than in psychotherapy, can often point the way only to the general, while for the more specific cognitive and historical elements both analyst and patient depend on the patient's traumatic memories and unconscious fantasies reconstructed by the analytic work. Psychotherapy can more characteristically lead to approximate, inexact, or general insights. These sometimes take the form of a screen acceptance of an approximate interpretation which, as any screen element, a screen memory, or a screen affect or mood (Greenson, 1952), can be true but incomplete. Further precision is more typical and possible with psychoanalysis.

INFANTILE TRAUMA IN ADULT LIFE AND ANALYSIS

A secondary focus of this paper is the subject of how infantile trauma and its derivatives are reflected in adult life. Analytic reconstructions of early life, rapprochement, and other preoedipal determinants occur from phenomena visible in adult analyses as well as analyses of younger patients. The recent interest resulted in a number of panels and discussions devoted to the links seen in the psychoanalytic process between infantile experiences and adult life.

I have pointed out how, in addition to reconstruction being available from verbal associations, nonverbal aspects of analytic work with adults can also be utilized in the service of early reconstructions (Rangell, 1984a). Postural, gestural, vocal, other than verbal, and other indirect modes of behavior and communication, when analytic attention and interpretations are turned toward them, may lead to verbal anamnestic material which points the way to more specific therapeutically useful interpretative reconstructions.

Many examples occur routinely to any psychoanalytic clinician, al-

though frequently overlooked and left out of psychoanalytic sur-
veillance and understanding. In my own psychoanalytic practice, I
have pointed to many of these clinical instances of infantile manifestations reflected in the adult state as seen in adult analysis, and have
linked them to the various arcs of the intrapsychic process which I have
described in psychoanalytic theory. One patient's periodic stretching,
yawning, and sighing on the couch represented an attempted discharge of the tension state, a phase of the intrapsychic sequence indica-
tive of a beginning, mounting traumatic state. Another patient's repetitive patting and rubbing of his thighs, or playing with his fingers or
toes, represented the motor equivalent of masturbatory activity. Another stretched her hands behind her head toward the analyst, opening and clasping them repetitively, in an unconscious gesture expressing the desire to have her hands held for security purposes by the
nurturing parental figure, now the analyst. Starting from these gestural phenomena, verbal associations led to the unconscious fantasies
underlying them, and the anxieties, dangers, and situations of psychic
trauma feared and defended against in earlier life.

In keeping with my thesis of the closeness and frequent confluence
between anxiety and trauma, one patient can easily feel the subjective
difference between anxiety states, anticipated danger, and the "ache"
in his chest during the suffering of the trauma in the here-and-now as
he fantasizes being rejected and abandoned by his love object. He has
had experiences with this sequence, and togetherness, of psychic se-
quelae during particular developmental periods and in specific relationships at various ages of his life.

Here too, in adult observations and analysis, as they relate to earlier
states, the questions of specific and nonspecific are to be kept in mind.
The currently admired direct observers of newborn infants add minute observational phenomena of earlier ego-responsive states in infancy than previously thought. Yet in the flush and excitement of the
immediate aftermath, and the challenge and appeal of interpreting
these in analyses, premature and ill-considered specificity needs to be
avoided or treated with caution. These new observations do not necessarily lead to or make more available specific reconstructions of such
early stages in later analysis. While some think that the observations of
Stern (1985) make for earlier differentiation and individuation than
Mahler found—usually analysts who said the same about having other
new observations and ideas immediately replace the old—these new
observations, in my opinion, add further data without obviating or
outdating the old. It is unlikely, from these studies of "the observed
infant," that an early, independent, inborn self as agent, which needs

no autistic or symbiotic phase, will replace Mahler's later-differentiated self, or be substituted for Hartmann's (1939, 1964) inborn ego appa-ratus, or perform differently from the pre-ego functions noted at this stage by Anna Freud (1981) and Greenacre (1971). Harley (1978) finds herself "incapable of comprehending how structural conflicts may be divorced from those developmental disturbances which date back to preverbal times yet which have entered into the very formation and texture of the later intrapsychic conflicts."

I will end with clinical examples from quite routine adult analyses which demonstrate the points and cautions I have been making. The derivatives of infantile trauma in adult life as seen in adult analysis also stem from the specific to the nonspecific, and span the spectrum of early etiologic foci. Rapprochement, which has been the subject of our special interest, does play an important part, but the temptation to isolate it is to be tempered with an openness to all levels and an awareness of the continuous developmental line. The following is an excerpt from an adult analysis typical of the derivative level at which presenting analytic material appears. It also demonstrates the facility and appeal of being part of a theoretical group, in this case of the theory of rapprochement.

A man in his 60s returned home from a business trip. It was close to midnight. On his way from the airport to his house, he found himself becoming inexplicably angry. The thought behind this feeling was that his wife would be waiting for him in bed, not at the door. He came in irritable and surly. His wife was awake, waiting anxiously and lovingly. The patient felt guilty, as he did again the next morning relating this incident to me.

Is this not temptingly simple, derivative, and corroborative of rap-prochement anxiety, especially when linking material is amply forth-coming? His wife-mother was not waiting for him (technically as he wished it) when he chose to return, his fears were confirmed, rap-prochement had failed again. The relevant history, known from the analysis (and I return to the surface now), included the following mem-ories and associations. The patient remembered his coming home from school as a young boy, after running anxiously to escape the other boys, who would chase and beat him on his way home. The patient was small, the only Jew, out of step, frightened to the point of terror. In these memories he came into the house, his mother was never there, he was alone through the afternoon hours. He was anxious and angry. He remembered playing alone in the backyard, making believe he was Clyde Beatty, the lion-tamer, imitating what he had seen in the circus. In many early associations, we came to think of the mother as working at the store with the father, i.e., the picture of her was of a hardworking, downtrodden, self-sacrificing mother. This picture was corrected in later memories of her being quite self-indulgent, playing cards and mahjong with her friends during these afternoons.

After an interpretation linking the present with the past, to the effect that he was reliving the feeling of his mother not waiting for him, not wanting him, rejecting and abandoning him, the patient reminded himself and the analyst, "No, she idolized me." He was in fact considered by all to be triumphant over the father and sisters; the sisters still spoke of how he was always the favorite one. Mother loved him better than any of the others. "Why don't I remember the positive but only the negative?" he plaintively asked. Because danger and the possibility of trauma came first; defenses and all means of guarding against these took precedence.

There were intermediate related events in his life history. In his 20s and 30s, he had a first marriage during which his young wife was cuckholding him with a neighbor man, the husband of a friend. The patient in retrospect tolerated this, after knowing it for several years. Both the patient and his wife went into therapy, but the patient continued to suffer and to accept repeated insults and betrayals. In an earlier period in his teens, he remembered a traumatic incident when he saw his first girlfriend, with whom he was in love and felt linked, come into a store with her mother, no longer wearing his track medal around her neck that he had given her. This was a crushing blow which was the beginning of the end of that relationship. In his current life, the patient did the same thing to his present wife as his girlfriend and first wife had done to him by conducting a clandestine love affair for a number of years.

In addition to these experiences of rejection and trauma, frustrated sexual longings, along with doubts about his masculinity, were characteristically present and repetitive during his developmental history. Intertwined with his sexual, parental, oedipal relationships, he reconstructed very convincingly an overt and conscious sexual longing for a maiden aunt, who sat on his bed in her nightgown while he was a young boy. This aunt overtly loved her older, successful brother; her nephew, the patient, could only look on; he remembered his excitement, frustration, and fear. There were overt, incestuous fantasies, dreams, and near-acts with two stepdaughters, and material suggesting similar instinctual wishes toward his own daughter, and in his early life his two sisters. The frustration and feelings of rejection behind these repetitive incestuous fantasies served as both fuel and brakes to them. Dangers in each developmental period, whether preoedipal threats against security or castration anxiety for sexual wishes during the overt oedipal period, took precedence over situations of safety and satisfaction and aroused defensive and protective activities.

The incident first reported connoted, in an exquisite and specific sense, a failure of rapprochement and its reassuring quality. His present wife idolized him as his mother had done. The bridge was the feeling of rejection and the need for her reassuring presence. She was not waiting at the door or the window. The total psychic flow, however, was from both before and after the specific rapprochement subphase, from the preceding phase of symbiotic union and the following oedipal stages and beyond. His mother had also warned him, taking a cue from a doctor's remark, that he had a small and weak heart, that he was never to play baseball or fight with the boys. These warnings and forebodings never left him, even though today, in his 60s, he jogged for miles. His masculinity always needed to be affirmed.

The same question put by another patient, "Why do I think only of the bad things? There were also good things that happened," elicits the same response and reasons. The traumatic state is the first order of psychic concern and awareness. The goal of anxiety and defense is to ward off the traumatic state, especially if it is already partially present, either chronically or intermittently. There is a variable anxiety-trauma-defense complex latent behind the surface character elements operative in everyday life.

The need to be wanted, the pivotal issue in rapprochement conflict, can be converted to a need to be needed, and anxiety when this is not forthcoming. This is the intrapsychic situation in some instances of retirement anxiety, an internal state more frequent than one would think. The anxiety and conflicts can be mild to severe, and can reach the proportions and dynamics of obsession or addiction. A patient not yet 65, who left a prestigious and important position and was engaged in part-time and temporary consulting work, felt anxious, far beyond the economic necessity, when he was not employed or in demand. The amount of money he told himself he needed to continue his way of life—he always made many thousands of dollars above what he actually had—was easily seen as a thin rationalization. Not being needed meant not being wanted, not being loved. If there was no follow-up employment, or if a friend did not call him, or called him on time, or called him unexpectedly, he had that nondescript feeling of anxiety and rejection, converted even into psychosomatic chest pains. This affective complex was continuous with a theme which had run through his life. He recognized that he was "fixed" on being wanted, and that any incident which did not supply this needed state resulted in immediate anxiety. The tracing of this complex during the analysis relentlessly went back through every stage of life, to his childhood and by extrapolation to his infantile state. Rapprochement anxiety was included but not exclusive in this continuum of anxiety and defense and the dangers these warded off. The patient also felt at this point that when he reached the magic age of 65, this would go a long way toward improving his condition, since this was the accepted time of retirement and thus would not signify his not being wanted.

Such an affective state is not limited to the mid-60s. A much younger person, in his 30s, a writer, could not write at home but did his best work when sitting over coffee, or at a meal in a restaurant during the day, when he was surrounded by other people. This atmosphere gave him a feeling of being in the stream of things and more wanted. This was not so at dinner; eating alone in a restaurant in a more formal way, without writing, he had feelings of anxiety, loneliness, separation, and rejection. The dynamics in this case were similar, although again with their own individual and idiosyncratic determinants. In this patient, rapprochement anxiety was actually more definitively evident in the analysis. The patient was alone with his mother for the first year and a half, after which his father, who had been on military duty overseas, returned from the service and deflected his mother's attention in a way which had repercussions for the rest of his life. Nevertheless, here too the subsequent line of development contributed a cumulative succession of traumatic threats from all levels of further development. Probably many instances of loneliness-depression in singles or in lonely married people stem from a chronic, diffuse, adult derivative of the infantile state of separation, aloneness, danger, and threat. The nature of the threat changes from one libidinal and ego phase of development to another, but a thread linking all of the subsequent stages to the earliest experience of ego insufficiency and infantile trauma exists through them all.

SUMMARY

The historical development of preoedipality in evolving psychoanalytic theory is traced. Particular reference is paid to the elaboration by Mahler of the separation-individuation phase and the specific rapprochement conflict and crisis within it. In addition to the valuable contributions these discoveries have brought about, the tendency is noted for every new locus of interest to be obscured by excessive claims, and distorted by overuse and reductionism to explain complex and multidetermined behavior.

This leads to the question of the specific and nonspecific in analytic reconstruction. Psychoanalysis invites a search for the specific superimposed upon the general. What I believe is nonspecific is the experience of the traumatic state, variable in degree, and the anxiety always adherent to it. The cognitive and historical data which initiated and maintain these affective states need to be arrived at with clinical accuracy and sustaining data, transference and historical.

With discipline and restraint, and effective clinical bridges for interpretation, rapprochement and other distant preoedipal determinants can be pointed to in analytic reconstruction with confidence and profit to the analysis. Clinical examples are cited of valid and therapeutically effective reconstruction of early infantile traumas, including rapprochement, as well as instances in which significant etiologic determinants from contiguous phases are fused and continuous.

Rapprochement plays an important role, but the temptation to isolate it is to be tempered with an openness to all levels and an awareness of the continuing developmental line. Such a wide etiologic spectrum is in keeping with the total range of observations and formulations made by Mahler, from the psychological birth of the infant, through separation-individuation, to phenomena and stages long after the attainment of object constancy.

BIBLIOGRAPHY

BAK, R. C. (1968). The phallic woman. *Psychoanal. Study Child*, 23:15–36.

BLUM, H. B. (1974). The borderline childhood of the Wolf Man. *J. Amer. Psychoanal. Assn.*, 22:721–742.

———— (1977). Preoedipal reconstruction. *J. Amer. Psychoanal. Assn.*, 25:757–783.

BOWLBY, J. (1969–73). *Attachment and Loss*, 2 vols. New York: Basic Books.

BRAZELTON, T. B. (1984). Why early intervention. In *Frontiers of Infant Psychiatry*, ed. J. D. Call, E. Galenson, & R. L. Tyson. New York: Basic Books, vol. 2, pp. 267–275.

DEUTSCH, H. (1925). Zur Psychogenese eines Tic-Falles. *Int. Z. Psychoanal.*, 11:325–332.

FERENCZI, S. (1921). Psycho-analytical observations on tic. In *Further Contributions to the Theory and Technique of Psycho-analysis*. London: Hogarth Press, 1926, pp. 142–174.

FISCHER, N. (1985). Anorexia nervosa and unresolved rapprochement conflicts. Read at the International Symposium on Separation-Individuation, Paris.

FREUD, A. (1968). Indications for child analysis and other papers. *W.*, 4.

———— (1981). Psychoanalytic psychology and normal development. *W.*, 8.

FREUD, S. (1905). Three essays on the theory of sexuality. *S.E.*, 7:125–243.

――――― (1933). New introductory lectures on psycho-analysis. *S.E.*, 22:3–182.

GALENSON, E. & ROIPHE, H. (1974). The emergence of genital awareness during the second year of life. In *Sex Differences in Behavior*, ed. R. C. Friedman, R. M. Richards, & R. L. van de Wiele. New York: John Wiley.

GREENACRE, P. (1971). *Emotional Growth*, 2 vols. New York: Int. Univ. Press.

GREENSON, R. R. (1952). The defensive function of some affective states. In: L. Rangell, Report of Panel on "The Theory of Affects." *Bull. Amer. Psychoanal. Assn.*, 8:300–315.

HARLEY, M. (1978). Observational studies and analytic reconstruction. Read at the Margaret S. Mahler Symposium, Philadelphia.

HARTMANN, H. (1939). *Ego Psychology and the Problem of Adaptation.* New York: Int. Univ. Press, 1958.

――――― (1964). *Essays on Ego Psychology.* New York: Int. Univ. Press.

HERMANN, I. (1935). Clinging—going-in-search. *Psychoanal. Q.*, 45:5–36, 1976.

KLEIN, M. (1925). Zur Genese des Tics. *Int. Z. Psychoanal.*, 11:332–349.

KOHUT, H. (1971). *The Analysis of the Self.* New York: Int. Univ. Press.

――――― (1977). *The Restoration of the Self.* New York: Int. Univ. Press.

KOVACS, V. (1925). Analyse eines Falles von "Tic Convulsif." *Int. Z. Psychoanal.*, 11:318–325.

KRIS, E. (1956). The recovery of childhood memories in psychoanalysis. *Psychoanal. Study Child*, 11:54–88.

MAHLER, M. S. & MCDEVITT, J. B. (1982). Thoughts on the emergence of the sense of the self, with particular emphasis on the body self. *J. Amer. Psychoanal. Assn.*, 30:827–848.

――――― PINE, F., & BERGMAN, A. (1975). *The Psychological Birth of the Human Infant.* New York: Basic Books.

――――― & RANGELL, L. (1943). A psychosomatic study of maladie des tics (Gilles de la Tourette's disease). *Psychiat. Q.*, 17:579–603.

RANGELL, L. (1954). The psychology of poise. *Int. J. Psychoanal.*, 35:313–332.

――――― (1955). The quest for ground in human motivation. Read at the American Psychiatric Association and the West Coast Psychoanalytic Societies.

――――― (1984a). Structure, somatic and psychic. In *Frontiers of Infant Psychiatry*, ed. J. D. Call, E. Galenson, & R. L. Tyson. New York: Basic Books, pp. 70–81.

――――― (1984b). Homage to Imre Hermann. Read at the Hungarian Psychoanalytic Society, Budapest.

――――― (1985). Discussion of "Anorexia nervosa and unresolved rapprochement conflicts" by N. Fischer. International Symposium on Separation-Individuation, Paris.

――――― (1987). A core process in psychoanalytic treatment. *Psychoanal. Q.*, 56:222–249.

――――― (1988). Seventeen: a developmental node. In *Frontiers of Adult Psychiatry*, ed. R. A. Nemiroff & C. A. Colarusso. New York: Basic Books.

――――― (1989). *The Human Core.* New York: Int. Univ. Press.

ROIPHE, H. & GALENSON, E. (1981). *Infantile Origins of Sexual Identity*. New York: Int. Univ. Press.

ROSEN, V. H. (1955a). Strephosymbolia. *Psychoanal. Study Child*, 10:83–99.

———— (1955b). Reconstruction of a traumatic childhood event in a case of derealization. *J. Amer. Psychoanal. Assn.*, 3:211–221.

SOCARIDES, C. W. (1979). A unitary theory of sexual perversions. In *On Sexuality*, ed. T. B. Karasu & C. W. Socarides. New York: Int. Univ. Press, pp. 161–188.

———— (1987). *Preoedipal Origins and Psychoanalytic Therapy of Sexual Perversions*. New York: Int. Univ. Press.

SPENCE, D. P. (1982a). Narrative truth and theoretical truth. *Psychoanal. Q.*, 51:43–69.

———— (1982b). *Narrative Truth and Historical Truth*. New York: Norton.

SPITZ, R. A. (1957). *No and Yes*. New York: Int. Univ. Press.

———— (1959). *A Genetic Field Theory of Ego Formation*. New York: Int. Univ. Press.

STERN, D. N. (1985). *The Interpersonal World of the Infant*. New York: Basic Books.

TYSON, R. L. & TYSON, P. (1982). A case of 'pseudo-narcissistic' psychopathology. *Int. J. Psychoanal.*, 63:283–293.

VAN DAM, H. (1989). A developmental approach to acting out. In *The Psychoanalytic Core*, ed. R. H. Blum, E. Weinshel, & F. R. Rodman. New York: Int. Univ. Press (in press).

DEVELOPMENT

Therapeutic Processes

A Longitudinal View

SAMUEL ABRAMS, M.D.

I WILL DESCRIBE A SERIES OF BRIEF THERAPEUTIC CONTACTS I HAD WITH A girl named Cindy from the time she was just 3 until she was nearly 16 years old. For the most part the presentation will be in the form of a psychotherapeutic dialogue or a clinical description of what went on. Everyone will be involved with the dynamic issues; some also with structural or organizational ones; others with the object-interactional system; others still with questions of development. The transference-countertransference axis will pique everyone's curiosity, as it did mine. Each of these factors influences the direction a treatment takes; sometimes one seems a more important source of the healing process, sometimes another. Psychotherapy cases, because they do not provide the depth and breadth of analytic ones, are generally not persuasive pools of theory-building about treatment action. However, a series of psychotherapeutic encounters with a child over a protracted time-span has one advantage: it provides a *longitudinal* perspective on therapeutic processes covering very different ages and phases. This presents an opportunity to consider what thread runs through all of them and hence what might be fundamental for a wide variety of successful psychotherapeutic encounters.

CINDY

Cindy Evans was one month shy of her third birthday when her parents came to see me. Mr. Evans was an agreeable young man, self-assured and soft-spoken. He was tender to his wife and concerned

Clinical professor of psychiatry, New York University Medical Center, New York.
The Maurice R. Friend lecture, the Psychoanalytic Institute, New York University Medical Center, October 8, 1987.

43

about his daughter. Mrs. Evans was openly fretful. Her voice almost quivered on occasion. A wide range of emotions were readily available to her. They were an attractive young couple; and the attractiveness was somehow enhanced by the fact that Mrs. Evans was very, very pregnant.

Cindy retained her bowels, they explained, sometimes for as long as a week and often accompanied by a good deal of crying. "I have to make doody," she would shout, "my stomach hurts, my belly hurts," but despite the pain and discomfort she would simply sit on her potty and strain as much to retain her stools as to release them. Bowel training, they volunteered, had begun in earnest some 5 months earlier. Cindy was given her choice of training pants or diapers, chose diapers, but screamed every time she moved her bowels into them. The pediatrician assumed that her stools were too hard and recommended some mineral oil to soften them up a bit. He also hoped that the ease of movement would make her more willing to go. Her stools began to leak and it looked for a while as if she were truly getting sanguine about the whole thing when suddenly she would start screaming in the toilet. She often required her father to sit with her and hold her hand, at the same time accusing her mother of not loving her like Daddy did.

Mrs. Evans was a sophisticated woman. She assumed that such accusations meant that it was Cindy who was the angry and unloving one, defensively turning the whole thing around. So she began to engage her daughter in "talks." She would say that people can love each other and still be angry from time to time. Cindy would reply, "Say it again." Despite her sophistication, however, it was not until recently that it had occurred to Mrs. Evans that the pregnancy might be contributing to the chaotic situation at home. Her anticipated delivery date was only one month off, but she had not looked pregnant for quite a while, so she had discounted it as a potential stimulus. When she finally brought her pregnancy into the "talks" between them, Cindy announced that her own belly was big too, and Mrs. Evans assured her that she would have a baby of her own someday. The mother repeated this reassurance often, assuming that there was nothing else Cindy had against her except envy of the pregnancy. Cindy became craftily evasive about the entire matter. Once she said she had a baby of her own in her "tum," and Mrs. Evans asked her how it felt to have a baby in the tummy. "No, no, no," Cindy replied, "in my 'tum,' my 'tum,'" indicating her *thumb,* and with that she moved quickly on to another subject. The bowel retention intensified. The scenes at stool times became more dramatic and more disconcerting. The pediatrician upped the dose of mineral oil. He proposed to loosen her bowels so much that she would no longer be able to retain them.

"It was so sad to watch her," Mrs. Evans volunteered. "She would lie down perfectly still in order to control her urge." Mr. Evans added, "She looked wasted and unhappy and her whole body would hurt her and there would be 20 or 30 false starts and you could do nothing to get her onto the potty, although she was asking to go." Mrs. Evans: "The false starts were bad, but it was even worse without the false starts." Cindy began to smell from leakages all the time, was getting to be a *persona non grata* at the daycare center, walked about with a tense, pained look, and was making everyone in the house pretty miserable. "We began to have our doubts about the mineral oil approach," Mr. Evans offered. "Even if it had worked for her bowels, something was bothering her and we assumed that it would only come out some place else." So when the suggestion was made that they consult with a child analyst, they accepted it with some eagerness.

Indeed, stool retention was not Cindy's only problem. She had become an "extremely hysterical unhappy child" in the past 5 months. She was easily disappointed by other children. A thread in her bathtub could ignite her terrors; if her foot was uncovered at night, she would begin screaming. Seven months earlier she had become aggressive at the daycare center, pulling at other children's hair and provoking fights. Her closest friend was Katie. She would begin punching Katie and even as she was doing it would insist that she wasn't. She would say to Katie, "I'm not hitting you, Katie." The daycare teachers, not to mention Katie, were hardly persuaded by such protestations. During those times, Cindy insisted that her parents beat *her* up, evoking a certain sympathy from the crowd.

Cindy also was afraid of loud noises and of bridges. On the positive side, the parents thought she was a very bright and alert youngster. She also had a lively imagination. She would learn a song and soon transpose the lyrics into something more personally relevant. She held frequent conversations with her cookie-monster puppet, even when it was not around. Separating from her parents had never been a problem. She loved the other adults in her life and freely visited with them. She went through an "It's mine!" phase with other children for a while, but recently had pledged herself to greater sharing. And, in general, although Cindy was hesitant whenever she faced a new task, she had always readily engaged new people, children or adults.

After our first visit, I met with each parent separately. I found out a little about their own lives, their backgrounds, their relationship to

each other, and both filled me in about Cindy's earlier years. Sib-
lingship seemed to be a problem for each of the parents, and Mrs.
Evans was also troubled about her relationship to her own mother. Her
pregnancy with Cindy had been "nice"; she described herself as being
in a cloud, smiling all the time. She was a librarian and worked until a
week before the delivery. The parents had attended natural childbirth
classes; looking back at it from a distance of 3 years, both recognized
that they had accepted everything about childbirth except the fact that
a baby would soon become a part of their lives. Each would probably
have preferred a boy. When Mr. Evans saw Cindy moments after her
birth, he said, half-kiddingly, "That's not a boy." Mrs. Evans was mildly
depressed following the birth. Cindy was an irritable baby, and Mrs.
Evans received conflicting suggestions about management. When Cindy was 6 months old, Mrs. Evans was besieged by such a severe attack of
claustrophobia that she rushed off into analysis and had been in treatment since. It was her analyst, in fact, who had finally urged that she
consult about Cindy. A feature of behavior that struck both parents
was Cindy's attitude about control or mastery. They first noticed it
when she began eating solids. She refused to eat what *they* fed her but
ate heartily once she was able to use her own hands to pick up the food.
They tried to let her do things at her own pace and in her own way. The
stool issue, however, had exceeded the limits of their tolerance. We all
agreed that my meeting the child directly might be helpful. Mrs. Evans
thought that Cindy would accept the idea of seeing a special doctor
who might deal with her doody problems, so a time and date was
arranged. It was July; my vacation and the second baby were just a few
weeks away. I hated the idea of a deadline and worried about how
much could be done.

The child who arrived was tiny; she had straight hair that was cut
short and she had large, pale-blue eyes. There was an expression on
her face that was halfway between a grin and a grimace. Her abdomen
protruded. She eyed me cautiously and slowly disengaged herself from
her mother. My first impression was that she was as cute as a button.

She came with a naked doll, a small bag with the doll's clothing in it,
and a toy swing. She began to advise me about the care of her doll, how
it was to be clothed and how it must be fed. She explained that her doll
was scared of monsters and especially of the cookie-monster. I grunted
a noise that conveyed the idea that it was a terrible thing to be afraid.
Once the doll was fully dressed, Cindy placed it in the swing and
pushed it back and forth in a gentle rhythmic manner. She called it a
baby. I noted aloud, more or less addressing the ceiling, that a baby was
soon coming to her house. "A brother," she said. She expected to feed

him once he came. As she said this, she inadvertently stuck her foot out and kicked the doll out of the swing in such a way that it shot halfway across the room. She stared at me blankly; then her expression took on an apprehensive cast. It was a tense moment.

I felt emboldened: "That looks as if it was fun." I was lucky. She laughed and did it again, then again. It became a game: doll in the swing, rock the baby, kick it across the room, retrieve it, and place it back into the swing again. Cindy was laughing heartily. She told me that her mom said she shouldn't hit Katie. All the time her mom said she shouldn't hit Katie. But she couldn't help it, sometimes she was mad at Katie. My success emboldened me even further. I said, "Maybe you're mad at the new baby who's coming, too. You want to be the only child in the house." "I must show you something," she replied in an apparent *non sequitur*. She scampered to the waiting room and came back with a magazine with a picture of an alligator in it. She pointed out the alligator, talked about cats and dogs, and imitated all of them. "Kangaroos have babies in their pockets," she noted, giggling playfully and darting about. Demonstrating some of her physical exercises, she did some sit-ups vigorously, pointedly touching her bottom, while assuring me that she was able to make "sissy and doody" by herself. She came to rest, happily smiling. She turned her attention to the doll across the room, still flat on its face on the floor. "The doll likes you," she said. I was all confidence now. I said, "Maybe the doll likes me, but I know that you like me too and don't want to share me with the doll." Retrieving the doll, she drop-kicked it to the other side of the room again. I suggested that she would just as soon not have that brother, either. She pulled out another book about animals and told me how they slept and how her parents slept in their own bedroom without her. She wanted to join them. She did some drawings for me, a figure that she called a person, and another that was a cookie-monster. When I asked her to draw a mommy, she drew the capital letter "H," explaining that it was a "mommy-H," and placed a "broken baby small-h" alongside. The session had proceeded at a fast pace; we were both a bit worn out as it came to an end.

I thought it had been quite an hour. Cindy must have thought so, too. Mrs. Evans called to tell me that Cindy spontaneously moved her bowels in the toilet when she came home.

I saw her two more times before I left for vacation. We talked about the expected baby. Bowel retention was no longer a problem.

In August, a sister, Emily, was born. Cindy returned in the fall and we had a few more sessions together. Something new was on her mind. She introduced another game. She assembled blocks and seemed compelled to put the blocks together in a way that created spaces. There were stables for horses or barns for cows or rooms for people. The ability to construct a space seemed more engaging to her than who or what would occupy it. She came upon a toy gun and gleefully shot up the office. Her attention was straddled between the spaces and the gun. (Making some assumptions about the symbolic meanings of spaces and guns, I hypothesized that she was struggling with gender assertion, a phallic phase conflict.) She sharpened a pencil as finely as it was possible to do and drew a family comprised of a mother, a father, and a baby. The baby was a boy. She giggled and confessed the baby was *really* a girl. She showed me how to change the boy into a girl by giving the figure larger eyes and longer hair. "That's the difference between boys and girls," she explained. She ended that meeting by telling me a little about her sister and her involvement with her caretaking. Emily was not as bad as she thought she would be.

A sense of stability, even tranquility, fell over the household. Both Cindy and her parents appeared to have completely forgotten her doody problem. This first period of treatment came to an end. I was a bit uneasy about stopping. I consulted a colleague who agreed that the treatment could be brought to an end, and advised me that Cindy would be back. He was right.

I heard from Mrs. Evans 2 years later. She phoned with this story. Cindy had been having more difficulties with her old friend Katie. They had both been promoted and were in kindergarten together, still scrapping. A few days earlier, Cindy, who had insisted on having her hair grow in long, had impulsively taken scissors and cut it short, and in rather a raggedy fashion too. Furthermore, she had been complaining about witches in the fireplace. Matters had been going quite well otherwise, and none of those issues would have been sufficient reason to call. The evening before, however, Mrs. Evans had been reading a bedtime story to Cindy when Emily, the new sister, now 2 years old, called out from her own room. Mrs. Evans excused herself, assuring Cindy that she would be back in a second. The second became many minutes and almost an hour until she returned. She found Cindy seated bolt upright in her bed, frozen with rage, staring rigidly at the wall. "What's wrong?" Mrs. Evans asked. Cindy's reply was rich in meaning. "I think I better go see Dr. Abrams," she said.

The Cindy who came at 5½ was a bit taller but every bit as appealing as I recalled her. Her hair bore traces of the recent impulsive cutting; her eyes were as big and as blue as before. She was obviously happy to see me. She entered singing.

Momma and Emily sitting in a swing,
    K-I-S-S-I-N-G.
First comes love, then comes marriage,
Then comes Emily in a baby carriage.
    Sucking her thumb
    Wetting her pants
Doing the hula-hula dance.

It was clear that the intrusive little sister, the rival for bedtime stories, was now very much on her mind. With the song, she caught me up with 2 years of indignation. But that was not the only issue in the song.

Halloween was close at hand. It provided her with an excuse to talk about witches and ghosts and monsters. She assured me that she did not believe in them, but sometimes they really did visit her house. Her sister did not believe in them either. Her pet rabbit, however, very much believed in them.

Something strange was happening in her house with her pets. Her dog Freddie, a boy, was in love with her rabbit, Snow White. But they found out that the rabbit was also a boy, so they changed his name to Prince Charming. Now Freddie and Prince Charming loved each other, but they were both boys! This evoked peals of laughter from her. Imagine boys loving each other, she said. She repeated the song about Momma and Emily as she sharpened a pencil. She thought about sticking the pencil into my mouth, poisoning me with some make-believe poison on its tip. She told me with mock seriousness that she had a brother born when she was 4 and he was stuck with a pencil and died. I told her that love and having babies were very much on her mind these days. She gave me a look that all patients reserved when it occurred to them that the analyst was listening just a little more atten-tively than they had imagined and she promptly closed the topic by insisting we play "concentration." She was very good and almost beat me.

Cindy came several times in the next few months. The latent themes of family, loving, homosexual and heterosexual relationships, and babies interwove. It was difficult for her to represent the themes in words that were manageable, so I did my best to help her. She invented a story of a family comprised of mother, father, and daughter. Father left and mother and daughter lived happily ever after. She was strug-gling with what seemed to her as an absurd but intriguing relationship between mother and daughter. The rivalry with sister for one kind of love *from* mother had changed into a rivalry with father for another kind of love *for* mother. She talked, she drew, she played, and I tried to identify her feelings and help her articulate her unrecognized thoughts. As in the first period of treatment, Cindy settled down and the parents suggested that we stop. I was even more reluctant this time than before. Cindy was in the midst of a major phase conflict and it was not clear how it was resolving. The pathways of identification seemed clouded. But the restoration of stability at home proved decisive for the family; her parents withdrew her.

Six years later, Mrs. Evans called again. Cindy was 12. She had transferred to a new school and did not seem to be doing as well as the parents had hoped or expected. She charmed the teachers and got good grades without doing much work. Mrs. Evans saw her as manipulative and controlling. Cindy's fear of witches had long since passed; however, she was a bit fearful of burglars these days. Someone had broken into the house a few months back, but the fear antedated the event, although it had intensified since. None of the old symptoms were around. The anal retentive problem truly had left long ago; however, Cindy was overly attached to her bathroom. She often made phone calls from the toilet and entertained friends there. Mrs. Evans reiterated that school was most worrisome: her daughter was not living up to her potential. Cindy was reluctant to meet with me over what she viewed as such a trivial issue, but would I see her?

Cindy had become a big girl. Her eyes still dominated her face; her hair was long and neatly trimmed. But she was broad, big-boned, even strapping-looking. The tomboyish effect was further accentuated by the fact that she came to my office wearing a football jersey. She brought a book with her; it was an interesting book, she explained, a mystery story, but every few pages the reader was offered the choice on how to proceed. If you decided the story should go in one direction, you were directed to page so-and-so; if you wanted it to go another way, then you went to a different page. There were many paths the story could take, but the paths were completely in the control of the reader. She liked the book. I silently recognized her message. She must be in control or it was no deal. Coming to see me was strictly her mother's idea, not hers. The image of Cindy, the infant, who would not eat solid foods until she could handle it herself, returned to me. This feature of acting upon persons and things in the service of control seemed to be a dominant feature in her character. She reminisced. She took the same chair she used when she was little. She recalled hiding from me at times in the waiting room. She smiled, recalling her fear of witches in the toilet. I commented that I could not recall her having been afraid of witches in the *toilet*. She explained that that was why she retained her stools when she was little, because she was afraid they were in the bowl. Didn't I realize that? Later, they moved on to the fireplace. She laughed at the memories of her childishness. I recalled to myself that the fear of witches was an age 5 phenomenon. I was silently struck with this example of retrograde distortion arising from subsequent phase reorganization; her aggressiveness was not available in the reorganization, only her anxiety and the displacement. She volunteered that she was currently afraid of robbers; but someone *really* did break into the house recently. She was not afraid of them stealing anything—oh, it was true that she had some cash hidden in a box and her stereo *was* valuable—but her main concern was that robbers sometimes killed. Occasionally, she had trouble falling asleep thinking of the robbers and had to call to her mother for solace. This irritated her mother, so she made Cindy come to see me to do something about those nighttime awakenings. School was okay. She wanted to be a journalist. She did a report on *Flowers for Algernon*, about a mental defective who was cured and then became dumb again. I sensed the transference in the comment. Her father traveled a lot; her mother was back in the library; her sister was a snot. The rules of the house were that she could not hit Emily unless Emily hit first. Their old dog died, but they had a new one. She had three close friends, all tough girls like her. One could beat up her brother. They even rode on subways. She liked to be with people who could take care of themselves. She had a bird and a hamster, but her parents were insisting that she take better care of them, so she may get rid of them. She once had two turtles; one got diarrhea, so she got rid of *them*. I silently recognized the continuity of the repressed original hostility, not so subtly displaced. She went on: there were no problems in her life. In the future she would not call out to her mother in the middle of the night quite so often. And, thank you, but she was not coming back.

The parents came to see me a week later. They reviewed their concerns about Cindy. She could do a great deal, but she always had to be pushed. She needed approval too much. She was less fearful at home since her visit to me. They decided to provide her with a tutor to enhance her "potential" and Cindy seemed responsive. After the phone call to me, Mrs. Evans thought about Cindy's excessive involvement with the toilet and decided to speak to her about it. Curiously, Cindy immediately renounced the habit. They had another conversation recently where Mrs. Evans, despairing about having to push Cindy so much in everything, asked her what she would do if something happened to her parents? Cindy reassured her mother: she always had Dr. Abrams. I told Mr. and Mrs. Evans some treatment might be useful at this time, but that Cindy was simply too reluctant to go ahead. In any case, it looked as if the consultation had been enough to pull things back into place in a way that pleased everyone.

Three years later, Cindy phoned for an appointment herself and arranged for a visit. Her hair had more of a reddish cast than I had ever noticed before, setting her blue eyes off in an attractive way. She smiled easily, but her face also revealed some sadness. Her voice was in a low register and it was throaty. She was broad and slightly overweight. She explained she was having repeated quarrels with her mother. Emily, thank goodness, was now an ally. Father had been known to lock himself up in the bathroom to retreat from the quarrels, which were usually over school matters. Mother regarded her as irresponsible. Cindy was secretly dissatisfied with her performance, but her mother was even more dissatisfied. Cindy felt worse about her mother's disappointment than her own dissatisfaction. The school was a difficult one; the academic standards were high. She was considering a transfer to a place that would allow her to concentrate on her artistic side. She liked to draw, especially with charcoal or acrylic paints. She usually did still lifes; nonrepresentational art, she explained, required you to feel a "certain" way about life and she did not feel that way. She enjoyed dancing. She loved piano and played the viola in the school orchestra. Classical music moved her. Ordinarily, she hated practicing her scales but when she got them all right, she had a very satisfying feeling.

There was no one in the house she could talk to these days, with the possible exception of her sister. When she felt lonely, she talked to the pictures that hung in her room, or sometimes carried on a dialogue in her mind. It was especially bad when she was restricted from the phone. (I remembered the little 3-year-old who loved to chat with her imaginary cookie-monster.) Her best friend was Lisa, a nice girl. She had no fears. She laughed at the memory of her childhood anxieties. She could not remember the stool retention at all now, but the witches in the fireplace were still vivid in her mind. She would like to see me for a while.

This time we spent nearly 6 months together. She complained about her distant father and her quarrelsome mother. She was on the edge of quitting her school with its demanding academics, when she turned it around and began to do well. She decided to remain, while intensifying her artistic interests at home and extending her friendships. She was ready to give up on her mother. They had violent quarrels over school, weight, and friends. Cindy rebelled: she told her mother she must be allowed to pursue her own interests and find her own direction. Mother could not cut her off from her friends just to punish her; she was as upset about her grades as her mother and would try to do better. Emily became a real sister, siding with her openly; she was a good kid, after all. When finals came and she did well, Cindy told me that it was time to stop again. Mr. Evans phoned me. He said things were much better at home and he thanked me. Once again the treatment concluded with the appearance of greater stability in Cindy and within the family system.

DISCUSSION

The mind attempts to maintain psychological stability in the service of adaptation by dealing with a host of changing outer and inner stimuli. That sentence is even more complex than it seems to be; inherent within it are certain assumptions about psychological aims, about what "outer" and "inner" actually mean, about the mind's many functions and how they are distributed within different agencies, about the concept of adaptation. From a clinical point of view, distressing symptoms or signs of an unsettled struggle within the object-interaction system suggest that the mind is failing at its task and that some interventions are indicated.

The interventions can be conceptualized from an operational point of view or from an intrapsychic one. Operationally, an analytically oriented therapist or an analyst helps sort out meanings or discover unrecognized ones in order to promote a psychological system less encumbered by unconscious pathogenic components. He does this by questions, confrontations, clarifications, and principally by interpretations. Conceptualizing operationally focuses on the relationship as a transaction or an encounter or as a setting for transference-countertransference exchanges. The intrapsychic point of view focuses on what goes on within the mind of the patient in response to the interventions, i.e., what personal meanings the patient assigns to the relationship or to the proposed interpretations in his or her pursuit of a restored psychic equilibrium. The distinction between the operational and the intrapsychic is clinically useful. Sometimes a therapist says one thing, while the patient understands it as something else. If a remission of symptoms results, the therapist may feel confirmed in his operational propositions without bothering to recognize that the patient has placed a different valence or understanding upon what has been proposed. At the same time, the patient may reaffirm the foundations of his own personality, with many of the pathogenic components intact, without needing to recognize that the therapist has been offering something very different. This may readily occur, particularly if the patient has a compelling need to control and has well-developed synthesizing and organizing capacities.

There may be a group of patients characterized by such capacities. They are able to utilize the perceived relationship or the proposed offerings in ways that permit them to restore outer and inner stability along previously laid-out paths. Some may do it by finding support for defense; others by viewing an intervention as a fresh myth and simply substituting it for an old personal one; others still by turning self-directed guilt into outer-directed blame. The restoration of stability is a valuable achievement, sometimes an essential one in children if the disruption threatens to impair the developmental pull forward. It is also frequently useful in adults, allowing many patients to bring order to their lives and relationships so that they may engage in new tasks or experiences. For the clinician engaged in the study of the determinants of clinical results, it is important to try to differentiate the therapeutic processes that are activated within a treatment setting, e.g., the restoration of stability on the one hand as contrasted with the discovery of unrecognized meanings on the other.

This frame of reference helped me understand some of the benefits and the limitations of Cindy's treatment. I think she had competent organizing, synthesizing, and integrating capacities. For one thing, her need to act upon stimuli in the service of control suggested such capacities. For another she had a strong pull forward toward new organizations which further reflected this area of competence. In all four contacts, relief resulted: relief of symptoms, relief of family tensions. The first encounter appeared to have succeeded once she recognized her hatred for the unborn child in a therapeutic setting where such hatred was tolerated, even encouraged. I think I felt uncomfortable about her leaving so soon, because the anger against her parents, especially her mother, seemed insufficiently engaged. Cindy could make what I offered work for her: she took the interpretation about hating the unborn sibling and used it to overcome her major symptom and ease her parents' dissatisfaction with her. She probably did this through further repression of the aggressivity against her primary objects. Nevertheless, the next phase came forward, even if it was not so sharply demarcated from antecedent ones.

Something similar happened in the second encounter, where the oedipal engagement was so evident. She was in a setting of intense conflict and the homosexual elements were quite prominent. Looking back at it now, I suspect that the prior unsettled hatred of her mother was an encumbrance to some of the feminine identifications needed to move the oedipus complex toward a more felicitous solution. But, as before, the therapeutic interaction served her well; or to approach it from an intrapsychic framework, what she did with the interaction served to restore stability along a path that worked for her. Empirically, her phobias diminished and the family interaction became smoother.

In the very brief third encounter, Cindy was centered in a preadolescent phase. The tendency toward regression that characterizes this phase was simply too much of a threat for someone who relied so much on a control system, so she rejected any extended contact. Nevertheless, she found elements in her mother and me that allowed her to reinforce the threatened stability and she brought those elements together. She agreed to work harder at school and stop her socializing in the toilet.

Finally, in the fourth period of treatment, she used the interaction as a springboard toward "object removal," toward a new sense of autonomy, and self-development, tolerating the discomfort of the concomitant feelings of isolation and depression. She was able to achieve this even while accepting her parents' values about school and work—although she made them her own values. During this time, the organizing capacity helped her negotiate the pull forward in the service of development.

The continuity of her relationship to me over time and through different phases struck me as remarkable, something that went beyond transference-countertransference concepts as they are generally understood. How I was represented in her mind (a primary object as well as a displaced one, a persistently magical object as well as the voice of reality) stirred my curiosity no end. I cannot be sure what features of my behavior were most important and what she did with those features. I know I was kindly, interested in helping her feel better, committed to enriching her understanding of who she was, and I always liked her. Those are my conscious contributions to the *operational* issues. Her translation and representation of me and my offerings are on the *intrapsychic* end of the conceptual spectrum, an area far more difficult to explore. Yet for an analyst, it is most vital since it is an area that could provide core answers to questions about treatment processes. Regrettably, because of the limitations of depth and breadth in such brief contacts, I cannot propose a satisfactory scheme that bridges the operational and intrapsychic in this instance. However, it is my impression that the use of her inherent synthetic, integrative, and organizing capacities appeared to be a unifying and perhaps a fundamental factor in all her improvements. Her psychotherapies were effective since they allowed her to restore inner and outer stability. These hypotheses about therapeutic action are less dramatic than those ordinarily expected from psychoanalysts, because they underscore structure and function rather than meanings. But I believe they may be usefully applied in clinical work and in theory-building. I would like to contrast the work of restoring stability in psychotherapy with what goes on in psychoanalysis, where, I believe, the analyst imparts a continuing *disequilibrating* effect, precisely in order to reach pathogenic components ordinarily not accessible by other techniques.

SUMMARY

1. Psychic equilibrium serves work, love, and play.
2. When such equilibrium is disrupted, symptoms occur.
3. Psychotherapy is effective when the equilibrium is restored. The restoration of such equilibrium may be a unifying feature of many psychotherapies.
4. The actions undertaken to restore the equilibrium may be viewed within an operational framework or an intrapsychic one.
5. The operational framework is more readily inferred from observable features. It describes the relationship the patient and doctor make with one another in pursuit of their avowed aims. It highlights technical features.
6. The intrapsychic framework attempts to describe and explain what goes on in the mind of the patient as the treatment proceeds, and what goes on is often very different from the avowed aims of either participant. It highlights individual structure, organization, and meanings.
7. There may be a class of patients who very easily restore their psychic equilibrium within a therapeutic setting, independent of the theoretical assumptions of the therapist or the avowed goals of the treatment. They are people with compelling synthesizing, integrative, and organizing capacities used in the service of development, mastery, and control. There may also be a class of therapists with similar capacities who apply them in conjunction with their authority in order to facilitate such a restoration. The restoration of stability is a valuable treatment goal for many children and adults.
8. Attention to these capacities may be useful for furthering clinical work and for appraising various theories of therapeutic action, especially those theories that rely heavily on positive clinical results for evidence. It may also be one of the starting points to distinguish the treatment process in analysis from the treatment process in other therapies.

The Reality in Fantasy-Making

SHLOMITH COHEN, Ph.D.

PSYCHOANALYTIC INVESTIGATIONS INTO HUMAN EXPERIENCE HAVE RE-
vealed the complex relationship between inner experience and outside
reality. The contributions of reality to experience are manifold. They
range from the physical characteristics of the body with its strengths
and weaknesses, through daily events of child care, family structure,
and environmental conditions, to traumatic events such as abuse, accidents, illness, and death. These impacts of reality on experience and
behavior captured the focus of attention in psychological research for
almost a century. At the same time, psychoanalytic research focused on
the other side of the issue—the ways by which inner reality affects
experience and shapes outside reality. Many issues are related to this
topic, for example, discharge of drives, the yearning for objects, the
need for defensive devices for the protection of oneself and others
from inner sources of danger.

In trying to address these issues, we are recurrently faced with the
problem of the interplay between the perception of reality and fantasy
life. The sexual abuse of children may serve as an example of the
problem. Clinical experience tells us how difficult it is to untangle
components of reality from the components of fantasy in such alle-
gations. What is perceived as an assault from the outside may turn out
to be a production of fantasies, motivated by drives at a certain stage in
development. Yet, some fantasy products are believed to result from
actual confrontations with an abusive person in reality. The difficulty
in sorting out reality from fantasy in these cases is evidence of the
ambiguity in the formulation of the relationship between the two.
These matters have long been at the center of disagreements and
debates inside the psychoanalytic school and between this school and
other disciplines.

Department of psychology, Hebrew University, Jerusalem.

This paper was written while I was a visiting scholar at the Yale Child Study Center. My
thanks to Albert J. Solnit for his many contributions in preparing this paper. I also wish to
thank Sidney Blatt, Judy Freed, and Rita McCleary for their helpful comments on earlier
versions of the paper.

57

Relating inner experience to reality is not only a problem at the level of theory. A playing child who is engrossed in a pretend play, who is putting a doll to sleep, or who is attacking with a hand puppet a herd of animals, will reveal to the observer the complexity of the process involved in accommodating his inner experience to the reality of the play situation. The choice of play materials is not totally arbitrary. There is always a process of choosing, checking, and matching of objects for play. Issues of reality and fantasy are daily matters for the young child, and this period of life seems to deserve the term "magic years" coined by Fraiberg (1965). Yet, is it satisfactory to assume that the ambiguity and complexity of the relationship between reality and fantasy are overcome by the end of early childhood with the victory of the realistic attitude in adaptation to the environment? In this paper I want to explore developmental aspects of the relationship between inner experience and the perception of reality. More specifically, I shall look from a developmental perspective at the concepts of reality and fantasy, exploring some implications of these concepts to psychopathology and health. In particular, I want to focus on the construction of fantasy, which I shall call *fantasy-making* and look at its developmental course and significance. A clinical example may serve as a starting point, and will help clarify the issues at hand.

A CLINICAL VIGNETTE

B. was 6½ years old when he came to treatment. He was in kindergarten, a year behind in his academic course. At the age of 3, B. was diagnosed as suffering from delay in linguistic development, both receptive and expressive. His vocabulary was limited, and he spoke unclearly and in very brief sentences. The diagnosis resulted in placement in a nursery school that specialized in rehabilitating children with language problems. The referral to the child guidance clinic was initiated by the school because of B.'s severe behavior problems; he hit other children, demanded total attention from his teachers, and did not concentrate on his work or play. It was felt that without improvement B. would not be able to adapt to the regular school system and would need to be placed in a school for children with special needs. Despite quite a disturbing presentation, B. was diagnosed at the clinic as suffering mainly from a conduct disorder of a neurotic nature. This conclusion was based on the appreciation of his ability to play and to communicate with the therapist during the evaluation, and on the content of his fantasy that revealed him to be an anxious, little boy who suffered from castration anxiety. Psychotherapy was recommended, and B. started therapy once a week in the clinic.

Within a few months a pattern emerged in B.'s activity in the therapeutic sessions. He showed two ways of using the toys and the therapist.
One was the way of reality, in which he would try to build constructions
out of pieces of cardboard or wood. He had plans, mainly to build a
house, for which he needed real materials and tools like nails, a ham-
mer, paste, and the like. In this engagement B. approached the therapist almost solely to ask for things that he felt were missing, and occasionally for help. It was more typical that if B. needed help, he would
not ask directly but would make it clear through nonverbal gestures,
leaving the therapist to rely on guessing and approximating. Being
with B. in those hours felt like being with an electively mute child, with
all the frustrations and anger that this state entails. But there was
another way for B.—the way of fantasy. In the second hour he built
mountains and valleys in the sandbox; he had a father, mother, and
child in the scene, and buried the mother, declaring, "Our mother Sara
is dead."[1] He engaged in imaginative play, in which the preferred
instruments were plastic materials like sand, play-dough, human and
animal dolls. In this mode B. expressed rich contents, which were
conveyed through a wide variety of verbal and other playful vocal
expressions. The fantasies that B. developed in his play were not only
pleasant and secure; they were true reflections of B.'s conflicts and
contained elements of danger and anxiety. For example, there was a
young horse that was peeking into his parents' house, and then hopped
on top of the roof to find himself struggling with a dangerous monster.
His mother came to rescue him and they both went galloping, but again
they were caught by monsters who possessed both of them. Only the
appearance of the father horse could free mother and son from the
monstrous hold, and the family could return home safely. In another
fantasy play the family of horses was trotting around in a circle, so that
no one was the first and no one was the last, but one young horse
decided to leave the circle and started to run away. At first nobody
could compete with his speed, but eventually the mother managed to
catch him and bring him home, back to a status of dependency, passivity, and nurture.

The therapist was not invited to take part in the imaginative scenes,
but these were clearly made for me to watch, and my efforts at clarification were willingly accepted up to a certain point. The main difficulty
for me in trying to navigate my way through the therapy was the
dichotomy between B.'s two ways of relating in the sessions. He was not
ready to verbalize his thoughts and feelings outside the context of the

1. This was understood as referring to the Biblical Sara, but it could not be further
clarified.

fantasy play. This state of affairs raised a question with important technical implications: Did the mode of real action in constructing and building serve as a defense against the material that was expressed in fantasy, or was the setting of fantasy a defense against the frustrations of the more realistic attitude? An answer in either direction would lead to different interventions regarding B.'s choices of action in the sessions. Judged by the affective atmosphere and by my countertransference reactions, the trials at mastery of real tasks were the more painful of the two modes for B. His disappointment when his constructions fell apart, his fury when he lost, his sensitivity to insults from children outside the therapy and from me in the sessions, his fear of rejection and humiliation when he was not performing well—all were impossible for him to talk about, and hard for me to probe. It was in the realm of fantasy that B. seemed much more sure of his ability to attract me, to maintain his relationship with me, and to experience pleasure. Bridging the gap between the two ways of relating became the challenge of the therapy. It seemed that B. was expressing his libidinal oedipal wishes through fantasy, while experiencing guilt and inadequacy in his more realistic encounters. However, such understanding opened up another question concerning the relationship between the realistic attitude and fantasy life for B. In order to attend to this question it seemed necessary to look more generally into the issue of the interrelationship between fantasy and reality in the course of development.

A Developmental Perspective

Psychoanalytic theory draws a developmental line from a state of little awareness of and concern with reality toward a mature, consistent, realistic orientation. In the first stage the main concern is with the internal states, as expressed in the pleasure principle. During early childhood critical developmental achievements allow the child to move gradually outward and to take into consideration more and more aspects of reality. Cognitive achievements such as understanding of constancy, formation of concepts, and acquisition of language enhance the child's ability to learn about reality and adapt to its demands. Developmental research has been widely engaged in describing stages in the development of functions that are involved in perception of reality. Piaget's (1973) theory of cognitive development relates directly to that issue and has generated extensive research. Flavell et al. (1986) concluded that the perception of what is real has a developmental course; its first stage, reached around 3 years of age, is the differentiation through action of real and pretend. The capacity to interpret more abstract perceptual cues that allow a finer differentiation of the real from the apparent evolves only later, around the age of 6.

But while we concentrated so heavily on the issues of adaptation and adjustment, much less attention has been paid to another aspect of this developmental achievement—the capacity to create fantasies, that is, to construct scenes that are different from the immediate reality. This capacity of the human mind fascinated Freud and had a special place in his psychoanalytic thinking from its inception. Dreams, jokes, artistic productions, and play served as an invaluable reservoir of clues to both the inner structure of the mind and early experiences with reality. Analyses of these matters have been focusing mainly on what fantasies express of the inner experience and have not paid much attention to their developmental aspect. A developmental account of fantasy life needs to follow the ways of construction and function of fantasies in various stages of development, in order better to understand pathological expressions of fantasies and their use in the therapeutic process.

Anna Freud (1936) attended to the relationship between fantasy and reality in her discussion of the role of denial. Using some examples of young children's fantasies, she wrote:

> The ego's capacity for denying reality is wholly inconsistent with another function, greatly prized by it—its capacity to recognize and critically to test the reality of objects. In early childhood this inconsistency has as yet no disturbing effect. . . . It seems that the original importance of the daydream as a means of defense against objective anxiety is lost when the earliest period of childhood comes to an end. For one thing, we conjecture that the faculty of reality testing is objectively reinforced, so that it can hold its own even in the sphere of affect. . . . At any rate it is certain that in adult life gratification through fantasy is no longer harmless [p. 80f.].

In the course of development, then, the capacity for reality testing becomes more refined and efficient, and eventually it becomes a dominant factor in adaptation. As a consequence of this development, the child gradually gives up the emphasis on creating fantasies as a major adaptive and defensive measure, and he or she may even relate critically to old fantasies that were useful at an earlier stage of development. It should be noted, however, that Anna Freud referred to the denial of reality as a capacity in its own right and not necessarily as a weakness in reality testing. She was also hinting at a developmental course in the relationship between the denial of reality and reality testing.

From this perspective, the young patient B. can be seen to be on the verge of giving up the familiar fantasy-making as a dominant way of achieving gratification and comfort concerning his oedipal wishes. We may see in B.'s oscillations between fantasy and reality an expression of his difficulty and anxiety involved in reaching the level of recognition of the reality of his oedipal situation. This achievement would entail a recognition of his oedipal ambitions and an acceptance of the limitations of his abilities as a small boy to fulfill these ambitions. Yet, B.'s ability to construct rich fantasies was an expression of his ability to cope with reality in creative ways, which might have been significant in his development.

The dynamic relationship between fantasy and reality seems to be most accessible in the oedipal period, when the child moves freely from one mode of relating to reality to another and is ready to share this move with others. This phenomenon is most clearly observed in children's play.

FANTASY-MAKING IN PLAY

The child's ability to play and to be engaged in fantasy has been widely accepted as a major indicator of well-being, both emotionally and intellectually. This view was maintained by Neubauer (1987) and by Solnit (1987). In his formulation of the psychoanalytic view of play, Solnit emphasizes the role of play in adaptation as a way of "trying out" motoric and physical, mental and affective faculties. Yet, in the criteria that he set for recognizing play behavior, he points to another essential component of play—the ability to be nonrealistic in a deliberate way (p. 217). This component of play invites further exploration of its meaning and function. In this formulation there are in effect two active components in play behavior: one is the overt aspect that involves the practice of various skills—motoric, such as running, climbing, and building; social, such as separating and cooperating; and intellectual. The other active element is a more subtle one. It involves some sort of mental activity that perceives what is real and what is not real, and then actively chooses to dwell on the nonreal. This action is fantasy-making; it seems to be an inherent part of the action of playing and of its adaptive quality. This mental activity seems to be most intimately connected with the affective component of play. Let us look at an example for further clarification of this point.

A little girl takes a spoon and "smokes" it as a cigar. In doing so she demonstrates some remarkable achievements. Beyond the fine perceptual-motor integration, beyond the capacity to imitate, and beyond the capacity to differentiate the "real" use of the spoon and the playful, invented one, she shows that she can orchestrate and be the master of all these capacities, commanding the unreal as well as the real. The little girl could look for an object that is more like a cigarette, or she could say, "I am grown-up," or "I want to be a grown-up." All these would indicate her perception of reality vis-à-vis her need to express her wish to be a grown-up and to partake in the forbidden pleasures. In this hypothetical example we cannot specify whether these realistic options are available to the little girl, but we can feel quite comfortable assuming that she is aware of the unrealistic nature of the act that she chose to perform. I daresay that we may adore the many great achievements in the little girl's performance, but it is the playful quality, her command of the unreal, which attracts us the most. Very soon this play becomes a social game, either through adoration of the "little adult" or through sharing the pretend act in one way or another. The little girl may go on playing pretend games while being alone, exercising her capacity and need to command wishful acts. But pretend games are by no means isolating activities for young children. In fact, children seem more often than not aware of the great appeal that their fantasy play exerts on others, and the ability to engage the other via the creation of fantasy may involve some of the invaluable adaptive value of pretend behavior and fantasy-making. The child seemed to communicate something through creating fantasy, and in so doing she is likely to find an eager audience. Anna Freud observed this unique quality of adult interaction with children: their readiness to suspend reality and to participate in the young child's pretend acts and fantasies (p. 84). Indeed, we feel sorry for those adults who cannot respond to such attractive maneuvers, and we admire those who can share in the creation of the fantasy in appropriate ways.

From a developmental point of view, we ought to address this behavior not only as a source of meaningful content but also in terms of the capacities and limitations that collaborate in creating such rich varieties of sometimes unpredictable and surprising, but very often enchanting outcomes. We also need to understand the changing function of fantasy-making along the line of developmental tasks.

Within the psychoanalytic school, Winnicott was the first and the strongest believer that play and fantasy-making are capacities that develop in the child, and have a constructive and adaptive function throughout life. Winnicott emphasized particularly the unique position of this function vis-à-vis reality, and conceived of the field of active fantasy-making[2] as mediating between inner experience and outside reality. This mediation can be successful only if it incorporates aspects of reality at the same time that it adheres to inner experience. In Winnicott's view, as long as the function of fantasy-making is intact, that is, as long as a person can play, mental development can continue its natural course. The therapeutic implications are clear—the task of the therapist is first and foremost to enable this function to be active. This is more important than the task of deciphering the secret codes of play in order to penetrate to the deeper layers of the unconscious (Winnicott, 1971).[3] Winnicott's interest in *what* the child was trying to work out through playing is clearly shown in his clinical work. However, guided by his unique approach toward playing and fantasy-making, he showed little interest in transforming play into another mode of expression and communication.

In order to elaborate further on the relationship between fantasy-making and play, let us look at another example.

A little boy, 5 years old, pretends that he is a lion. He goes around roaring and attacking visible and invisible targets. At one point he attacks his younger brother and bites him; the bite really hurts. Is this painful bite still part of fantasy play? I would answer in the negative. The common consequence of such an episode would be play interruption and some signs of distress in the "lion." Not only is the wishful determination obviously there, but so are the concrete elements of the real situation. However, what is missing in this episode is the element of pretense, which would stop the act of biting before it really hurts. It may be that the little boy can fantasize being a lion, but he is not able to fantasize inflicting pain. He is not able to appreciate the real effect of his biting; therefore he is not able to create a pretend act, that is, to enjoy the fantasy-making of biting. Learning about the reality of his power will precede the boy's ability to enjoy some more lion play. In accordance with Solnit's definition of play as nonconsequential, in order to create a nonconsequential act, the boy has to have a notion of the consequences of his biting in reality before he can deliberately avoid them.

I believe that fantasy-making, far from being divorced from consid-

2. My concept of "fantasy-making" is in accordance with Winnicott's term "illusion." Winnicott reserved the concept "fantasy" for the stored early structures that populate the unconscious; see Davis and Wallbridge (1983, p. 67f).

3. It should be noted that Erikson also is a great advocate of play as an important developmental vehicle. Yet his view resembles Piaget's, in that he sees play as a precursor of full-fledged reasoning. He is less interested in its special qualities with regard to reality (Erikson, 1950, p. 222).

erations of reality, is a mental capacity that involves a mechanism of monitoring reality as one of its specific qualities. We are familiar with the conception of reality as constant and given. The concept of reality testing is derived from this idea and is correctly perceived as a cardinal achievement in mental development. Yet, in the activity of fantasizing there is evidence of the need and the capacity to take an active position with regard to the laws and restrictions of the perceived reality, that is, to exercise mental freedom from reality testing. This type of activity is by no means a sign of inadequate functioning of the ego or the higher mental functions. On the contrary, its absence is more alarming. It is our task to strive to understand how this capacity serves to enhance development, and determine what are its unique qualities in relation to drives and affects. In concluding his exposition of the psychoanalytic meanings of play, Solnit offered the idea that there exists a play-state, which is analogous to other mental states (p. 219). On the basis of the present analysis I would speculate that such a state is characterized by the capacity to monitor reality. This capacity controls the duration of the play-state and its quality.

FANTASY-MAKING AND METAPHOR

The relation of fantasy-making to the reality-oriented approach seems to be analogous to the relation of metaphors to literal language. The words composing a metaphor are commonly associated with meanings and contexts of occurrence which differ from the ways they are used in the metaphor. That is the literal meaning of a word or a phrase. If the literal meaning of a word or a sentence is totally unrecognized, then it will be understood not as a metaphor but rather as a novel linguistic material and may not be comprehended at all. The relationship between the literal meanings and the nonliteral meanings of linguistic utterances has maintained a central interest for researchers in that field. They have addressed such questions as how do the shifts in meanings of words and sentences occur, and how a meaning of a sentence or a word is influenced by the context in which it is embedded. If we look at metaphors from a developmental standpoint, there is clear evidence that the ability both to produce and to enjoy metaphors has a developmental course, which depends upon the growing ability to differentiate between the literal use of a word (or an object) and its nonliteral use (Winner et al., 1976). These results corroborate Piaget's theory of how the attitude toward reality develops. But the investigation of metaphoric language offers us an additional view of this cognitive achievement.

In the case of metaphors, after a person has reached the level of differentiation between the literal and the nonliteral, he does not discard what is recognized as nonliteral or unreal; rather, he tends to be motivated further to engage in the process of its understanding and appreciation. Unfortunately, this attitude toward reality in the use of metaphoric language has not yet been looked at in its own right, but it has been studied in the context of theories of brain functioning (Gardner, 1975). From his work with patients who suffered brain damage, Gardner concluded that the capacity to create metaphors is a function of the healthy brain and is a precondition for the adequate perception of the self and of others (pp. 294–297).

Research in the field of metaphors illuminates the intricate relationship between the perception of reality and unreality. It allows us to conclude safely that the interest in unrealistic expressions is based upon the ability to differentiate the real from the unreal. Even after such differentiation is achieved, nonliteral and unreal expressions maintain an active role in the healthy functioning mind.

In clinical practice, we are always aware of the fact that any instance of behavior is embedded in a context, as is true for any linguistic utterance. A child who takes toys from the shelves at the beginning of a therapeutic hour is understood to be doing something quite different from a child who performs the same act as he is about to leave the room. We would assume that both children are aware of the reality of the dimension of time and that in their actions they elaborate on this awareness. As in the case of metaphors, we cannot understand behavior as separated from its context. Fantasy-making may be one of the main tools available for creating and changing the context of behavior, so that it will become more meaningful and acceptable to the person himself and to others in his environment. Fantasy-making may be as communicative to others as is metaphoric language. It may be regarded as no more inferior to reality-oriented behavior than metaphors are to literal language.

FANTASY-MAKING IN ADULTS: THE CASE OF ATTACHMENT

In our culture the interest in the capacity for fantasy-making in adult life has been reserved to a few and relatively special situations: to the creative process and its connection with artistic or scientific products, to psychopathological states, and to the psychoanalytic situation and its derivatives. In any other context, the evidence of fantasy-making has been treated as a deviation from the naturally expected adaptive behavior and has been commonly neglected or condemned. Only lately has it become acceptable and even fashionable to harness this process and use it as a coping mechanism in situations of stress (Lazarus, 1977).

I want to shed some light on one area of adaptive behavior that seems to meet the criteria of fantasy-making and at the same time is a most common and essential feature of everyday life situations. I am referring to the parents' contribution to the social attachment created between them and their child.

In her investigations of the mother's internal experience and its effect on the formation of mother-infant relationship, Bibring (1959) followed mothers through their pregnancies into their first period of motherhood. She concluded that the acute disequilibrium that often accompanies pregnancy should not be interpreted in terms of earlier psychopathology; rather, it should be seen as a normal developmental crisis, whose outcome profoundly affects the early mother-child relationship (see also Bibring et al., 1961). Although widely accepted and applied, this notion has not stirred much psychoanalytic research into the nature of the processes and mechanisms that are activated in the mother during pregnancy and postpartum. In this context, I wish to stress, the process of fantasy-making has a significant role.

It is of interest to the present discussion to look at how parents become involved with their children. Loewald (1980) compared the analyst at work to a parent who helps the child through the developmental process. Describing the special state of mind of the analyst with regard to his patient, Loewald referred to Freud's comparison of the analyst to the sculptor. He wrote:

> The analyst in actuality does not only reflect the transference distortions. In his interpretations he implies aspects of undistorted reality which the patient begins to grasp step by step as transferences are interpreted. This undistorted reality is mediated to the patient by the analyst, mostly by the process of chiselling away the transference distortions. In analysis, we bring out the true form by taking away the neurotic distortions. However, as in sculpture, we must have, if only in rudiments, an image of that which needs to be brought into its own [p. 225f.].

Loewald compared the analyst to the good parent who always aims a little higher, beyond the present stage of his developing child. Thereby the parent directs his child forward in his development, helping him to evolve expectations that he can rely upon and be happy with. "The parent ideally is in an empathic relationship of understanding the child's particular stage in development, yet ahead in his vision of the child's future and mediates this vision to the child in his dealing with him" (p. 229).

What serves the parent as the guiding line in his expectations of the future? Clinical work with parents offers a wealth of information about and insight into the processes that are activated in their becoming attached to their infants and in developing images and expectations that guide them in caring for their children. One situation that particularly allows a closer look at this matter is the case of adoptive parents. Adoptive parents are often more conscious than biological parents with regard to the process that they undergo in becoming attached to their babies, probably due to the fact that they have to make extra efforts in achieving that goal. This issue undoubtedly deserves a separate discussion, but I shall look at such material in order to illuminate the function of fantasy-making.

L. was a 14-year-old boy who had been adopted when he was 9 months old. He was an active, easily irritable baby, who turned into a highly active toddler and a very hard-to-manage child. Some years later the mother sought help for L. This resulted in psychotherapy for the child and counseling for both parents. The focus of the work with the parents was their difficulty to see their adopted son as their own. Although fully committed to care for him and be responsible for his wrongdoings, they maintained a certain detachment that could turn their child very easily into "this" child. After three years of painful work the mother expressed her feelings about the change that she underwent in a pair of metaphors: She used to resent the way L. used her and their home, feeling like in a train station, where he would come and go with no real contact with her. Now she felt it was more like a nest, where the young ones fly out and return when they need refueling.

She became aware of her doubts about her own part in L.'s growing up. Then, by association, she went back to the first period with L., the new 9-month-old baby. She had had a hard time getting to know him; she was never sure whether he ate enough or was tired. She remembered how she had been fascinated by his vigilance and fine motoric ability, which reminded her of a beloved older relative. That older relative was very capable with his hands and had a special talent with watches. She knew that L. would be like her uncle, and this "knowledge" helped her face many moments of rage and anxiety, when other images of this baby and his origin were about to take over.

Why did she need to liken her new baby to any person that was part of her family experience? Would she not be better off by learning how to handle him from the experienced nurses? Their advice was available all around, but this was not what she was looking for. This was not what she was lacking. In order to become attached to the baby in a meaningful motherly way, she had to appropriate this new and real baby through incorporating him into her memories and fantasies. She needed to turn away for a moment from the external reality to her own internal reality as a measure of mastering this new real situation. We cannot describe accurately what the mother was going through by contrasting a realistic attitude toward the baby with an unrealistic one. She was trying out images and making fantasies in order to cope with a new reality. Some fantasies were horrifying, others were comforting and reassuring, but they were all part of her efforts in adjusting to a new reality. Actually, she was doing what a child does when he deals with reality via play.

This suggested formulation of the mother's mental activity seems close to Piaget's notion of assimilation as one facet of the intellectual process that leads to adaptation (the other facet being accommodation). It also seems to fall within Loewald's definition of internalization. What the present formulation of "fantasy-making" seems to offer at this point is a more concrete and specific way of discussing these important theoretical concepts. If we are able to observe more specifically and identify the processes that are responsible for making fantasies, we may be able to achieve a better understanding of their relation with reality. We may recall Bibring's discussion of the psychological processes in pregnancy. She asked whether the modern scientific attitudes toward pregnancy and birth have deprived some women of the channels of organizing emotions and anxieties. These channels had been available in irrational, magical, and superstitious customs that surrounded pregnancy in earlier ages. Without being nostalgic, we can rephrase this question in the terminology that is offered here: What can be the outcome of delegitimizing or blocking the adaptive function of fantasizing, for the mother and for the mother-child relationship? We need to know much more about the conditions in which the capacity for fantasy making develops and functions beyond childhood, through adult life, before we can address these questions.

CONCLUSION

In this paper I discussed fantasy as an ongoing, vital, mental activity that is involved in our relating to reality and to others. Calling this process fantasy-making, I attempted to trace its marks in various situations at different stages of development.

Most commonly, fantasy-making is connected with the play situation in children. In the present account I followed Solnit's emphasis on play as a nonconsequential, deliberately nonrealistic activity, and suggested that we view fantasy-making as a major process through which the person prepares to approach reality. Fantasy-making is based on the ability to monitor the meaning of behavior. When we create a fantasy, any behavior can acquire different meanings both for the creator of the fantasy and for an observer, who momentarily participates in the activity and shares the fantasy. Interruptions of play, for example, when play becomes too loaded with anxiety, suggest that fantasy-making can serve as a defensive measure against happenings in reality, but it might also be blocked by defensive reality-oriented maneuvers.

Research into metaphoric language highlights the role that a non-realistic stance plays in development. The ability to enjoy nonliteral use of language is enhanced with the development of the differentiation between real and nonreal; it is not weakened by this achievement. Development is not a unidirectional movement, from a stage in which we are unable accurately to perceive reality to a stage in which we fully accept reality and abide by its laws. Rather, the mastery of reality develops and expands through the capacity to be nonrealistic. Fantasy-making is analogous to using metaphors in the playful, active control of the realistic context, which lends new meanings to these expressions.

The model of unidirectional development from domination by inner forces toward reality-orientation has been disputed by a few theoreticians in psychoanalysis. Loewald (1980) challenged the notion that drives and the primary process are inherently opposed to the ego and have no contact with the outer world (p. 235f.). Recently, Eagle (1984) discussed extensively and critically the notions of "innate hostility" and of "primary antagonism" between blind forces that need to be controlled and the controlling agency that is in the service of the reality principle (pp. 116, 212). The function of fantasy-making, as formulated here, may serve as a process of linking inner experience and the outside world. Fantasy-making seems to be a case of *becoming unrealistic in the service of reality.* I offer this notion here as a variant of the formulation of "regression in the service of the ego." If we are ready to accept that the process of fantasy-making is active beyond early childhood, then the concept of "regression" becomes problematic. What takes place here seems like a motion inward rather than a motion backward.

The adaptive function of fantasy-making in adult life is evident in the formation of attachment in parents. Parents are faced with the task of incorporating a new infant into their very intimate experience. This task has especially dramatic qualities for adoptive parents and may be easier to study in their case. In the process of getting attached to their babies, the parents evoke many images and memories associated with the situation. While they actually handle the baby, the activity of fantasy-making enables the parents to "try out" images on the baby and to project their wishes and goals for the baby into the future. This process, shaped by the reality of the infant, further shapes the reality of parent-child relations.

Due to its special relation to reality, the process of fantasy-making can be best observed in conditions that are neutral in their demand for accurate reality testing. For that reason, the psychoanalytic situation seems to be the best context in which the activity of fantasy-making can be observed and understood. Indeed, in the clinical situation there is little doubt that the ability to be engaged in fantasy as an ongoing activity is an essential ingredient in a fruitful therapeutic process. Looking at fantasy-making as a process and as a developing capacity, one can see the achievement of integrated experience that occurs in therapy as dependent upon the restoration of the function of fantasizing, with its special relation to the perception of reality. If we wish further to advance those issues and their relationship to pathology and to therapy, we need to look for new observations that will enable us to clarify this very unique human capacity.

BIBLIOGRAPHY

BIBRING, G. L. (1959). Some considerations of the psychological processes in pregnancy. *Psychoanal. Study Child,* 14:113–121.

———— DWYER, T. F., HUNTINGTON, D. S., & VALENSTEIN, A. F. (1961). A study of the psychological processes in pregnancy and of the earliest mother-child relationship. *Psychoanal. Study Child,* 16:9–72.

DAVIS, M. & WALLBRIDGE, D. (1983). *Boundary and Space.* Harmondsworth, Middlesex, England: Penguin.

EAGLE, M. (1984). *Recent Developments in Psychoanalysis.* New York: McGraw-Hill.

ERIKSON, E. H. (1950). *Childhood and Society.* New York: Norton.

FLAVELL, J. H., GREEN, F. L., & FLAVELL, E. R. (1986). Developmental knowledge about the appearance-reality distinction. *Monogr. Soc. Research in Child Development,* no. 212.

FRAIBERG, S. (1965). *The Magic Years.* New York: Scribner's.

FREUD, A. (1936). The ego and the mechanisms of defense. *W.,* 2.

GARDNER, H. (1975). *The Shattered Mind.* New York: Knopf.

LAZARUS, A. (1977). *In the Mind's Eye.* New York: Guilford Press.

LOEWALD, H. W. (1980). On the therapeutic action of psychoanalysis. In *Papers in Psychoanalysis.* New Haven: Yale Univ. Press, pp. 221–256.

NEUBAUER, P. B. (1987). The many meanings of play. *Psychoanal. Study Child,* 42:3–9.

PIAGET, J. (1973). *The Child and Reality.* New York: Grossman Publishers.

SOLNIT, A. J. (1987). A psychoanalytic view of play. *Psychoanal. Study Child,* 42:205–219.

WINNER, E., ROSENTHAL, A., & GARDNER, H. (1976). The development of meta-phoric understanding. *Develpm. Psychol.*, 2:289–297.

WINNICOTT, D. W. (1953). Transitional objects and transitional phenomena. In *Collected Papers*. New York: Basic Books, 1958, pp. 229–242.

——— (1971). *Playing and Reality.* London: Penguin Books, 1980.

From Protomasochism to Masochism

A Developmental View

JULES GLENN, M.D.

I WILL APPLY THE DEVELOPMENTAL POINT OF VIEW TO CLARIFY CONFU-
sions that have arisen about masochism. First, confusion arises from
the multiple meanings analysts have given to the term masochism.
Second, it also arises from the fact that masochism, even conceptualized narrowly as a phenomenon based on conscious or unconscious
sexual fantasies in which suffering is necessary for the individual to
achieve sexual satisfaction (Arlow in Panel, 1956), comprises a variety
of psychic structures with a variety of determinants.

Protomasochism during the preoedipal period should be differentiated from masochism, which can appear only with the achievement of
the oedipal stage. At that time and later, oedipal fantasies may organize
and transform preoedipal experiences so that masochistic sexual fantasies occur. Failure to differentiate masochism from its precursors
and labeling as masochism many determinants of masochism have
muddled our thinking.

Masochism per se can be definitively diagnosed only when conscious
or unconscious sexual fantasies which include pain or painful affect
are demonstrated or reconstructed. These fantasies are *compromise formations containing ego and superego elements as well as aggressive and libidinal drive contributants.* (I underline the fact that nonlibidinal aspects
contribute to and are part of sexual fantasies.) Although psychoanalysts have demonstrated that sexuality starts in the preoedipal period (Freud, 1905), it will be recognized that mature sexuality, i.e., with
sexual fantasies, consolidates in the oedipal period.

Clinical professor of psychiatry and training and supervising analyst, The Psychoanalytic Institute, New York University Medical Center.

Maleson (1984) and Grossman (1986) have studied the precision and usefulness of the term masochism as it is employed in psychoanalysis. The fact that masochism comprises not one but many configurations (Glenn and Bernstein, 1990) has led some to deprecate it as a grab bag of superficial and deep concepts erroneously viewed as a unitary structure. On the other hand, clinicians find it a compelling and useful entity which cannot be discarded. DMS III R includes Self Defeating Personality Disorder under pressure from clinicians who want to bring masochism back into focus while isolating its conscious or unconscious sexual component. Analysts have used the term masochism loosely to encompass the capacity to find pleasure in pain, or broadly to signify any self-destructive behavior or fantasy, or more strictly to mean particular perverse sexual activities or fantasies. The fact that one cannot know without extensive analytic work the genetics, dynamics, and structure of a variety of "masochistic" disorders casts doubt on the validity as well as the utility of our labels, especially when they are applied prematurely.

Freud (1924) described three types of masochism (moral, feminine, and erotogenic masochism) with quite different determinants, and then revealed that the determinants may overlap, that erotogenic masochism lies behind the other forms. We know that masochism can result from the factors he described (and others) in a variety of combinations. Studying the development of masochism, Freud (1919) distinguished precursors from full-blown masochistic beating fantasies. However, he applied the term masochism to preoedipal as well as oedipal configurations. Writing about the fantasy "'A Child Is Being Beaten,'" Freud emphasized the role of development:

> It is in the years of childhood between the ages of two and four or five that the congenital libidinal factors are first awakened by actual experiences and become attached to certain complexes. The beating-phantasies which are now under discussion show themselves only towards the end of this period or after its termination. So it may quite well be that they have an earlier history, that they go through a process of development, that they represent an end-product and not an initial manifestation.
>
> This suspicion is confirmed by analysis. A systematic application of it shows that beating-phantasies have a historical development [p. 184].

It is apparent that this development starts before the oedipal period, with the fantasy becoming transformed as oedipal desires ensue.

The failure to distinguish preoedipal antecedents from oedipal masochistic fantasies continues to be a frequent failing in our discourse and conceptualization. For instance, passive wishes for pleasurable pain during the anal stage and those accompanying genital sexual fantasies are both called "masochistic." I will use knowledge of development to clarify the many determinants of masochism which should be differentiated from precursors which have been labeled premasochism or protomasochism (Loewenstein, 1957; Galenson, 1988).

THE DEVELOPMENT OF MASOCHISM

THE DEVELOPMENTAL POINT OF VIEW

The developmental point of view (Abrams, 1977), a subspecies of the genetic point of view, cannot be isolated from the other metapsychological aspects in studying the personality. Development implies the unfolding interaction of biological maturational forces under the influence of the environment. As development proceeds, structures form and become more elaborate, and conflicts of different types occur. Earlier configurations become transformed and integrated into more intricate structures. The ego becomes more complex in its autonomous and conflictual aspects; drive configurations change from predominantly oral to anal to phallic and genital, each succeeding level containing at least certain of its predecessor's altered characteristics. During the oedipal phase, pregenital urges and conflicts still appear in modified form under the aegis of genital primacy (Freud, 1923). The superego becomes more complicated as well. Development includes changes in the ego, id, and superego working together, the interaction of which can be studied as developmental lines (A. Freud, 1965). Early development is to a great extent internally nonconflictual, but sets the stage for preoedipal and oedipal conflicts and for psychic solutions—including masochism. These preoedipal and oedipal stage conflicts are further complicated, reorganized, and transformed in later stages, including adolescence. This view of development differs from that of some who emphasize nonconflictual areas when they discuss development.

PROTOMASOCHISM AND MASOCHISM

Masochism per se has been differentiated from early experiences that lead to masochism and from protomasochism (Loewenstein, 1957). I define protomasochism as a conflictual or nonconflictual structure or pattern of interaction with others that may later be incorporated into a masochistic fantasy in which sexual pleasure and pain are linked. It does not include a full-blown conscious or unconscious genital sexual fantasy. Extending this line of thought, I consider the appearance or reconstruction of such a fantasy essential to diagnosing masochism (Glenn, 1984a, 1984b), a point Grossman (1986) has emphasized. The appearance of an unequivocal masturbation fantasy of course facilitates the diagnosis. Hence, when we see a patient who is provocative and thus gets people to attack and hurt him, we may guess he is masochistic and tentatively make that diagnosis, but we cannot be sure until the sexual fantasy appears. Early protomasochistic states do not yet include such fantasies. In overt sexual masochism, in which the person requires conscious pain, humiliation, or even torture in reality or fantasy to enjoy the sexual act, the diagnosis is clear-cut. When the patient suffers from unconscious masochistic desires without an overt perversion, as occurs in a wide range of clinical disorders, the definitive diagnosis may await extensive psychoanalysis. Clinically we can be less stringent in our criteria and rely on our guesses that the provocative person will turn out to harbor unconscious sexual fantasies of being injured. But analytic scientific rigor requires more careful standards of diagnosis. A clinical definition of masochism such as this is necessary because metapsychological definitions fail to establish it as a unitary structure.[1]

Galenson (1988), who regards protomasochism as "precursors of masochism" and emphasizes the development of aggression, defines masochism broadly, quite differently from me, as "the capacity for experiencing pleasure in unpleasure or pain." Since we define masochism differently, our views on preliminary stages, although they overlap, are at variance. I consider what she calls masochism an aspect or precursor of the condition.

With this as background, I will discuss observations by analysts that indicate some form of masochism and protomasochism at different developmental levels. The factors I describe do not comprise a developmental line leading to masochism: rather they are experiences that occur in a developmental context. A developmental line implies a compelling progression from early experiences to later end points (Grossman, 1985). However, protomasochistic experiences and other determinants which appear prior to oedipal organization do not inevitably lead to masochism. Certainly not all children become masochists after they traverse the anal libidinal stage or the rapprochement subphase, perceive the primal scene, are teased, or have any of the experiences to be listed.

---

1. This line of reasoning is consistent with the principles of medical diagnosis. A clinical diagnosis is a tentative one which requires confirmation after the physician employs verifying examinations and tests. A final definitive diagnosis may even have to await postmortem examination.

PREOEDIPAL AND OEDIPAL DETERMINANTS

Loewenstein (1957) appears to have coined the term "protomasochism" (and as a synonym "premasochism"), but applied it only to a pattern of interaction in early childhood which he called "seduction of the aggressor." He described "a little girl of eleven months being jokingly scolded by her grandmother for putting her thumb in her mouth. The baby would, with visible fright, observe the stern face of her grandmother; but as soon as she saw the grandmother smile, she would start to laugh and put her thumb back into her mouth, with a naughty and provoking expression. And so the game would go on. When the prohibition became serious, however, i.e, when the grandmother's face remained serious, the child burst into tears. Needless to say that she would try to transform every prohibition into a game of this sort, to elicit the smile of the grownup, to create that affectionate complicity which undoes the prohibition and eliminates the danger of not being loved" (p. 214). This defensive maneuver intended to prevent anxiety or sadness requires the cooperation or encouragement of the adult. It also requires sufficient perception of the adult's expression by the child to recognize the grownup's emotions.

Adult sadism may be important in this and other teasing games. The child will learn that he or she can attain the parent's love by enjoying the parent's sadism. The child may also react to his parent's nonsadistic aggression (Galenson, 1988). When the child is allowed no other outlet for aggression, or limited use of objects for such purposes, he will become prone to attack himself. Spitz and Wolf (1946) have observed such behavior, which I label protomasochistic, in infants deprived of caring objects.

Mahler (1966), without using the term, has observed protomasochistic outcomes during separation-individuation. She stated that a toddler may experience "impotent resignation and surrender (in some cases with marked masochistic coloring)" (p. 163), but did not describe a *universal* protomasochism.

The child's concurrent passage through the anal libidinal stage may facilitate a sense of subservience during the rapprochement subphase. Freud (1905) emphasized the "sadistic" nature of the anal stage. Of course, as Abraham (1924) noted, the oral stage can carry a "sadistic" cathexis as well. When the oral or anal sadism is turned against the self, *masochism* appears. However, in accordance with my terminology, the aggressive-libidinal attachments of the oral and anal stages should be called protomasochistic and, to be consistent, protosadistic. Further, protomasochism appears as the toddler submits to his parents during toilet training.

Freud described two additional phenomena that facilitate later masochism: (1) the appearance of a sibling and (2) primal scene experiences. These can occur in the preoedipal period or later.

Freud (1919) underlined the importance of sibling rivalry in the development of masochism. The child wishes to be the sole lover of his parents, even in a disguised way, through being beaten. He wishes his siblings were attacked, needs to be punished for these wishes, and therefore imagines himself beaten for his evil desires.

In "'A Child Is Being Beaten,'" Freud (1919), who used the concept of protomasochism but not the term (he suggested preoedipal precursors of the full-blown beating fantasies of the oedipal stage), distinguished three stages in the development of that fantasy in girls. In the earliest version, the girl imagines that her father is beating a child, most often her brother or sister, whom she hates. This initial fantasy, which may appear as a memory, signifies: my father, whom I love, does not love the other child; he loves only me. The girl thus gratifies her jealousy and its erotic underpinnings as well as her narcissism.

Freud observed that in the second period the fantasy is transformed into a highly pleasurable one, which the analyst must reconstruct. It becomes: I am beaten by my father. The girl, now guilty because of the successful achievement of her wishes for father's love, which have become incestuous and perhaps masturbatory, punishes herself by a reversal of the triumph. The "sadism" expressed in the first beating fantasy is converted into "masochism." At the same time, the forbidden libidinal desires appear in disguised form as a regressive substitute for the genital feelings toward father. The beating now signifies sexual activity.

In its final form, a man, such as a teacher but never the father, Freud said, beats a number of children, most often boys the girl does not know, as the girl looks on. The achievement of this form of the fantasy is complicated indeed. The teacher is the father in disguise, and the boys being beaten stand for the patient; hence the masochistic gratification of the second stage maintains itself. Simultaneously, the girl continues to express her hatred for her rivals and, for the first time, Freud says, gives vent to her hatred of boys whose masculinity she envies. Although Freud did not use the term "defense," we can see the patient's use of repression, regression, displacement, identification, and reversal.

We have entered with Freud into the oedipal stage with masochism appearing as a disguise, a compromise formation (Brenner, 1959). We should note that the first stage Freud describes involves protomasochism, a preoedipal precursor of the later oedipal beating fantasy. In the first stage the girl's beating fantasy, as Maleson (1984) observes, signifies that father loves her, but not in the genital sense. In addition, sibling rivalry can and does occur prior to the oedipal stage (Neubauer, 1982). Similarly, penis envy, which Freud says appears later, actually occurs in the preoedipal days as well (Roiphe and Galenson, 1982). Further, the penis envy generally occurs in the context of male envy in a society that favors males, and in families that do the same. The girl's perception of the boy's special status can occur quite early in his life as well.

In the boy, Freud (1919) observes only two steps. The first stage consists of the fantasy: I am being beaten by my father. This is a disguised passive homosexual fantasy. In the second stage, the homosexuality is repressed, but the passivity remains. The fantasy becomes: I am beaten by my mother. We are clearly in the oedipal realm with a prominent oedipus complex. In the first masculine stage, the negative oedipus complex manifests itself. In the second stage, a positive oedipus configuration may mask or develop from the negative complex. Freud wondered whether preliminary stages occur in boys. They do.

As the boy in the rapprochement subphase (Mahler, et al., 1975) tries to separate from the mother with whom he feels fused in a symbioticlike union, he becomes furious at her for seemingly deserting him and frightened because he imagines he has lost her protection. He then clings, but again becomes angry because he feels his independence interfered with. Among the defenses he uses are reversal and erotization. Splitting may temporarily prevent a protomasochistic or later a masochistic outcome insofar as it prevents fusion of aggression and hostility by directing such emotions toward different self and object representations.

I now turn to the influence of the primal scene in the preoedipal and oedipal periods. The interpretation of the experience will change when the child is in one or another of those stages, and the interpretation of remembered early primal scene experiences changes when the child enters the oedipal stage.

Primal scene experiences in their purest form consist of perceiving or imagining the parents engaged in sexual intercourse (Freud, 1918). The experience may result in shock trauma or have milder immediate repercussions. The child may see or hear his parents or other adults engaged in actual sexual relations, or interpret fights and arguments as sexual in nature. Because of his immature state or correct observation of his battling parents' pleasure, he usually understands the interactions as protosadistic and protomasochistic, involving fused aggressive and libidinal interchanges. It will seem to the child that the parents are attacking each other libidinally. Identifying with both partners, his sadistic and masochistic propensities are enhanced.

Once the oedipal stage appears, the primal scene takes on a new significance either retrospectively with regard to early events or in relation to current occurrences. In the child's view, it is the oedipal parents that are engaged in intercourse, with the child being excluded from genital sexual pleasure. The child feels left out, but longs to engage in and be included in the sadomasochistic pleasures.

In brief, the oedipus complex becomes the organizer of the masochistic fantasy. It incorporates and transforms preoedipally based precursors of masochism. Through defensive regression as a result of castration anxiety or superego pressure, precursors may become active determinants with a life of their own, but they retain the oedipal cathexis. The formation of the superego enables it to enter into the masochistic fantasy as a self-punitive agency.

In some patients the preoedipal factors may play the larger role, while in others the oedipal organization dominates the clinical picture. For the most part, both preoedipal and oedipal determinants overlap and are entwined. A person may use masochistic fantasies to overcome feelings that he is incomplete (Reich, 1940; Kohut, 1977). The fantasy of deficiency can stem from an unconscious conviction that the preoedipal mother must be present to complete him, or from a feeling of genital inferiority, or from a wish for genital oedipal union.

ADOLESCENT DETERMINANTS

With the advent of adolescence there is a restructuring of the personality and an alteration of sexual fantasies and feelings. Drives become more intense and cognition more complex. The superego consolidates, accommodating to the new and more mature urges and adapting to societal demands (A. Freud, 1958; Blos, 1962).

The teenager finds himself in a situation that is perilous as his drives are both heightened and directed toward his parents. In addition, his wishes for intercourse or murder may actually be realized because he has the physical ability to execute them. As the adolescent is faced with the incest taboo, he invokes a number of defenses. Using a form of reversal, the adolescent in part replaces his love with antagonism. The adults, confronting urges that are complementary to their children's, often do the same. As adult and child start to provoke and battle each other in these defensive maneuvers, their love often finds expression in a sadomasochistic interaction. Regression to early narcissistic states, another defense against incest, may reinforce the sadomasochism.

The ego ideal, based on the adolescent's new capacity for formal operations (Piaget and Inhelder, 1969), encompasses goals that are new, more complex, and often unobtainable. The superego will wax and wane as it is being reformed, but since the teenager's capacity to achieve his ideals is often wanting, he will find himself attacked through this punitive agency. These attacks, which may encompass a fantasy of being beaten by a moral parent, frequently become incorporated into the masochism. The more mature ego ideal of the teenager or adult may involve wishes to achieve idealistic goals even if sacrifice is involved (Blum, 1987), a dynamic which may or may not be incorporated into a masochistic fantasy.

The teenager's newly developed biological state often produces displeasure and lack of comfort, especially when drive discharge becomes restricted because of superego pressure. Physiological concomitants of sexual excitement may appear in intense, overwhelming, even traumatic forms, creating pain which gratifies and often propels masochistic wishes (Glenn, 1985).

CLINICAL ILLUSTRATION

There is more than one road, more than a single dynamic, to masochism. Masochism is the final common denominator of a variety of preoedipal and oedipal trends that vary from individual to individual. It encompasses defenses as well as drives and superego elements. Just as the oedipus complex incorporates and transforms preoedipal urges and patterns (Freud, 1923; Abrams, 1977; Silverman et al., 1975), so masochism contains altered early configurations in an oedipal mold.

A clinical abstract will illustrate how a variety of factors, including preoedipal protomasochistic elements, may interact to produce a masochistic sexual fantasy. The patient's oedipal masochistic sexual fantasy was uncovered during analysis when he was 9 years old. I suspect that an oedipal masochistic fantasy was present earlier, but no direct evidence for this appeared.

Bill's fantasy manifested itself after his mother, seeing a scab on his foreskin which he had produced while masturbating, offered him a circumcision as a birthday present. Delighted, he agreed to the procedure for a number of reasons. The operation would enable him to become a man, be more like his father. He considered the foreskin a feminine organ equivalent to a vagina. Its absence would make him more masculine, he imagined. In actuality his father was not circumcised, but in fantasy the father was manly because he had no foreskin. Boys said Bill looked like a girl because he was uncircumcised, he told me. The operation would also serve as a punishment for his masturbating with an attendent fantasy and serve to protect him from full castration. It gratified his wish to please his mother. His masturbatory fantasy became: I will please my (sadistic) mother who wants me to undergo a painful castration.

The form of Bill's masturbation reflected its content. The patient defended himself against the imagined ill effects of stroking his penis with accompanying oedipal feelings and imagery by stimulating his testicles and scrotum. He sought painful and passive experiences through testicular and scrotal masturbation (Glenn, 1969). He would squeeze his testicles to produce pain, thus attempting to master through repetition a painful recent scene (testicular pain after injury) and one that might soon occur (the circumcision). The pain also served as a punishment for his tabooed wishes.

Derivatives of the patient's protomasochistic-masochistic propensities appeared in his relations with children, his play during analytic sessions, and his autoerotic practices. At school he teased other children provocatively until they attacked him verbally and physically. In analysis he acted the victim when he played war; he would be the soldier who fired his rifle, and then, as the soldier who was shot, he fell to the floor wounded. At times he wanted me to shoot him in play, but he did not press his demands when I declined.

In one session he told me a fantasy story which he said was secret. If his friend David's mother found out about it, she would hit David with a brush for doing a bad thing. At this point he became excited as he started to hit himself on the behind with an imaginary brush. He then told me the story. David and the patient were walking in the woods in an area where one was not allowed to trespass when they came upon a tommy gunner. They saw a truck with keys in it, but when they came back later gunner and truck were gone. They figured that whoever was in the truck was a crook and that if they caught him, they would get a reward. But David would not be able to claim the money because his mother would get angry if she knew he was in the forbidden area. Hence, Bill, my patient, would have to obtain the bounty and give half of it to David. There was, however, some doubt as to whether he would share the money with his friend. In this story Bill fantasized venting his wrath on his friend by imagining him beaten and by depriving him of the reward money in addition. Identifying with David, Bill was punished for forbidden entrance and activity; and found satisfaction through picturing himself beaten by mother.

Eventually Bill informed me of his masturbation which included "tickling" his penis and scrotum and squeezing his testicles to produce pain and discomfort in his upper and lower abdomen. Through these practices he could punish himself for his aggressive and sexual wishes and transform a painful experience into a pleasurable one.

Bill's oedipal sexual fantasy had roots in the preoedipal period as well as later. Early painful experiences appeared to have contributed to his seeking pain. He had suffered from colic and projectile vomiting of unknown cause briefly in his first month. When he was 2 years old, he passed an ascaris worm anally, thus explaining previously puzzling periods of crying. Toilet training, according to the history his parents gave, went smoothly. He was toilet trained at 3, but at 6, after he saw his mother attempt suicide, he became enuretic. The wetting stopped during the consultation prior to the start of analysis at 8. Later, during the analysis, he engaged in battles with his mother because he didn't wipe himself thoroughly after defecation and often let a drop of urine soil his underwear after micturation. His mother's upset about cleanliness suggests that toilet training had not been as uneventful as the history indicated.

Bill's parents displayed both masochistic and sadistic traits throughout the boy's life. The mother pictured herself as her husband's victim and often provoked him until they attacked each other verbally. The father, constantly wary of his wife's malice, also portrayed himself as a victim. In one session with me he covered his genitals in a protective gesture as his wife railed and roared. The two, especially the mother, were often bitterly critical of their son. We can reconstruct the mother's having encouraged Bill to submit to her angry demands even in the preoedipal period.

Bill had repeatedly seen and heard his parents fight with one another. Even when he was in early infancy, they would challenge and scream at each other. The father was calmly and coolly cruel, while the mother was for the most part loudly and actively aggressive. For instance, around the time of the threatening circumcision, she was angry at her husband because she felt he was the cause of her recent appendectomy. Her wanting her son to be circumcised was in part a displacement of wishes to murder her husband. She also wished to curtail her rage and anxiety by being the active aggressor (the arranger of the operation) rather than the passive victim (the one operated on). However, her rage could not be sufficiently abated. In her fury she wanted to castrate her husband and even chased him about the house with a knife. Bill watched this battle, as he had many such encounters, through the preoedipal and oedipal periods and the time of latency.

He recognized his parents' excitement and correctly understood its sexual nature. He identified with both of his parents in their sadistic and masochistic aspects.

Another childhood scene was incorporated into the boy's self-destructive tendencies. At the age of 5 he observed the commotion in the house after his mother had attempted suicide by ingesting pills. Horrified, as he correctly assessed the situation, he identified with the woman he almost lost and wished to save the woman who attacked herself.

The early desire to please his sadistic mother, his anal and intestinal experiences, his repeated identification with the parents of the primal scene and elsewhere, the need to seek and master painful stimuli were significant in themselves. In this case the oedipus complex served as the organizing factor. The desire for genital pleasure with mother could be expressed and defended against through the masturbation fantasy mentioned above: I will please my (sadistic) mother who wants me to undergo a painful castration. The affectionate wish for mother and the desire to be manly like father through circumcision appeared disguised in the masochistic fantasy. The pain and planned surgery served as punishment for the oedipal crimes as well.

SUMMARY

A developmental view may help clarify confusions that exist regarding masochism. Following Loewenstein, I suggest that protomasochism be distinguished from masochism. Protomasochism comprises conditions prior to the oedipal period which may lead to masochism. Preoedipal precursors of masochism are organized and transformed during the oedipal stage and later. A conscious or unconscious genital sexual fantasy in which pain is an integral part may appear at that time. The demonstration of such a fantasy is essential for the definitive diagnosis of masochism. It is overdetermined and may result from a variety of dynamic configurations and genetic origins. In making those suggestions, I assume, following Freud, that erotogenic masochism is basic to all forms of masochism.

BIBLIOGRAPHY

ABRAHAM, K. (1924). The influence of oral erotism on character-formation. In *Selected Papers on Psycho-Analysis*. London: Hogarth Press, 1949, pp. 393–406.

ABRAMS, S. (1977). The genetic point of view. *J. Amer. Psychoanal. Assn.*, 25: 417–425.

BLOS, P. (1962). *On Adolescence*. New York: Free Press of Glencoe.

BLUM, H. P. (1987). Discussion of this paper at the Long Island Psychoanalytic Society, June 1.

BRENNER, C. (1959). The masochistic character. *J. Amer. Psychoanal. Assn.*, 7:197–226.

FREUD, A. (1958). Adolescence. *Psychoanal. Study Child*, 13:255–278.

―――― (1965). *Normality and Pathology in Childhood*. New York: Int. Univ. Press.

FREUD, S. (1905). Three essays on the theory of sexuality. *S.E.*, 7:125–243.

―――― (1918). From the history of an infantile neurosis. *S.E.*, 17:7–123.

―――― (1919). 'A child is being beaten.' *S.E.*, 17:175–204.

―――― (1923). The infantile genital organization. *S.E.*, 19:141–145.

―――― (1924). The economic problem of masochism. *S.E.*, 19:157–170.

GALENSON, E. (1988). The precursors of masochism. In *Masochism*, ed. R. A. Glick & D. R. Meyers. Hillsdale, N.J.: Analytic Press, pp. 189–204.

GLENN, J. (1969). Testicular and scrotal masturbation. *Int. J. Psychoanal.*, 50:353–362.

―――― (1979). The developmental point of view in adult analysis. *J. Phila. Assn. Psychoanal.*, 6:21–38.

―――― (1984a). A note on loss, pain and masochism in children. *J. Amer. Psychoanal. Assn.*, 32:63–74.

―――― (1984b). Psychic trauma and masochism. *J. Amer. Psychoanal. Assn.*, 32:357–386.

―――― (1985). Inner bodily sensations, trauma and masochism. Read at the Fall Meeting of American Psychoanalytic Association.

―――― & BERNSTEIN, I. (1990). Sadomasochism. In *Psychoanalytic Concepts*, ed. B. Moore & B. D. Fine (in press).

GROSSMAN, W. I. (1986). Notes on masochism. *Psychoanal. Q.*, 55:379–411.

KOHUT, H. (1977). *The Restoration of the Self*. New York: Int. Univ. Press.

LOEWENSTEIN, R. M. (1957). A contribution to the psychoanalytic theory of masochism. *J. Amer. Psychoanal. Assn.*, 5:197–234.

MAHLER, M. S. (1966). Notes on the development of basic moods. In *Psychoanalysis—A General Psychology*, ed. R. M. Loewenstein, L. M. Newman, M. Schur, & A. J. Solnit. New York: Int. Univ. Press, pp. 152–168.

―――― PINE, F., & BERGMAN, A. (1975). *The Psychological Birth of the Human Infant*. New York: Basic Books.

MALESON, F. G. (1984). The multiple meanings of masochism in psychoanalytic discourse. *J. Amer. Psychoanal. Assn.*, 32:325–356.

NEUBAUER, P. B. (1982). Rivalry, envy and jealousy. *Psychoanal. Study Child*, 37:121–142.

PANEL (1956). The problem of masochism in the theory and technique of psychoanalysis. M. H. Stein, reporter. *J. Amer. Psychoanal. Assn.*, 4:526–538.

PIAGET, J. & INHELDER, B. (1969). *The Psychology of the Child*. New York: Basic Books.

REICH, A. (1940). A contribution to the psychoanalysis of extreme submissiveness in women. *Psychoanal. Q.*, 9:470–480.

ROIPHE, H. & GALENSON, E. (1982). *Infantile Origins of Sexual Identity*. New York: Int. Univ. Press.

SILVERMAN, M. A., REES, K., & NEUBAUER, P. B. (1975). On a central psychic constellation. *Psychoanal. Study Child*, 30:127–257.

SPITZ, R. A., & WOLF, K. M. (1946). Anaclitic depression. *Psychoanal. Study Child*, 2:313–324.

Music of the Self and Others

Longitudinal Observations on Musical Giftedness

KYLE D. PRUETT, M.D.

There is only the dance.

T. S. ELIOT

SKILLED AND TALENTED MUSICIANS MUST FACE A CONUNDRUM EARLY IN their professional lives, if their art and person are to remain mutually supportive, lifelong companions. How is the performer to render his or her own, unique creativity publicly without violating or distorting its intimate, private origins and meanings?

This dilemma demands different solutions at each new developmental threshold. The natural exhibitionism of the prelatency child seems far removed from the image of the talented but addled adolescent who frets about the correctness of his attire, the obviousness of his perspiration, and the acniform eruptions on his chin. This image is in its turn equally remote from the warm, relaxed, expectant presence of the mature, acclaimed, adult performer whose entry on the stage simultaneously comforts and excites the audience. The adolescent tableau elicits a parental worry over the young artist's ability to control his art, his anxiety, and his technique. A successful performance engenders appreciation and relief. The latter image of the accomplished adult invites the audience to attend and enjoy, if not enjoin, a dialogue between artistic form and creative intimacy.

Clinical professor of psychiatry, Child Study Center, Yale University, New Haven, Connecticut.

An earlier version was presented in Aspen, Colorado on July 30, 1987, to the Fifth Annual Symposium on Medical Problems of the Performing Artist.

My thanks to Steven Marans for his helpful suggestions on the text. My thanks to Blake Stern for his gifts. This paper is dedicated to him.

My interest in the relationship between the artist's art and his developing self over time led me to an ongoing observational study of musical giftedness as it was being actively experienced by talented and skilled young music-makers at various developmental stages. It has been obvious to me as a clinician and observer of children that children experience their own giftedness quite differently from the way that same giftedness is experienced by the adults around them.

My purpose here is to articulate a sampling of children's experience over time of the simultaneous exhibition, enjoyment, and expansion of the musical gift while dealing with the unique problem (and opportunity) of the child's body serving as the medium of expression of that gift. Notions of the self, the role of significant others, "play" in the playing of music, creativity as generativity, and the role of normal narcissism in the life of the young musician will serve as points of discussion.

An anecdote articulating some of the internal events at work at the music stand will set the stage.

As a musician I have occasionally been called upon to serve as judge for vocal musical competitions. On one particularly memorable occasion, an especially gifted 8-year-old pianist was to accompany the singing, by her 17-year old sister, of a piece of her own composing. This was a family well known to me as I had had the opportunity to perform with various other family members previously. The audience was eagerly anticipating this duo's arrival on the stage, when a note was passed to me requesting my presence backstage *urgently.*

The young composer/accompanist was sobbing inconsolably in the wings. In the words I could make out she said she was "too scared to go out there unless mommy comes." I was surprised, as I knew Anna was the veteran of many solo public performances. Between her whimpers and further information supplied by her sister, the following story emerged. Anna had known previously that her mother could not attend the competition and had said she would "be okay without her." Missing a performance was unusual for this family as both parents were quite supportive of their children's artistic endeavors. However, Anna and her mother had had "words" over the dress Anna had chosen for the performance earlier that afternoon. Though her sister reported that her mother and younger sibling had "parted friends," *rapprochement* still sounded rather incomplete to me.

Anna desperately wanted her mother here to hear her piece. She seemed paralyzed by any alternatives. With the help of her teacher, I quickly organized two reality interventions. The first was a phone call to her mother from the stage door telephone. The second was the borrowing of a small tape recorder, which Anna was to carry on stage, place on the piano bench, and turn on to record the performance especially for her mother "from close beside her." The phone call soothed, the tape recorder recorded, and a lovely performance of this "musical gift" ensued.

After the performance was over, Anna requested a third intervention. She asked that a photograph be taken of her at the piano, with her sister at her side, holding her music and tape recorder, and "looking really neat in my dress." Her earlier distress was now ancient history.

The distressing preperformance conflict between Anna and her mother had increased her anxiety about performing without her mother present, something which her ego could easily have accommodated without the burden of the preceding conflict. Consequently, the need to document and *realize* her composition as a love gift to her mother increased significantly. It served the dual role of peace *and* musical offering.

Anna certainly had not lost the capacity technically to perform her music, but the emotional climate in which she was to play did not feel "right" to her. There is a great difference between the making of music publicly and its conception in private. Anna was distressed that the audience out there, watching and listening to her make music, was missing a critical object. The absence of that ingredient at this point in her life rendered that group momentarily menacing. But with a few simple arrangements, the important internalizations were reinforced, the balance between fantasy and enactment was reestablished, and the show went on—*in public*.[1] Playing, singing, even dancing in solitude may be quite beautiful and richly creative. Its artfulness and its value as communication, however, erode quickly if other hearts are not attuned in reality or fantasy.

This communication aims to counteract an adultomorphizing trend in the study of the experience of growing up musically gifted and talented. Hence, this nonclinical observational study of a normative population focuses on children who tell their own stories while they are still living them, not as recollections from an adult, selectively remembering.

The gift of musical talent is the earliest of the performing art gifts to emerge. Music seems so biologically embedded because its tools originate in the intimacy of the nurturing dyad. Witness the common lex-

---

1. This could have been a preview of what may be ongoing low levels of conflict over exhibitionism that seems to plague many performers, a not insignificant factor in the evolution of certain performers' performance anxiety as adults.

icon used in music and in the description of the successfully nurturing, mutually satisfying dyad—*rhythm, pitch, tone, tempo, resonance*. We take it for granted that the gift presents early in those children most talented and gifted. By the age of 8 or 9 the truly gifted child is already under the influence of the special pleasure and preoccupations of musical schemas.

Phyllis Greenacre (1957) defined the characteristics of talent according to four basic attributions; (1) a greater sensitivity to a variety of sensory stimuli; (2) an unusually keen capacity for the awareness of relationships *between* various stimuli; (3) the predisposition to an empathy of wider range and deeper vibration than usual; and (4) the intactness of sufficient sensorimotor equipment to permit the building up of projective motor discharges for expressive functions, i.e., an earlier and broader responsivity to both form and rhythm.

The study of the development of creativity in children is difficult because of the problem of identifying the population early enough to acquire prospective data. One exception to the weaknesses in the research to date is that of David Feldman (1980) who used Piaget's notions of development to articulate certain processes at work in the child prodigy. Whereas Feldman would agree with the necessary endowment articulated by Greenacre, he adds a further proposition. He speculates that rather than being wholly different from the normal population, children with prodigious talent move through certain "special domains" at an accelerated rate. He describes the prodigious child as one who passes through typical developmental progressions in "overdrive." He also acknowledges that the environmental response must be of the most supportive, solicitous, and fertile nature. Rosen (1964) amplifies the picture with his insight that the most important coefficient for the development of giftedness is the presence of "a special sensory endowment which determines the perceptual organization of the individual" (p. 4).

Because of my long-standing connection with the musical community where I live, I have had the opportunity to be involved with a number of performing musical children and their families over an extended period of time, not as a clinician, but as a fellow performer. This has permitted unique access across time to some 18 children who have eventually developed into the condition usually described under the rubric of musically gifted and achieving. Vocally gifted musicians were usually encountered around the age of 8 or 9, whereas the instrumental musicians were generally encountered somewhat later.

I have previously described the earlier observations (Pruett, 1987) and would like to focus here on the transition from the musically gifted adolescent to young adulthood after clarifying some concepts and de-fining some terms. Navigating one's musical gift safely through adoles-cence is a complex task, especially with regard to the art of making music in public. The longing for peer acceptance renders the adoles-cent especially vulnerable to anxiety over the way he *appears* to be making his music. Privately the adolescent may be feeling quite in love with his music in a very exposed, but driven way. Publicly he must be seen, however, to be exactly the opposite—cool, in total control, invul-nerable regardless of the medium of his music, be it jazz or high ba-roque. Such conflict makes heavy demands on the young ego's reper-toire of defenses and coping strategies. Jean Bamberger (1986) refers to this developmental dilemma as the musician's "mid-life crisis," when familiar, separate expressive musical dimensions seem to float free of their moorings in musical *representations*. This less integrated, but po-tent liberation forces the personality to come up with a strategy to protect it from overwhelming anxiety.

Two vastly different paths present themselves. One is a highly ide-alized, narcissistic preoccupation with music and the musical life as privately experienced by the musician. The other is one of an identifi-cation with the important musical adults and peers in his life, most of whom are already involved in the musical and personal life of the musician. The danger for the young musician in choosing the first path is the precarious reliance on the image of the self which is grandiose and totipotent. Self-esteem becomes anchored to the possession of certain *qualities,* such as musical success or talent, rather than the more enduring authenticity of one's own perceptions and affects. He be-comes addicted to admiration and adulation. This path generally is not chosen consciously, and is frequently the heir of a deeply rooted web of troubled early object relationships. The fortunate adolescent may ex-perience its tug only transiently, and then pushes ahead more forceful-ly, with the aid of friends, supportive teachers, and parents, to move along the path of joining rather than trying to transcend the more ordinary, less promethean life. This second option assists the adoles-cent through identification with peers and teachers to work through the struggle over the ownership of his musical talent, i.e., the gift is ultimately his or hers to nurture or abandon as he or she chooses and is neither a parental nor a publicly held property. The adolescent can then admit periodically to ambivalence about his music, without threat-ening his value as a human being. He will eventually be able to develop artistic autonomy without attacking or coming into conflict with the important internalizations in his life.

A loose correlation exists here between these two alternatives and what Winnicott (1988) described as the "false" and "real" selves. The "false self develops on a compliance basis and is related in a passive way to the demands of external reality" (p. 108). The true self is "the theoretical position from which comes the spontaneous gesture and the personal idea. The spontaneous gesture is the true self in action. Only the true self can be creative and feel real" (p. 106).

Winnicott (1988) goes further to help us understand why the successful performer succeeds in pleasing us. "The artist has not only produced something recognizable to others, but also something which is individual to the artist's true self; the finished product has value because we can appreciate the struggle that has gone on in the artist in the work of drawing together elements originally separated" (p. 109), including the previously separate artist and audience.

For the maturing adolescent, personal revelation runs many gauntlets. Increasing awareness of what his peers think (as well as the important adults in his life) augments his anxiety over the enactment of his musical (and nonmusical) fantasies. Normative adolescent processes promote self-consciousness. Meanwhile, repression arrives as a bulwark against the raucous, instinctual claims which threaten equilibrium—not an easy time to stay in touch with the core of one's artistic creativity.

Sublimation as buffer and filtration system urges the adolescent to move further away from direct involvement of the body in sensual gratification, especially in public. There may be a subtle difference here between the metapsychological experience of vocal and instrument musicians. Whereas the vocalist's "gift" emanates directly from deep inside the body and passes through the vocal (oral) orifice to the outside world, relatively unadulterated, the instrumentalist's "gift" passes through a peripheral apparatus which at least begins life as an inanimate, separate object. The latter route seems to offer somewhat more protection from unintended revelations. It is hard for an adolescent to believe that a "beautiful voice" can emanate from anything other than a "beautiful body." For the instrumentalist, normative drive derivatives of exhibitionism must expand to embrace the musical instrument which touches the performer's body. As such, the performer, his exhibitionism, and his instrument (if applicable) progress through various developmental stages together.

If this developmental integration of artist and instrument (including vocal chords) fails—and it frequently does, especially during periods of disappointment in one's performance and art—and regression ensues, a temporary disequilibrium between the cathexis of body parts may follow, frequently accompanied by a transient dip in self-regard.

Mack (1983) articulates this dilemma: "the representation of the self-as-a-whole is much more than the sum of images of the body parts . . . the assessment of self remains throughout life intimately tied to the state of the body and its parts" (p. 27). The young musician who thinks of his music as just one of several of his important "parts" has a far better chance to "get it together" later on.

The importance of making music with (and not just for) someone during this developmental era cannot be exaggerated. Whereas I agree with Gedo (1988) that a "fantasied other" is not indispensable to the creative process, it is for the adolescent especially playful to make music with friends, particularly those who share similar sublimations. This gives the adolescent the opportunity actively to play *out* certain rhythmic, instinctual derivatives with peers rather than with more conflict-ridden internalized objects on whom he cannot safely be too dependent. Most music schools and conservatories heavily credit small-group vocal and instrumental ensembles for helping the adolescent successfully weather talent's "mid-life crisis." The need to belong, to be part of someone else's experience, is as useful in the second individuation stage as it is in the first.

Sarah was an 8-year-old flute player when I first encountered her in a chamber opera as one of several instrumental music cast members. The oldest of four children from a middle-class family, she was memorable for the vitality and forcefulness of her personality and musicianship, somewhat overwhelming the other children in the cast. Neither Sarah's mother nor her father were musical, though her paternal grandfather had been concert master of a well-respected community orchestra in England before immigrating to America at the close of World War II. Her parents marveled at her musical skill and provided her with good instruction and support.

Sarah was 14 when we met next, and I was surprised to learn that she was now playing the piano. She had moved from public to private school, with the assistance of an academic scholarship which made it easier for her to study music as well. She explained her reasons for changing instruments rather casually: "The flute was beautiful—clear, clean, and pretty, always pretty—even when I tried to make it strong, or sad, or angry, and not sound so pretty. But you can make a piano do anything—loud, soft, pretty, ugly, happy, sad—anything!" Her father did not seem to be troubled by the change in instruments, but did wonder why she needed to play it "so loud all the time." Sarah: "I love fast forté passages. I hardly ever touch my flute anymore."

Our paths crossed next when Sarah was 17 just after she had won a regional piano competition. She spent most of her time talking about her relationships with her nonmusical friends, being careful to explain that she "didn't make a big deal" of her musical talent in conversations with her nonmusical friends. It was not that she was not deeply committed to her musicianship, but she had learned through a variety of painful experiences not to speak only of music. Sarah did have a special place in her life, however, for her friends who really did understand her music. She seemed to wish to perfect her playing to present it as a gift to those who mattered most deeply to her, reminiscent of Phyllis Greenacre's description of the artist's "love gift to the world."

Two years later, Sarah had left college after one year to go to a conservatory. She had begun thinking about playing the organ, because it gave her an opportunity "not only to make beautiful music and noise—and lots of it. But you get a chance to sit *in* the music, rather than just in front of it." She also explained that she had become particularly concerned about her public appearance in performance. "I do get nervous about memory lapses, fingering mistakes, but most of all looking like I don't know what I'm doing. I'm so critical of people who *look* lost when they sit down at a keyboard. They make the audience nervous, their mistakes make the audience feel bad, like they're supposed to feel sorry for the performer. I hate that."

Sarah had also learned to manage some of her preperformance anxiety by the development of several "mind games, finger and breathing games." She had the habit of stealing a look at the audience from behind the curtain or stage door. "I don't want to have to face them first when I walk out to sit on the bench."

My last encounter with Sarah was just before her twenty-second birthday. She had begun to run afoul of her own success. She was no longer considered young and undiscovered. She felt "tremendous pressure" from the younger competitors in her field and described herself as "middle-aged." She had become quite preoccupied with her own practice techniques, feeling that they were not as productive as they used to be. "I'm getting all tangled up with whether or not to practice hands alone or hands together. I've lost a little confidence in my teacher. I'm tempted to shop around. I can't seem to find anyone who speaks my language—they all want to speak theirs."

The only thing "really working" in her life was her "love life." She'd fallen in love and loved it! What's *it?* "Being in love." Is it affecting her music? "Very, very much. Certain pieces have become magical, especially the ones we both like. Some of my old favorites I can't play at all anymore. My teacher is distressed with me now and says that I better get myself together. My personal goal now has to do with trying to get elegance and power to cooperate in my music." Can you still work with your teacher? "Yes, but he's not flawless anymore. I still love his ideas, but some of mine are pretty good too. I'm going just a little bit nuts over these technical problems and he can't help me very much with them. Oh, well, I know I'll work it out. He keeps telling me that I'm getting out in front of the music, whatever that means. But the critics still seem to like me."

Sarah's teacher seemed to be aware of something she was conveying to me as well about the changing relationship between herself, her music, and the emotional, creative intent of her music. While she was anxious as a maturing young adult to integrate "elegance and power," two highly valued qualities both in her music and her personality, she seemed to have momentarily lost her bearings in that place somewhere between composer and audience where the musician lives *in performance*. Her "new love" seemed to be changing the symmetry and shape of her own musical holding environment. Her loves were changing partners in the dance.

Joan was 9 years old when we first met as soloists in a choral production. She was an energetic, ebullient redhead envied by the other children in the cast for the sheer volume and decibel level of her voice. She could sing in tune, stay on pitch, and seemed to have reasonable tone quality in a raw, wholly undisciplined voice.

Joan was the oldest of three daughters born to an Australian father and a French mother. Her father was a professor of piano and her mother taught violin. Hers was a family of intellectuals and gifted people who felt some obligation to "improve the lives of others through music and art."

Upon meeting Joan's family I heard an anecdote which Joan was later to call "part of my family's musical mythology about me." As an infant, she babbled and cooed rhythmically with complex "recognizable" tonal contours while alone in her crib. Her family seemed convinced that certain of the rhythmic and tonal patterns resembled certain fragments of nursery songs sung to her by her mother.[2] Could we be hearing the description of vocal, *musical* transitional phenomena in which the infant is allowed to claim magical control over external reality, prolonging the omnipotence implemented originally by the mother's adapting to the infant's needs (Winnicott, 1988; see also McDonald, 1970)?

---

2. Dowling (1982) reports that by 6 months of age normal infants notice subtle changes in tonal contour of comparative musical passages and can match pitch. Joan's family was uncertain as to the actual timing of her skill, but guessed it was somewhere in her third month that this began.

Joan was 13 at our next meeting, and she informed me that she was studying music "professionally," but theater interested her more than music, complaining that her singing lessons were "work."

Two years later, I was somewhat surprised to learn that Joan had abandoned her singing and had taken up the viola. She chose this instrument "because it sang." She took particular pleasure in the deep resonance of its tone, and her capacity to "make one line different from another—to make a temper, a mood, or a line." Joan had also become somewhat disaffected with singing because of the struggles she had had as a singer noticing the difference in the quality of text settings and the quality and complexity of the musical settings. "You run into a lot of lousy poetry set to really beautiful music when you try to expand your repertoire fast. The viola doesn't have that problem. Words get between you, the music and the audience."[3]

At 19, Joan and I met again and she had changed considerably. She was dealing with her musical talent and gift more intellectually and had given considerable thought to her musical experiences. She talked about feeling successful as a musician: "You've got to have the technical facility actually to *make* music the way you want to, at least most of the time. I decided to stop singing so I could focus my whole musical life on viola. Next, you need discipline. A lot of people who aren't musicians can't believe the discipline that it takes. Then you need a confidence that borders on arrogance." Joan had just won a 4-year tuition musical scholarship to a college of her choice. For her it came at a timely, fortuitous juncture because she had recently had a major falling out with her family. Her parents had "driven me nuts with their ambivalence about my music. We spent a lot of time talking about how special it was, but then they seemed to want me both to get better at it and quit at the same time."

At 22 Joan was attending college only half time as a senior to provide more room in her life for music. She had all but abandoned her viola, and had begun an active career as a conductor, producing regionally acclaimed chamber concerts with pick-up groups of "old friends." What happened to the viola? "I was always plagued with the idea that though I played well, even naturally, it was never natural enough. My singing—now *that* was natural." Why conducting? "I've played for so many *bad* conductors. A bad conductor *takes* the music from you. You

3. Kohut (1987) describes the intrusion of words in intimate contacts such as comforting or holding. "Words stress the otherness of the other. They stress a distance . . . a difference between human beings when what is needed . . . is participation in the security of another person" (p. 70).

feel tense, and angry, alone in the midst of so many musicians. You really begin to hate the instrument. You become more afraid of the mistakes you make. The public may not know, but you do. It was like I turned into a ball bearing—you bear a lot of weight and try not to cause any friction.

"I found out that I was hardly alone. I met a large number of disenfranchised string players. I decided to get 15 or 20 together. We got so good so fast, we scared ourselves. We're frightened now of taking the next step. We make this beautiful music together, and it's like this precious jewel in our otherwise messy little lives. We're really reluctant to go further. The idea of competition sickens many of us.

"About two years ago I suddenly began to feel *old* as a performer. I decided I couldn't bear the idea of being a solo performer for the rest of my life."

Was it a hard transition? "No: it was liberating!" What is liberating about conducting? "I get so *up* for a performance. When it's working, I feel as though I'm up and out of my body somewhere. Some place apart where the composer, musicians, audience, and conductor all meet. It's not in the conductor, although a lot of bad conductors think it is. They uniformly kill the audience's impact on the performance. But when it's done right, it's like listening to a dance. I've really finally found my place to make music—but I'm still not sure what to do with it. We're reluctant to develop a concert series. It's like we're afraid of what happens when we *have* to do it. I'm so confused."

I responded that she sounded confused and excited about what she was doing. "Well, I am mostly confused. I've been doing some editing and producing of recordings for a small company owned by my grandmother. It's raised a lot of questions in my mind about whose music is it anyway! Digital supertech gives the editor/producer enormous power over the final product. My God! I'm a god—muse, scribe, and lyre, all wrapped into one. I can delete, add, change; I can make it better or worse than it actually was! This became very clear to me when I was fooling around with my own recordings. Now I've stopped editing my own work. I really don't like listening to my own stuff that much anyway. Too many warts which I alone can hear. I'm not alone here either. Lots of musicians are squirrelly about listening to their own performances. They're aware of how far from perfect the product is from the intention. I don't feel that way about my vocal stuff. That's still fun to listen to."

In these selected anecdotes, not remembrances, by Joan and Sarah, we hear young adults emerging from the search for and insistence on self identification, eager and willing to fuse that identification with others—other people, other musicians. They are both ready for a kind of intimacy between their art and selves which resonates with the intimacy they are seeking in relationships. They can now commit this intimacy to partnerships, even, to quote Erikson (1950), when it "may call for significant sacrifices and compromises. [Risks are taken] in the solidarity of close affiliations . . . friendships, . . . in experiences of inspiration by teachers, and of intuition from the recesses of the self. The avoidance of such experiences because of fear of ego loss may lead to a deep sense of isolation and consequent self-absorption" (p. 263).

As we listen to these stories over time, we hear less about teachers and mentors as role models and more about them as catalytic agents or midwives. The musician's experience of his own creativity fills the gap left by the receding mentorship. Musical ideas can now exist and be fulfilled both in public and in private, apart from the teacher who may have initially assisted in their birth and delivery.

Both of the musicians who have spoken here (and they are representative of most of the children I have been following) seem to feel that their music aptitude is still evolving. It is also important to note that these young adults do not necessarily see the ultimate goal in the making of music as the elimination of stress or conflict. It belongs there as a fellow traveler, right alongside skill, sensitivity, and ambition.

Finally, it is clear that the drive to *make* music has profoundly shaped the life of these children—now adults. It is a drive which is so compelling that it is difficult to believe that environmental influence alone is sufficient to fuel the journey. Children do find that experience difficult to articulate verbally, but they have no trouble articulating it in the making of their music. It seems unique to the process itself and does not appear in other areas in their life. They are able to concentrate intensely on their unique version of the musical experience to the exclusion of competing stimuli, occasionally even of human contact. Prior to adolescence, the performance of music often is seen as a love gift.

Many talented children do not initially view themselves as particularly worthy or valuable human beings. They are merely doing what they *need* to do. They are often aware of the expensive, negative aspects of owning significant talent. We are privileged to see a developmental continuum that leads in the gifted child's experience from performing in the mode of his or her teacher (and the Suzuki method is the paramount example here) to performing the way he feels he *must* as an independent adult artist.

What seems to sustain the vitality and integrity of the musical gift is its capacity to endure and adapt to changes in sources of gratification demanded by the differentiation of the child into the adult over the entire developmental continuum. It is so pleasurable (and occasionally so maddening) over a long period of time because each new developmental era simultaneously demands and provides new choreography for the dance of self, its music, and their most intimate friends—teachers, nurturing objects, composers, and audience. Erikson (1950) clearly articulates the energy source for this task. "The strength acquired at any stage is tested by the necessity to transcend it in such a way that the individual can take chances in the next stage with what was most vulnerably precious in the previous one" (p. 263).

The study of the understanding of the child's experience of his own giftedness and talent is essential to our ability as adults to nurture to full and healthy fruition. But there are limitations to the application of such understandings. As adults we glibly muse over a child's *intentions* with regard to his music. In the end, however, it may well be the *instinctive* that really counts in the musical rendering. What the musician *intends* to do or say in and through his music may be one of the less important factors in his and its expression. More important is what is being said *through him* or, in some cases, in spite of him.

As to the ultimate value of learning the dance, it may not be serendipitous to note that concert musicians and conductors outlive their fellow professionals by a statistically significant margin (Wassersug and Wassersug, 1986).

BIBLIOGRAPHY

BAMBERGER, J. (1986). Cognitive issues in the development of musically gifted children. In *Conceptions of Giftedness,* ed. R. Sternberg & C. Davidson. New York: Cambridge Univ. Press, pp. 388–413.

DOWLING, W. (1982). Melodic information processing and its development. In *The Psychology of Music,* ed. D. Deutsch. New York: Academic Press, pp. 126–142.

ERIKSON, E. H. (1950). *Childhood and Society.* New York: Norton, 2nd ed., 1963.

FELDMAN, D. (1980). *Beyond Universals and Cognitive Developments.* Norwood, N.J.: Ablex Publications.

GEDO, J. (1988). Some differences in creativity in performers and other artists. Read at the Sixth Annual Symposium on Medical Problems of Musicians and Dancers, Aspen, Colorado.

GREENACRE, P. (1957). The childhood of the artist. In *Emotional Growth.* New York: Int. Univ. Press, 1971, vol. 2, pp. 479–504.

KOHUT, H. (1987). *The Kohut Seminars on Self Psychology and Psychotherapy with Adolescents and Young Adults,* ed. M. Elson. New York: Norton.

McDonald, M. (1970). Transitional tunes and musical development. *Psychoanal. Study Child,* 25:503–520.

Mack, J. (1983). Self-esteem and its development. In *The Development and Sustaining of Self-Esteem in Childhood,* ed. J. E. Mack & S. L. Ablon. New York: Int. Univ. Press, pp. 1–44.

Pruett, K. D. (1987). A longitudinal view of the musical gift. *Medical Problems of Performing Artists,* 2:31–38.

Rosen, V. H. (1964). Some effects of artistic talent on character style. *Psychoanal. Q.,* 33:1–24.

Wassersug, J. D. & Wassersug, R. J. (1986). Fitness fallacies. *Natural History,* 3:34–39.

Winnicott, D. W. (1960). Ego distortions in terms of true and false self. In *The Maturational Processes and the Facilitating Environment.* New York: Int. Univ. Press, 1965, pp. 140–152.

——— (1988). *Human Nature.* New York: Schocken Books.

Comments on Phobic Mechanisms in Childhood

ANNE-MARIE SANDLER

IN JULY 1976 A SYMPOSIUM WAS HELD IN LONDON BY THE INTERNATIONAL Association for Child Psychoanalysis, on the topic of "Fears and Phobias in Childhood." At that meeting two cases of the analysis of young children were presented.[1] There was, in addition, a panel discussion on the subject, and the meeting ended with a summing up by Anna Freud (1977). It is the remarks she made then that I want to take as the starting point for this paper. In spite of the excellence of the presentations and discussions in 1976, I (as well as many others) did not feel substantially wiser in regard to phobias after the meeting than we had before it. Anna Freud herself indicated her disquiet by starting her final comments with a criticism of the title of the symposium. She suggested that a title "Fears, Anxieties, and Phobic Phenomena" would have been more appropriate than "Fears and Phobias." Psychoanalysis, she said, had always distinguished between fear and anxiety, fear relating to a person's attitude toward real dangers threatening from the outside and anxiety being a reaction to internal threats arising from, as she put it, "clashes between the drives and internal opposing forces." Fears do not develop into phobias, she said, but anxiety can do so. To ignore the distinction between fears and anxieties, and "to treat the effect of external and internal threats under one and the same terminological heading is not a step forward in our theoretical position, but rather implies the reverse" (p. 86).

Thus the alternative title she proposed, "Fears, Anxieties, and Phobic Phenomena," spanned "the whole range from reactions to deprivation, frustrations, losses, injuries, accidents, attacks, disasters which threaten safety from the outside to the reactions to conflicts, guilt

---

Marianne Kris Memorial Lecture presented to the International Association for Child Psychoanalysis, New Orleans, 1988.
1. One of these cases was subsequently published (Tyson, 1978).

feelings, and so forth, which upset the mental equilibrium for internal reasons" (p. 86).

Anna Freud then turned to her specific criticisms of the cases described at the meeting. She took the view that neither of the child patients should be regarded as a classical case of phobia. Both children had fears and anxieties from external as well as internal sources, anxieties which were dealt with by a whole variety of defensive measures. Where the defensive measure involved a *phobic* mechanism, the phobic anxiety was only one of a number of different forms of anxiety. By phobic mechanism in this context Anna Freud certainly meant a mechanism involving displacement and externalization (or projection) used to create an external phobic object or situation, as exemplified by Freud (1909) in his case of Little Hans. Further, Anna Freud pointed to the need for an additional process to be taken into account in the formation of the phobia. This was *condensation,* a process which she saw as preceding externalization. She said, "This means that fears and anxieties do not remain diffuse but are compressed by the child into one encompassing symbol which represents the dangers left over from preoedipal phases as well as the dominant . . . oedipal conflicts. It is then this symbol (animal, street, school) which, as a supposed part of the outside world, is dealt with by avoidance" (p. 87f.).

Yet, although neither of the cases presented at the symposium could have been regarded as *classic* in the sense that Little Hans was, I have no doubt in my mind that they were *typical.* A search through the Hampstead Index before that meeting produced no case in which there was a monosymptomatic phobia—and in no case were phobic phenomena unaccompanied by other forms of anxiety. Perhaps the closest example found in the Hampstead Index might be a case recorded as follows:

> Six-year-old Tracie was noted by her therapist as having a fear of dogs which amounted to a phobia, yet Tracie tried to be brave and to placate dogs she encountered by giving them her sandwich. Fear that a dog might be at a party prevented her from going to it. In her play, beds had to be built very high and enclosed to prevent dogs jumping up. Tracie related this to a real incident when she was one year old and lying in her pram when a dog jumped up at her and scratched her face. She had been told of this incident or had overheard talk about it around her fourth year.

Tracie's therapist also reported that there were fantasies of terrifying animals which made nighttime miserable for her. The most dangerous of these was a mother wolf, especially dangerous when Tracie had been cross with her mother during the day. Wolves would jump up onto her bed, as would other animals—occasionally lions or foxes took the place of the wolves. The resemblance of this description to Freud's account of Little Hans makes it possible to argue that the mechanism in Tracie's fear of animals was phobic in the classic sense.

Consider now the case of Michael, who was described in the Hampstead Index at the age of 10 as having fears of bodily damage as a predominant symptom.

> Throughout the first year of treatment he was reluctant to touch the room heater or any part of the electric wall sockets. He was afraid he might get severe burns or be electrocuted. These fears were related to conflicts over masturbation and gradually diminished through interpretation. The displacement and projection of aggressive wishes played a role in his fear of body damage. For example, he wanted to purchase a punching bag, but he imagined that if he hit the bag, it would bounce back and hurt him. He was reluctant to play football at school because he was afraid he might get kicked and injured. While there was some reality to this fear, it also contained the projected wish to kick the boys in his class who were more competent at sport. For similar reasons he was also reluctant to engage in almost any rough play with his schoolmates.

In both the cases of Tracie and Michael the fears were related, among other things, to the projection or externalization of their own aggressive wishes. However, there is a distinct clinical difference between the two. Tracie's fears were focused on real or imaginary animals; i.e., there was a higher degree of condensation of her anxieties in that they related to a subclass of dangerous animals which included dogs, wolves, lions, and foxes. Michael, on the other hand, seemed to be ready to react with fear or anxiety to a much wider range of objects and situations.

What of Jimmy, aged 6, who, according to the Index record, displayed marked phobic traits? The therapist wrote that at 2½, when his mother was pregnant, Jimmy externalized his hostile wishes toward her and became frightened of cranes breaking, lamps coming off lampposts, and pneumatic drills. These fears were still present during treatment. For example, one of his fears of the bullies at school was that they might take off his glasses and break them. While Jimmy had a number of other fears as well, many belonged to the general class of "fears of things breaking." Do we say that condensation occurred here as well? One could, I think, argue both ways.

Clearly it must be of clinical value to distinguish between the various *mechanisms* entering into different sorts of fears, anxieties, and phobic phenomena, but I want to approach the problem by taking the view

that the use of these various terms interchangeably is here to stay, and
that we may have to look at the problem of differentiation in a somewhat different way than in the past. It is striking that throughout the
cases indexed in the Hampstead Index therapists used the terms "fear"
and "phobia" more or less synonymously—an indication that whatever
theoretical distinction could be made between fears and phobias, from
a descriptive point of view it is not at all easy in our child cases to
distinguish between the two. It is worth reminding ourselves that
Freud continued, after the publication of his paper on Little Hans, to
use the term phobia in the general psychiatric sense of "an irrational
fear." Even in his masterly revision of the theory of anxiety in 1926, the
distinction between fear and phobia is not consistently adhered to. For
example, Freud says, "The anxiety belonging to the animal phobias
was an untransformed fear of castration. It was therefore a realistic
fear, a fear of a danger which was actually impending or was judged to
be a real one" (p. 108).

One of the features of the 1976 meeting was a report from the
Hampstead Index Project (presented by Maria Kawenoka Berger) in
which it was suggested that children's phobias could be classified according to whether they were "extrusive" or "intrusive." Although I
am not entirely happy with these terms, I shall use them in the sense in
which they were introduced in 1976. The mechanism of the extrusive
phobias corresponded to the classical form for which Little Hans was
the paradigm. The internal danger was extruded onto the external
reality, and the avoidance or flight from the external danger provided
the illusion that the internal threat had been dealt with. It was pointed
out that in this case the phobia had a *function*, that the child *needed* the
phobic object or situation in order to cope with an inner conflict. Little
Hans's aggressive wishes toward his father were externalized onto the
horse, so that they could in some way be disavowed by Hans. Then the
little boy could avoid the horse by developing the phobia and could
experience an external conflict, i.e., one between himself and the
horse, instead of an inner conflict which was intolerable to him. It
followed that for inner reasons at that time Hans *needed* to be concerned with the horse, even when it was not present, needed to be
preoccupied with the possibility that he might be confronted with that
dangerous and threatening animal. Such a preoccupation can be obscured, of course, by the relief felt by the child who has been able to
distance himself from the dangerous external reality. Yet the underlying hostile wishes dealt with by the phobia do not disappear with avoidance of the phobic object. A *relationship* can be said to have developed to
the phobic object, and this relationship can be lived out in fantasy in

which the child deals with hypothetical or anticipated encounters with the phobic object. I believe that the concept of a "phobic relationship" may prove to be an important one.

It will be recalled that Little Hans, when his anxiety was strongest, expressed the fear that a horse would come into his room. Later, for a while, his fear of horses "became transformed," said Freud, "more and more into a compulsion to look at them." Little Hans had said: "I have to look at horses, and then I'm frightened." That horses were constantly present in his fantasies is reflected in his wish to ride on the back of a new maid while she cleaned the floor, calling her "my horse," holding onto her dress with cries of "Gee-up"; and so on.

In her discussion Anna Freud (1977) expressed her doubt:

> . . . children who suffer from phobias not only flee from the object of their anxiety but also are fascinated by and compulsively drawn toward it. Even though this may be so in some instances, it is certainly otherwise in the majority of cases. School-phobic or agoraphobic children can be seen to be quite unaffected so long as leaving home is not enforced; the same is true of the animal-phobic ones when the dreaded animal is out of sight. In short, there seems to be overwhelming clinical evidence that the truly phobic defense is effective in blotting out any positive seductive aspect hidden behind the anxiety and in leaving the child peaceful and not agitated in the absence of the phobic object [p. 88].

Anna Freud here appeared to disagree with herself, because in contrasting restriction of the ego with phobia she had said that "the wish has to stay alive in order for the phobic avoidance to be there. . . . [In the phobic process] the investment remains firmly attached to the avoided activity or situation, and an anticathexis has to remain in place just as firmly" (J. Sandler and A. Freud, 1985, p. 360f.).

I said that Anna Freud *appeared* to disagree with herself, but in fact there was no real contradiction, because it would seem that she inadvertently extended the concept of phobia in 1977. While there is little doubt that children whose phobias are structured like Little Hans's are preoccupied by the phobic object, Anna Freud was quite correct to doubt whether this is always so, because it is not a feature of *all* phobias, using the term in the wider sense of irrational fear. The argument put forward in the Index report was that the impressiveness of Freud's description of the processes occurring in Little Hans had placed restraints on the subsequent psychoanalytic understanding of fears and phobias, leading to a sort of "double think," i.e., a tendency to see, on the one hand, all phobias in terms of the mechanisms described by Freud in 1909, and on the other to call all irrational fears "phobias."

There are a large number of fears, anxieties, and phobic phenomena which are, in a sense, "situational." If we think, for example, of a person who suffers from a fear of flying, and who is not required to fly regularly, then we have a good example of what is meant by "situational." The person does not dwell on the anxiety about flying unless he or she is confronted with the demand or necessity to fly. Such a demand disturbs the equilibrium which the person has reached, and the fear is *intrusive* in the sense that anxiety is aroused *by the situation,* and that this anxiety is dealt with by avoidance. In no way can it be said that such a fear of flying performs an ongoing *function* in maintaining the internal equilibrium of the person. Rather, the equilibrium is *disturbed* by the impact of external reality. I shall return to this point later.

Many of the fears labeled as phobias in our child patients do not involve a constant preoccupation with the phobic object; in fact, for the bulk of the so-called phobias observed and described by therapists at the Anna Freud Centre the child *does* experience relief, does appear to be relatively unaffected when away from the phobic situation or object. The view put forward in the Index report was that the mechanism which *is* at work is often that of a panic reaction to specific sorts of "intrusion" from the external world, an intrusion which upsets the child's internal equilibrium.[2]

Let me try to be a little more explicit, as I believe that the distinction between the two sorts of mechanism is of crucial clinical importance. In the case of the "classic" phobia, the function of the phobia is to deal with an internal conflict by condensation, externalization, and avoidance. The phobic object is *needed* for this mechanism to work. In contrast, in the "situational" phobias, i.e., the intrusive phobias, the phobic object or situation is needed, to put it colloquially, "like a hole in the head." It is the *last* thing the child needs and wants.

Of course, what I have done so far is to draw attention to two extremes. Clinically the distinction is not at all clear-cut, although I believe it to be of analytic importance to keep these two dimensions of the concept of phobia, the two different mechanisms involved, in mind. What muddles the clinical pictures is that, on the one hand, a classic Little Hans type of phobia, an extrusive phobia, can follow a panic and a threat of being overwhelmed resulting from an intrusive experience. In commenting on Little Hans's phobia, Freud remarked, "We have

---

2. The entire area of the relation between phobias, panic states, and the fear of being traumatically overwhelmed is a complex and fascinating one, outside the scope of the present paper.

learned the immediate precipitating cause after which the phobia broke out. This was when the boy saw a big heavy horse fall down; and one at least of the interpretations of this impression seems to be . . . that his father might fall down in the same way—and be dead" (p. 51f.). One could say that the experience of witnessing the horse falling intruded into an unconscious fantasy of the father dying. The panic occurred because the wishful fantasy was suddenly reinforced by reality. In Little Hans the intrusive experience formed the basis for the subsequent extrusive phobia.

It is clear that not every intrusive phobia leads to the classic extrusive one exemplified by Little Hans. What may happen is that the child, following one or more frightening experiences, may become afraid of exposing himself to the unexpected, and as a consequence may restrict his activities in order not to expose himself to the situations which have frightened him, and which caused him panic and afterpanic, so that he is not helplessly overwhelmed by anxiety he cannot control. Here Max Schur's remarks, although they were made in connection with adult patients, are most pertinent. Schur (1971) said, in regard to the experience of utter helplessness in the phobia,[3]

> This helplessness becomes one of the most important sources of *danger.* . . . When we ask a patient what he actually fears in a given situation, he will answer, "I am afraid that I will get frightened." We treat this statement as resistance; we try to show the patient the hidden dangers. . . . However, such patients are not *only* "resisting"; they are also right. They are not *only* afraid of the danger of a disguised instinctual demand, they are also afraid of their own ego regression which would result in what I call "uncontrolled anxiety" in the situation of traumatic helplessness [p. 101].

What may confuse the clinical picture is the fact that an overwhelming frightening experience can act as an important organizing agent for the child's subsequent fantasies, so that it may seem that the child is preoccupied with the phobic object or situation, in the same way as Little Hans was preoccupied with the horse—but on closer examination this can prove to be deceptive, because the preoccupation may be related to the demands being made on the child. Consider, for example, the case of George, aged 8; one of his major symptoms was a fear of having to go swimming, which showed itself as a fear of going near a swimming pool. This anxiety did not preoccupy him when he was not supposed to go swimming with his family or with his class at school. In the analysis the phobia was understood as relating to George's fear of

---

3. Schur uses the term "phobia" in its broad sense.

being near the bodies of boys and men in the pool because of his own homosexual conflicts and fear of homosexual seduction. A contributing factor was the fact that George's brother, 2 years older, had been severely hurt when George was 5 by falling off a rock at the seaside. George's ambivalence toward and identification with his brother contributed to his swimming pool phobia.

All this emerged in the analysis in the material brought by George in various ways, through his play, drawings, dramatizations, and enactments in the transference. The relevant and central conflicts were over his aggressive and homosexual wishes, which were active in his preconscious fantasy life. The swimming pool and the prospect of bathing with other males intensified George's anxieties by reinforcing his conflicts and creating an internal situation in which he feared loss of control. The swimming pool situation created, *through intrusive reinforcement from the side of reality,* a situation in which George's ego could not contain the dangers connected with his conflictual wishes and his identification with his brother in his fantasy life. As Schur (1971) put it, "the shift from 'controlled' to 'uncontrolled' anxiety signifies . . . the failure of the ego to restrict certain responses to the 'signal' level" (p. 101).

In a previous paper (Sandler and Sandler, 1986), what was called the "gyroscopic" function of unconscious fantasy was described as follows:

> The gyroscope of fantasy . . . is like a spinning wheel in more senses than one. It weaves the available raw materials into formations that may be quite complicated. . . . And like the spinning wheel of the gyroscope, they have an adaptive, balancing function for the individual, who is constantly threatened with being pushed off balance.
>
> The homeostatic, balancing functions of the fantasies . . . are directed towards doing away with unpleasure and the gaining of pleasure (to the extent this is possible), as well as safety and reassurance. . . . They provide "compensation in fantasy" (to use Anna Freud's term) and in particular bring about intrapsychic adaptation through the use of various mechanisms of defense and the creation of dialogues with fantasy objects rooted in childhood introjects. . . .
>
> What is organized into the sort of unconscious fantasy we are describing serves the function of creating and maintaining a feeling of self-preservation. In doing this, defenses are used in relation to the object representations so that aspects of the self-representation are attributed to object representations, and vice versa. What we see in the construction of unconscious fantasy in this context are all varieties of projections, identifications, and projective identifications, displacements and externalizations of one sort or another. (In projective identification, as we see it, aspects of the self-representation are attributed to the object, and the

object is then controlled so that one gets the illusion of controlling something in oneself, which is nevertheless dissociated from [oneself].)
[Sandler and Sandler, 1986, p. 116ff.].

At this point I should like to elaborate some aspects of the mechanisms involved in the so-called intrusive phobias. Most fears shown by
children result from their perception of an external situation or object
which reinforces a fantasied frightening figure or event which had
been kept under control by means of a scenario worked out by the child
in conscious or unconscious (preconscious) fantasy. The construction
of such a scenario is part of the "balancing" or "gyroscopic" function of
unconscious fantasy described above. Whereas in the extrusive Little
Hans type of phobia the child chooses or constructs an *external* object or
situation which can be dealt with by flight, in the phobias I am now
speaking of the objects which contain the projected conflictual and
threatening aspects of the child's own self—usually the instinctual
drive aspects—are initially *fantasy objects,* which have been controlled
by the ego by means of the scenario developed in that fantasy. Thus a
child may develop fantasies in which there are attackers, robbers, indeed "bad" people of all sorts, wild animals who threaten to maim or
bite, devouring monsters, and the like. In imagination the child may be
able to triumph over the bad and frightening figures, bring them to
justice, or may in some other way reassure himself that he is safely in
control. He performs the internal fantasy equivalent of controlling the
phobic object, *but does not have a phobic relationship toward a specific external phobic object or situation.* Through unconscious fantasy he reaches an
internal balance which may suffice to contain his anxieties;[4] but the
internal balance which is reached is often precarious, and the anxiety
may be just under the surface, breaking through from time to time in
waking life or in dreams. *When this child is confronted by specific situations,
objects or demands from the external world which directly reinforce the internal
conflicts or directly or symbolically reinforce the image of a frightening figure
created in fantasy, a disequilibrium and a state of panic may result.* For example, George, when not required to swim, could deal with his homosexual impulses and conflicts by externalizing them *within* his own fantasy
life and could then deal with the resulting threatening fantasy figures
in a way which was conflict-solving and reassuring. Thus he was constantly fantasying (and this emerged in the course of the games he

---

4. These fantasies may, of course, find expression in play, stories, enactments, and
other "derivatives of the unconscious," but such expressions can be differentiated from
the reactions of dread and panic which occur as a result of the use by the ego of the
"classic" extrusive phobic mechanism.

played in his analytic sessions) that he was being attacked by foreign soldiers armed with rifles and bayonets, and defeated them by a variety of strategies, so that he emerged as the triumphant victor. But, because the swimming pool situation upset the balance achieved through his fantasies, it became for him an intrusive "phobic" situation which he had to deal with by phobic avoidance.

It is my belief that one of the sources of confusion in the large area of fears, anxieties, and phobic phenomena is an underestimation of the way in which unconscious fantasies (in terms of the structural model, the products of the fantasying activity of the unconscious ego) have defensive and regulatory functions which involve mechanisms of projection and identification, and indeed of projective identification as intrinsic parts of unconscious fantasy formation.

A beautiful example of the processes involved in the formation of a defensive fantasy of the sort I have been talking about can be found in the case of John, a very disturbed 7-year-old, who came to treatment with multiple fears, especially fears of strangers. When forced to go to nursery school, his panic led him to be very aggressive to the other children. He came to a session one day, in the second year of his analysis, and during the session sat down in front of a mirror and began to make frightening faces. He said, "There is something terrible in the mirror." He attacked his image in the mirror with a sword, and went on to insist that he build a throne in front of the mirror, because he was the king. He then elaborated a fantasy that he and the therapist had to fight the devil and his army, and had to behead many people, to cut their hands off and then to hang them. They had to be buried, but then John became anxious in case they were resurrected as ghosts. He insisted that now he and the therapist had to sing very loudly in order to frighten the ghosts away.[5]

We can see how, in this fantasy enacted by John, the aggressive and violent aspects of his own self representation were projected onto a terrifying figure—in the session the image in the mirror—which was then conquered and punished. This fantasy and others like it were precarious solutions for John, and his phobic reaction to strangers was a reaction of panic at reality intruding into his fantasies, panic resulting from the fear that he could not contain the intrusion and maintain the intactness of his own self. From the side of the ego, the better and more effectively such fantasies are structured, the better the child will be able to protect himself or herself against sudden anxiety aroused by a threat from the outside. Conversely, the less well the child can maintain effec-

5. I am indebted to Mrs. Karin Backa for providing this account.

tive unconscious fantasy formation, the more readily his inner equilibrium can be destabilized. *The "intrusive" phobias are effectively "destabilization" phobias.* Further, if the ego is in some way defective in its capacity for distinguishing effectively between reality and fantasy, then the child is likely to be extremely vulnerable to intrusive destabilizations, and may consequently fall into the diagnostic category of "borderline" and be susceptible to repeated traumatization through an inability to restrict anxiety to its signal or token function.

The notion of destabilization through the perception of an intruding external danger situation can be carried back to our understanding of one of the earliest anxieties of the infant, i.e., the so-called 8-months anxiety. In a Spitz memorial lecture I pointed out that "before the appearance of eight-month anxiety, the infant who has not yet a fear of strangers may still react with fear of 'the strange'. This includes such things as loud noises, people behaving differently from what the infant is used to, or indeed any grossly unusual sensory experience" (1977, p. 196). I noted that if the child feels sufficiently secure, the appearance of a stranger does not normally disrupt the child's subjective feeling of well-being, but, as I said then,

By about seven or eight months of age he has reached a critical period in his psychological reaction to his mother, necessarily forced on him by the development of his self-object boundaries. Other persons, including the mother, have thus far been very much a part of his own self, but the to-and-fro of his psychological development leads him to a greater degree of awareness of separateness, and thus of the specific characteristics of the mother, the most important other person in his life. The ongoing and developing dialogue with the mother suddenly becomes much more important for him as a source of comfort, security and well-being, as a means of counteracting his growing awareness of her as a person separate from himself, and the resultant diminution in what has been called his 'infantile omnipotence'. He becomes much more aware than before of the mother's specific features and characteristics. . . . His perception of both himself and his mother becomes more acute and differentiated in order to enable him to carry on the dialogue with his mother across the growing barrier of separateness.

Now, when confronted with a stranger, he may react with a moment of utter disorganization, panic and distress, because the expectation of perceiving the familiar 'mother-who-is-distinct-from-but-was-part-of-me' is suddenly disrupted by perceptual information which does not 'fit'. It is unfamiliar, unsafe and 'strange'. . . . At this point his own ego development and his increased perceptiveness and capacity for differentiation render him extremely vulnerable. If one were to try to put the child's feelings into words, one might say that the experience of sensory disruption by the appearance of the unexpected and unwanted stranger is the feeling: 'this person does not belong to the world of my mother and me, and intrudes nastily into it' [p. 196f.].

What appears to be true for the young infant is also in a sense true for the child with intrusive phobias. Such children inevitably have multiple fears, and whereas it is the infant's perceptual organization that cannot cope with the strange and unfamiliar, what we see in the older child is an inability to tolerate the anxiety aroused by the intrusion of reality, an intrusion which upsets his inner psychic equilibrium through reinforcing a threatening component in his ongoing unconscious fantasy. The child becomes afraid of fear itself, afraid of being overwhelmed, so that he or she may become, as Ritvo (1981) has described it, hypervigilant, signal anxiety attaching itself to situations in which there is the danger of the unexpected.

In contradistinction to the child with intrusive phobias, in a so-called classic (extrusive) phobia the child certainly has unconscious fantasies which represent attempts to deal with conflict and to provide a feeling of security. But the externalization of the threatening aspects of the self into an object which can be controlled *within* the fantasy life of the child is not enough. What is needed for such children is an *external* phobic object or situation which serves the purpose of defensively *anchoring* the intrapsychic conflict in the external world. *The object needs to be externalized in order to be avoided.* Moreover, as I have suggested earlier, there is a constant *relation* to the external phobic object, and in a curious sort of way it can be regarded as a negative version of Winnicott's transitional object.

Unfortunately the way in which the external object or situation is distorted and made dangerous by the child's fantasies and beliefs tends to be called projection or externalization in both sorts of phobias, and this is confusing. In the true, classic, or extrusive phobias the child does indeed fashion the phobic object or situation in a symbolic way through his projections, exactly as described by Freud for Little Hans. On the other hand, the phobic situation in the intrusive phobia is threatening because it evokes dangers which have to be avoided because they threaten loss of ego control. The intrusive phobias testify to a precarious internal stability, which can lead to a variety of psychopathological conditions as development proceeds. It is well worth reminding ourselves, however, that the child may also be able to cope with such phobic anxieties (I use the term phobia in its most general sense) by ego modification, by the formation of character traits, as described by Wilhelm Reich (1933), who pointed out that behind every character trait there lies a phobia, and by Anna Freud in her description of ego restriction. In this way anxiety is avoided. Anna Freud put it thus:

> Restriction of the ego deals with unpleasurable affect that is aroused by external experience . . . once the child has had the experience that such an affect can be aroused, the easiest thing for him is not to enter the same situation again. . . . From the earliest time there is a more or less automatic avoidance of the disagreeable, and after all why *should* we have disagreeable experiences? The ego feels that there are other things that one can do instead [Sandler and A. Freud, 1985, p. 359f.].

In reply to a comment that this seemed to be specially relevant to the crucial distinction between phobic avoidance (used here in the narrow or "classic" sense) and ego restriction, she said,

> You know, I had great trouble . . . making people understand the difference. They didn't want to understand it. They thought I was destroying something that was a very good psychoanalytic concept, namely the idea of phobic avoidance. Actually, in the beginning an ego restriction looks very much like phobic avoidance, but the crucial question relates to what is avoided in the phobia. We know that what is avoided is an inner situation, an inner urge, which is projected outward, displaced outward, and then avoided in the external world [p. 360].

The addendum I would like to make to this statement by Anna Freud is that the childhood fears, of the intrusive sort, are often the driving force behind the development of restrictions of the ego, to the extent to which such restrictions are tolerated by the world outside the child.

In conclusion, let me say that I have tried to help throw some light on an area of considerable confusion, even though I am aware that I may simply have contributed to increasing that confusion. My main point has been to emphasize a distinction between different mechanisms which was, I believe, lost in the 1976 symposium in London, and which deserves to be resuscitated. The true or classic phobic mechanism, spelled out by Freud for Little Hans, has been written about by a great number of people, including outstanding child analysts. Unfortunately, in much of the literature, the two types of phobic mechanism have been treated as if they were one. In the writings of analysts, not excluding those of Freud and Anna Freud, there is what might be called a certain conceptual slippage, so that the term phobia is at times restricted to the Little Hans type, and at other times embraces all fears of various aspects of the external world. A distinction of the sort I have described may enable us to differentiate, for example, between the truly extrusive phobia, in which there is a sort of object relationship to the phobic object or situation, on the one hand, and the so-called intrusive phobias, fears, or anxieties—call them what you will—on the other. The latter are, as I have tried to spell out, situations which, when the child is exposed to them, evoke an internal danger situation, but the child does not develop the same relation to the phobic object or situation as in the extrusive phobias. His aim is to make what is unpleasant disappear.

This whole area is beset by many complications and difficulties. Yet the topic is a fascinating one, and I have taken the liberty of expanding on some ideas which have helped to clarify my own thinking.

BIBLIOGRAPHY

FREUD, A. (1977). Fears, anxieties, and phobic phenomena. *Psychoanal. Study Child,* 32:85–90.

FREUD, S. (1909). Analysis of a phobia in a five-year-old boy. *S.E.,* 10:3–149.

——— (1926). Inhibitions, symptoms and anxiety. *S.E.,* 20:77–175.

REICH, W. (1933). *Charakteranalyse.* Vienna: published by the author.

RITVO, S. (1981). Anxiety, symptom formation, and ego autonomy. *Psychoanal. Study Child,* 36:339–364.

SANDLER, A.-M. (1977). Beyond eight-month anxiety. *Int. J. Psychoanal.,* 58:195–208.

SANDLER, J. (1983). Reflections on some relations between psychoanalytic concepts and psychoanalytic practice. *Int. J. Psychoanal.,* 64:35–45.

——— & FREUD, A. (1985). *The Analysis of Defense.* New York: Int. Univ. Press.

——— & SANDLER, A.-M. (1986). The gyroscopic function of unconscious fantasy. In *Towards a Comprehensive Model for Schizophrenic Disorders,* ed. D. B. Feinsilver. Hillsdale, N.J.: Analytic Press, pp. 109–123.

SCHUR, M. (1971). Metapsychological aspects of phobias in adults. In *The Unconscious Today,* ed. M. Kanzer. New York: Int. Univ. Press, pp. 97–118.

TYSON, R. L. (1978). Notes on the analysis of a prelatency boy with a dog phobia. *Psychoanal. Study Child,* 33:427–458.

CLINICAL CONTRIBUTIONS

The Analyst's Visual Images and the Child Analyst's Trap

JOHAN NORMAN, M.D.

IN THE CONTEXT OF THE CONTEMPORARY DISCUSSION ABOUT COUN-
tertransference (Levy, 1985; Piene, 1983; Tyson, 1986; Loewald,
1986; Blum, 1986; Emde, 1988; Bernstein and Glenn, 1988), it can
be said that the "psychoanalytic study of the analyst's psychic activity in
the analytic encounter is still in an early stage" (Loewald, 1986). In this
paper I have two intentions: (1) to describe and discuss a phenomenon
observed in adult analysis and supervision which can be called the
analyst's own visual images; this is a phenomenon which does not seem
to appear in child analysis; (2) to examine the analyst's emotional state
and difficulty "to think" in the sessions with children. The technique of
child analysis offers many problems. Two elements that characterize
the analytic situation with a child combine to form a trap for the analyst. I want to describe this in the following way:

1. In the session with a child the analyst is often hampered in his
ability to be aware of what is going on inside himself.

2. At the same time the child is bombarding the analyst with urgent
demands. The material presented by the child can reach beyond the
analyst's defenses and actualize those infantile phase-specific problems
and feelings that were left behind in development and never
integrated.

The burden of being caught in this trap, of the actualization of the
own infantile phase-specific feelings in combination with the hampered ability to get hold of them in the session, may be one of the causes
which makes child analysts prone to leave the clinical child analytic
work for teaching and supervision.

My interest in the visual images emerged from my impression that

Training and supervising analyst; chairman of the Child and Adolescent Analysis
Committee of the Swedish Psychoanalytic Institute, and President of the Swedish Psychoanalytic Society.

something was missing in the analysis of children. I had worked for 10 years with adults before I began child analysis. I would at times have a feeling that my "analytic instrument" was out of function in the sessions with the children, and I tried to study this disturbing experience. At this point only I became aware of pictures appearing in my mind while listening to my adult analysands, the phenomenon which I describe as visual images, while this did not occur in the sessions with children. I could then establish one of the main differences between a child and an adult in analysis. I really missed the help and enchantment which the visual images brought me in the analysis of adults. I continued to look for visual images in child analysis, but the result was meager. What I began to recognize was that my own emotional state sometimes had a special quality in the sessions with children.

VISUAL IMAGES

The Concept. Visual image means a spontaneous appearance of a picture or sequence of pictures in the analyst's mind while listening to the analysand. I call this phenomenon the analyst's own visual image in accordance with Gardner's (1983) development of this conception.

Differences among Analysts. We are more or less different as analysts. Some unquestionably accept that the analyst creates visual images and sometimes uses them. But just as often, I have received answers which really fail to grasp my thoughts along these lines. We seldom devote ourselves to individual differences in analysts, since our main interest is to stress similarities. These are, after all, the prerequisites for being able to establish a dialogue and a theory. But when we do emphasize singularities of the analysts' working method, we can become attentive to phenomena which may not be very conspicuous but which nonetheless may be worth a closer examination.

LITERATURE

In the psychoanalytic literature there are only few studies of these phenomena. The psychoanalytic situation is most often described in terms of transference, countertransference, interaction, unconscious communication, projective identification, etc. The analyst's own visual image is a response evoked in the analyst by the analysand and can be viewed as one of the elements that constitutes the analytic relation.

Freud (1900) was interested in the phenomenon of visual images as they "constitute the principal component of our dreams" (p. 33). The abstract expression in the dream thought is in dream formation exchanged for a pictorial and concrete one which is capable of being represented (1900, p. 339). This transformation into pictorial language is in the service not only of representability but also of condensation and censorship.

Freud's discussion of hypnagogic hallucinations, even called "imaginative visual phenomena," is relevant. The hypnagogic hallucinations can turn up as lively images in connection with falling asleep, or in a state of "mental passivity, a relaxation of the strain of attention. . . . It is enough, however, to fall into a lethargic state of this kind for no more than a second (provided that one has the necessary predisposition) in order to have a hypnagogic hallucination" (p. 31). Freud (1912) conceptualized this as the "evenly suspended attention" which spares "ourselves a strain on our attention" (p. 112). People differ in their tendency to have hypnagogic hallucinations, a difference which, of course, exists as an element in the differences between analysts. Freud also believed that hypnagogic hallucinations were in content identical with dream images (1900, p. 49).

Freud also discussed the phenomena described by Herbert Silberer as the so-called functional phenomenon (p. 344). Silberer described how he was working on a philosophical problem which he could not grasp. During a moment of relaxation, the abstract thoughts which he was intellectually preoccupied with transformed themselves into a visual image. I would assume that there are certain similarities with the situation of the analyst at work. As analysts we are constantly trying to find a solution to the contradictions which we are confronted with by the analysand. Sometimes the analyst must really strain himself intellectually, alternating with periods of free-floating attention and so closer to the hypnagogic hallucinations.

It may seem somewhat odd that the analyst should be half asleep and hallucinating, and I must then underline that I have not even been near to falling asleep on any of the occasions I present as examples. I have been wide awake but not occupied by anything other than the ongoing analytic work, a feeling of restful concentration, and an absence of any definite intentions.

Freud (1893–95) regarded the visual images of the analysand as a help in the analytic work, especially with hysterical patients, but he never devoted any special study to the analyst's visual images appearing in psychoanalytic practice.

Greenson (1967) gives an interesting description. When he does not understand the analysand, he goes through what the analysand has said, places himself in the person of the analysand, and tries to see the different events through the eyes of the analysand. This gives him the possibility of seeing what the analysand is defensively avoiding to see. The analyst can then discover the affects which the analysand wishes to hide. Greenson calls this empathy—to share and experience the other person's feelings in order to understand that person. This usually occurs preconsciously, with the mechanism being primarily a partial and temporary identification with the analysand.

Empathy is a function of the experiencing self; it leads to emotions and images; and it encompasses a partial and reversible regression of the ego functions and object relations. Intuition is a function of the observing ego, a thought process which suddenly can make me aware of having come across something of importance.

A most valuable contribution to a clarification of the phenomenon of the analyst's visual images is Robert Gardner's *Self Inquiry* (1983). He describes how he is always searching for visual images and how they emerge when it seems to him that his thinking is best: when he slowly oscillates between waking and the more dreamlike procedure. It seems to be in the passages between the two different states that the visual images tend to emerge.

Gardner describes how he often ignores the images that emerge because they seem to be direct translations of what the analysand is saying, which Gardner regards as an expression of the analyst's wish to blunt his own vigilance. He compares this with the best way of producing a coded message, letting the coded message be an utterance which does not seem coded. Gardner describes how the visual images give a form to that which he has come to know about the analysand without knowing that he knew. In this way of working he attaches great importance to the "edge-of-awareness," which is what he calls the attentiveness directed toward the outer edge of consciousness. Gardner shows how the visual images help him to recognize what the analysand is talking about, thereby making it possible to understand the analysand.

Examples from Adult Cases

Visual images in analysis are peculiar phenomena which are seldom described; the concept is not established in psychoanalytic thinking. It is necessary to present some detailed examples so that it will be clear what I am talking about.

Case 1. Albert was a 35-year-old man. In a session he talked about his summer house in northern Sweden. It was built on his maternal uncle's land, his mother originally having received this piece of land to build on. My analysand built the house himself, but now he was worried that his brother would raise a claim to some part of it. It was Albert's intention to try to get the house and the land legally registered in just his name. He had barely mentioned the house before this occasion. While he was talking about the house, I became aware of a visual image:

> A landscape which is markedly hilly with two great ridges covered with forest; down to the right there is a glimpse of a lake and the road leading up to the house where it is lying in the valley between the ridges. The image has a title: Mother's body.

I was surprised when I realized that the image of the landscape had this title. I became attentive to and then fully aware of my visual image.

But where did all this come from? Had he told me? No. Did I have a memory of a place just like this? Perhaps, but I was not conscious of it. I was using all kinds of elements in constructing this image, using building blocks which belong to my own repertory.

Even when I connected landscape and body, I used elements which belong to my own unconscious, making it possible for me to symbolize my own mother's body with a landscape. It could also be a preconscious quotation of Freud (1900) who writes that the female genital organ and body are in the dream symbolized by a landscape.

In this session I did nothing more than note the visual image, but it became clear to me how much the analysand was preoccupied with his mother.

Albert lived alone with his mother during his first three years. The father did not want to have anything to do with either his wife or his child. He subsequently came more often on visits and when Albert was 4 years old, the father resumed his position in the family and a brother was born. This was a total catastrophe for my analysand; his feelings of loss and hurt were immense. He withdrew with a feeling of hating his parents. This relentlessness persisted even after his mother had died and still many years later when his analysis began.

Through my image of the landscape I perceived a level of the material of which I might otherwise not have become aware—that the house in the country was a remnant of a good, preoedipal relation to the mother which he had managed to rescue from his hatred. The house which he himself built was his way of restoring the relationship he had had before reality and the reappearance of his father in the family crushed his narcissism.

My analysand was not conscious of the fact that he had in this way kept a part of his love relation to his mother. Off and on during the analysis my own visual image of the house in the rolling landscape reappeared as a reminder of the direction that we were then taking in the analysis—nearer the mother, nearer the narcissistic catastrophe.

One year later, at the beginning of the semester, Albert had just accompanied his son to school, his first day in first grade. He noticed that he felt anxious about leaving the boy and knew that in his little son he saw himself as a child. He remembered a dream he had had a few days earlier:

> The house in the country is placed higher up on the hill; it is standing on high plinths, like long poles. I peek in under the house. In the middle, under the house, I notice a large lump of cement about one square meter large. It is the foundation to the chimney and the fireplace. It looks as if the lump is hanging under the house. I then become aware of dangerous black animals moving about at the edge of the forest. I flee in fear, with the animals after me, but discover that the animals are not chasing me; they are aiming at my children who are some distance further away. In terror I roar at them to get inside the car and take cover, and I awaken with anxiety when the black animal clutches the youngest child, the 4-year-old who had not made it into the car in time.

As he related the dream it became clear to him that it had to do with his mother's body. He was extremely curious as a child, a real Peeping Tom. He also remembered that once, as a child, he was frightened by some slimy, repulsive animal that had hidden under the staircase of his maternal grandmother's house. It had suddenly rushed away when they were all sitting in the kitchen. He had always felt angry that no one really seemed to want to tell him what kind of animal it had been that had frightened him so much. On the one hand, he was curious and angry that he could not understand; on the other, he was frightened by what he saw, the genitals, the menstrual blood, the primal scene. My analysand mentioned very briefly that the house stood on plinths, but he thought this looked so naked; so he gathered rocks from the forest and built them up, making it look like the house rested on a stone foundation. But only the frontside was given this wall, the backside was left as it was. The naked front of the house reminded him of the frightening difference between the sexes, while the backside of neither house nor man was any problem.

The lump of cement in the dream was like the scrotum; he thought of his mother's body and the scrotum, the chimney straight through the house—and so the analysis went on, again with the house as a point of departure, but at that time it appeared as an element of his own dream, his own mental world.

Case 2. Bo, about 30 years old, had a devastating problem of rivalry. He was 11 months old when his sister was born. He seemed to have experienced the changes of the mother's body and the arrival of the sibling as a loss of the mother. He felt pushed out of the nest and was constantly preoccupied with the mystery of the female body and envy of it. The father's access to the mother's body and his own inability to reach the position he demanded created an admiration for big men, but also rivalry so intense that it was nearly impossible for him to learn anything from men. This had serious consequences in the analysis and threatened its progress for a long time because every step forward was seen by him as a sign of my power and therefore defended against. I thought of breaking off the analysis because I could see no way out of the negative therapeutic reaction.

One day during a session the following image presented itself to me, or rather, I recognized that something was going on "at the edge of my awareness":

> A small bird is flying with wings fluttering, a sparrow or a young bird having difficulty to lift. It rises a bit toward the left corner of my visual field and is crushed by something. I feel very distressed and turn my eyes toward the upper left-hand corner. There I see a metal object which looks like a huge metal clip, and it is this clip that had crushed or devoured the bird.

It immediately became clear to me what the analysand was talking about: the wish to fly before the wings are strong enough can be associated with a notion of a totally destructive, monstrous, internal attack. A few days earlier I had seen a wild life program with some scenes from a water hole in Africa. Thousands of small birds, called blood-billed finches, were flying with fluttering wings close above the water's surface. Many were caught by tortoises, eagles, and other wild beasts. The scene with the undisguised struggle among the animals for survival held the perspective of both the sparrow and the eagle, two sides which were both possible to think and to feel. I used this scene in my visual image, perhaps in a similar way as the day residues in a dream.

My own visual image frightened me for a moment. I was startled and at once became attentive, and I suspected myself of wanting to put Bo down. This I had already thought many times before, and had been attentive of, but now this aspect of the interaction received a new affective dimension. When I had a closer look at my image, I found that it was the perspective of the sparrow which engaged me and frightened me. I could imagine how huge and frightening the eagle was for the sparrow, and I could see myself as a sadistic giant for Bo. Apparently I had a resistance to being emotionally involved in his projection of his own sadism onto me; perhaps it could be called a resistance to a projective identification. "What I could not yet tell my-self in words" (Gardner, 1983) was that in spite of my attention, I saw myself as overwhelmingly sadistic to him. This forced itself on me in the visual image.

My empathy with Bo was increased. The visual image made me more sensitive to the difficult position he held in the analytic situation.

Case 3. Caroline was a middle-aged woman. She told me that while she was out jogging, she started fantasizing about playing a game with me, yet telling herself, "He'd never go along with it." Well, then she'd play it with *öjvind* instead, she thought; *öjvind* is a male Christian name and is also a combination of several words: *ö* = island, *j*(i) = in, *vind* = wind; *Vind* may also mean attic.

To *öjvind* she had different associations: being sent away, aban-doned, frightened of what may be lying in the attic of the cottage. She played with the word *öjvind, ö i vind* ("island in the wind"). It was apparent that she was searching for something she could not find. I myself had no idea. It was windy outside this early summer day, I saw the trees moving in the wind. An image emerged:

> The blue sea with some small islands far off, as it is in the Archepelago on a wonderful, very clear, somewhat windy day—"island in the wind."

Usually I keep my visual image for myself, but in that session I made an exception and asked my analysand if she had any pictorial image associated with what she was thinking about. "Oh, yes, a wonderful image of the sea, completely blue." In this image she could recognize the place where she used to go swimming with her sister and her father. The sea was beautifully blue, "just like father's eyes and his best suit." That was the place where she was supposed to learn how to dive, but everything went wrong because she couldn't do it and her father only cared about her sister who always managed everything. She was now aware of her love for her father but refused to accept this feeling. She was overwhelmed by her hatred of him and intense feelings of guilt because of this hatred.

The intense ambivalence toward the father prevented her at first from getting hold of the affects which were associated with *ö i vind.* Her joyful playing with the word awakened in me a pleasant visual image and affect, a sense of recognition. When I became aware of this, I realized that in spite of her "He'd never go along with it," she had managed actually to take me along; in a way she had seduced me. The implication of my question to her, which drew her attention to her own visual image, was that I knew more than the words. She had prepared me to contain the storm of ambivalence toward her father and in the transference to me. She was then able to get hold of this chain of associations which contained so much pain.

Case 4. Visual images may also occur in supervision. The candidate told me that her analysand (they are both women) was occupied by the oedipal problem of being triumphant over the analyst. One day the analysand announced that on her way to the analysis, she thought of going to a solarium, something she had never done before. Immediately after the session the analysand actually went to a solarium and the next day she very briefly mentioned that it had been unpleasant. She was supposed to lower a lid over herself; she was not able to look around, became frightened when she heard footsteps, and started thinking that someone could steal her things or attack her sexually. In the session the analysand was completely different from the way she had been the day before, much more controlled, and the oedipal triumph was gone.

During the supervision the candidate said that she very well understood the analysand's feeling of discomfort, but above all she attached her own attention to an intervention the day before which she thought was clumsy and which she took to be the reason why the analysand was so controlled. When we studied the solarium situation more closely, it turned out that the candidate had a visual image which she had been unaware of:

A compartment with a drapery out to a corridor, small windows high up under the ceiling, worn out and unpleasant; and she recognized the feeling of distress when one cannot see the surrounding room and the sense of threat connected with someone being able to walk about out there.

The candidate had created her own visual image of the solarium situation, an image which contained details not given by the analysand. The candidate responded to her own visual image with a feeling of discomfort which made her avoid the analysis of the analysand's discomfort. The candidate's avoidance to talk about the solarium situation was a defense against the reappearance of unconscious, repressed material activated by the analysand. There was a neurotic problem which the candidate had to explore in her own analysis. But the supervisor had to help her see if her avoidance was partly conscious or preconscious and had to do with the "analytic instrument" not yet having received its own intrapsychic space and integrity in relation to drive impulses and superego attacks (Blum, 1986). One's own visual images can be a helpful tool in becoming aware of such thoughts which are not just a sign of unsolved pathology. This allows for the meaning connected with the image to be referred back to the work with the analysand.

Visual images are only one element among many which together comprise the analytic instrument. The awareness and use of visual images can be a tool for the analyst in becoming aware of undercurrents in the material. "At edge-of-awareness I seemed to have told in visual image what I could not yet tell myself in words" (Gardner, 1983) contains the question why I have to tell myself in a visual image and why not in words. This question contains two aspects.

1. We have in analysis an unconscious communication, or at least moments of unconscious communication, between analysand and analyst. The analyst is listening with his unconscious directly to the unconscious of the analysand. In Albert's case I certainly was engaged in his Peeping Tom curiosity without knowing that this was going on; with Bo my unconscious was engaged in the omnipotent sadism; and in the case of Caroline my unconscious was involved in love and hate of primary objects. The analysands reminded me in this way of different aspects of my own mental biography and world; I became tuned in. The visualized thinking was the form of thought connected with this unconscious process. The production of visual images was continuous. The thing presentation and word presentation were occurring parallel to each other. Sometimes the thing presentation which belonged to the unconscious rose a bit above the surface, sticking up like the top of an iceberg, making it possible to catch a glimpse of it in the form of a visual image "at the edge of awareness." I directed my attention to the visual image which then was connected with affect and word and became conscious.

2. The way from unconscious to conscious is always connected with defense and that is of course valid also for the analyst. I defend myself against my unconscious. The visual image may evoke a defense when I become aware of it. And I have a better chance not to defend so much when I use the visual image in the analysis of myself, which is a part of my analysis of the analysand.

The images remain in memory. They may occasionally reappear. I need only to remind myself of some detail for the original image to present itself again. Further details are added, other parts of the scene are revealed, the image develops.

It is not always obvious who is creating the image. I follow what the analysand is talking about—descriptions of people, events, rooms, landscapes—and often have the feeling that what I "see" is actually what the analysand is describing. This visual commentary may not seem to hold anything outside of what the analysand is saying. Even then it is quite clear, when scrutinized, that the analysand has just given me a fraction of all the details which make up the visual commentary. I create a visual image which makes that which the analysand is talking about comprehensible. By literally "placing myself in" the tale the analysand is telling, I become acquainted with the world of the analysand.

This is probably the same process that occurs when we read a novel. In Virginia Woolf's book *To the Lighthouse* it all stands out for me so clearly that I could make a drawing of the house, the terrace, the hedge in the garden, the sea, people in spatial relations to each other—but nowhere in the book is it possible to find the description. The signs which the reader can use as elements in the visual image are woven into the whole text and only faintly hinted at. The talented writer reaches the unconscious of the reader with only a few signs, thereby making the reader create an inner scenery, the author managing to take the reader along with him in this mental work.

THE CHILD ANALYTIC SITUATION

As child analysts we are used to an emotional turmoil in the sessions, a turmoil that sometimes is inside the analyst. This production of emotions in the child analyst seems to correspond to the production of visual images while listening to an adult. The child analyst responds with feelings, the adult analyst responds with more visual images and thoughts.

The special quality in the child analyst's emotional response is connected with the child bombarding the analyst with phase-specific urgent demands. By placing myself in the world of the child, the child analyst sometimes goes beyond his own defenses and is caught in a developmental phase-specific emotional state. The child's urgent demands remind the analyst of what it is like to be a child—and that he himself was a child.

The emotional state that the child analyst sometimes is brought into can be experienced as a remarkable phenomenon and can be helpful for the analyst in his work with a child in the same way as visual images can be in working with an adult.

There is a difference between being in an emotional state and reading about it. The emotional state described in the following examples is not connected with visual images in the ongoing sessions, but the reader of the text can very well create visual images.

Case 5. Daniela was 5 years old when she began analysis. She was born in a country far away from Europe. Her skin was light brown. Her mother was put in a mental hospital three months after the delivery, and the girl was sent to an institution. At 5 months Daniela was adopted by a Swedish couple. During the first weeks with the new parents, she was in a very bad condition; she didn't move or respond in any way to them. It was a horrible experience for the new parents.

Daniela was very slow in her development, but it seemed to follow a normal path. When she was 3 years old, the parents adopted a boy from another part of the world. Daniela's reaction was very strong; she did not want the new member of the family. She was full of envy and regressed. When I met her, it was almost impossible to understand her language, even though she had had professional help. She had a way of clinging to her mother that made the mother exhausted. She was afraid of the dark and refused to go out after sunset; and inside the house she was afraid of ghosts and therefore could not be left alone in a room.

After half a year of analysis Daniela introduced a play. She was sitting on a shelf or under the table, fully visible, but we pretended that I could not see her. I walked around the room looking for her and talking to myself about how far I had to travel to see if I could find her, all over the oceans and all over the world. My efforts were in vain, but finally I got a sign, a scraping or knocking, or the table or a chair began to move, and then I found her. This play was repeated many times with only small variations.

In this way the ghost was introduced in the analysis. The ghost was an expression of her fear of all the feelings, wishes, thoughts, and fantasies connected with the mother in the foreign country who had born her; it was her "phantom mother" (Berger et al., 1980). After my interpretations of this, her fear of the dark and the ghost in the house disappeared.

One day we had a very ordinary session, with some play, drawing, and talk. We were sitting at the table and I had the following feeling:

> It is very strange that this little girl and I are sitting here. The world is strange, beautiful, and transparent, but there is simply no connection between us aliens. I have the feeling that I dare not move; I am sitting immobile and she does not move either. I fear that she can get lost if we moved, that she can get lost and never regain a feeling of security. It is better if we just wait a moment so that this can pass. In her brown eyes I see the bright reflex of the light from the window, I think that she feels the same as I do, and I am embarrassed and want to hide the dangerous feeling of estrangement.

I was caught by this feeling for a few minutes and thought that I had been told something about the core of her developmental difficulties, a fear of getting totally lost. It was so self-evident that all the connections that keep everyday life together were dissolved.

She had repeated the hide-and-seek play so many times that she had brought me to an emotional state in which I was reminded of the absurdity of existence and, in childhood, the everlasting struggle against the forces which dissolve the emotional bonds to those you need. Daniela had in her life met situations that may have been experienced by her as loss of emotional bonds. She was born by a mother who was so depressed that she was hospitalized and in her first three months of life. In the institution she may have found a substitute mother, whom she had to leave again when she was adopted by a new mother and father with totally alien appearances and voices. In the first weeks with the new parents she was in a condition of acute trauma. The adoption of another child when Daniela was 3 years old reminded her of her basic feeling of estrangement, which reappeared in my emotional state.

My emotional state somewhat resembled an oceanic feeling. It apparently was my own creation, but I have never had that feeling with another analysand. In the context of the analysis it is accurate to see the creation of this emotional state as connected with Daniela's mental state. It was dangerous for her to be a stranger for her new mother, who was the only reliable organizer of her life, the only structure and external reality. Disappointments and anger threatened her existence and had to be defended against.

Case 6. Erik was 5 years old when we began his analysis. He was a lonely boy with a lonely mother. The mother could handle the situation, however, and they seemed to have been happy the first year of Erik's life. He began at a nursery school at 11 months. After a few months he acquired an infection, the treatment was complicated, and he was hospitalized for three days. His mother tried to repair the relation by offering him her own bed and breast and since then they shared a bed and bodily proximity.

Very early he had a fantasy relation to his missing father, who lived in another country. Even when he was only 11 months, he paid such obvious attention to men that they recognized his approaches. When he was but a child of 1½ years and out walking with the nursery class, they would often pass a small statue of Master Palm (the founder of the Swedish Social Democratic party) standing in the park nearby. He would go up to it and hug it, saying, "Daddy." In fantasy he had his father; he had never to be alone. But this early "father" resembled a transitional object rather than a real object. He met his father only once, when he was 3 years old, and thereafter often played that his father was dead.

Erik was completely engulfed by his relation to his mother; it seemed as if no other object relation could ever find room in his world. Abandoning the mother meant extinction, but staying with her also meant extinction. At the nursery he subsequently came to be regarded as dangerous and possibly psychotic.

The first three months of analysis were characterized by his fear of and intense struggle with me. After some time, we found some space for us together where we could play cards, he could sit down and draw, talk about a dream, decide on some game. He often played that he owned me, I was his slave. He made a chain of clay which lay around my neck. The chain kept breaking apart, but he kept on repairing it unyieldingly. Many times he used small churches, which were among the toys we had, and built a construction together with a telephone. I thought this had to do with his father with whom he had spoken on the telephone a few times; and the church was connected with "Our Father who art in Heaven," the father he was missing and who didn't care about the son.

One session he became very gloomy, sitting quietly by himself, looking very lonely, and not saying a word. I attempted my usual "words," which had become my way of reminding him to try to find words for what he felt. But he was silent and sad. He used water colors to paint a picture of a church with a light shining inside it and barbed wire all around it. Very gloomily he said, "You can never help me, I know you can't." He said it with absolute conviction. I proposed that we try to talk about it, but he only repeated that he knew I could not help him. I said to myself: "No, I am not absolutely sure that I can help you." In that situation the following emotional state appeared:

> I am seized by a feeling of deep despair, a sense of total hopelessness. We are sitting here next to each other, quiet, and cannot find a way out. After a short while, I become aware of the scene: I am sitting here, together with this little boy and myself caught by my own strong emotion. I then get a hold of my feeling and I can recognize the desperation which I had felt myself as a 4-year-old child when I still did not have any answers, no idea of how things would work out for me; I could not know that I would manage to grow up into an adult. I could not, beforehand, see the way out which later on did turn up, after all. At this point, it is possible for me to find words for his feeling of desperation. I say to him: "It is a sad feeling you have of being caught and finding no way out, a very sad feeling you show in this picture." He replies: "It is impossible to tell you all that is worrying me; it will take 100 years to tell you all the thoughts I have about that picture." Our dialogue was reestablished.

Part of his problem was a conflict connected with development. At the same time as he felt such despair over not finding a way out, every way out meant that he must leave the symbiotic and incestuous relation to his mother. For months he kept finding arguments in favor of his locked position. In this attempt to convince me that it was impossible for me to help him, I naturally became an important external object, separated from his mother. He tried to gain control, thereby attaching great importance to me, charging me, and in that way turning back to the problems connected with his mother, but now in the transference.

The analysand had reminded me of my own gloomy feelings as a child which I had returned to in my own analysis and sometimes been reminded of during the analysis of adults. But there was one element which turned up with this analysand and which previously had not been as clear, namely, the feeling of a lack of perspective, of not knowing how the story will end.

Discussion

Children have a language of emotions that talks directly to the analyst's own experience of childhood. We call it empathy, to share and experience the other person's feelings. Empathy with the child brings the analyst beyond the integrations, compromises, and defenses. The unintegrated, phase-specific urgent demands and sometimes despair can reappear in this partial and temporary identification with the child. These emotions often have a high level and "any high level of emotion or drive opposes reason, intellect, and judgment" (Sandler and A. Freud, 1985). This is a burden for the child analyst.

In this context it is of interest to consider what is happening with emotional material in the sessions and afterward. In the session the child analyst is hampered in his ability to think because he is burdened by emotions. But in the same way as the reader may have created visual images while reading about the emotional states of the two children, Daniela and Erik, so the child analyst can after the session rethink what happened when his normal thought processes are reestablished.

The child analyst has to work with a time lag, very much as we work with dreams. We receive the manifest dream material in the session. Certain fragments immediately lead on to latent material, and subsequently other elements of the dream are clarified. Even after a long time there may emerge new fragments of understanding. The analytic instrument functions in this manner, independent of time and space, and especially child analysis often progresses outside of the actual session. It can go on during supervision, in a talk with the parents, during sessions with other analysands, while writing notes during a pause, etc. In this way the analytic instrument manages to keep up, although with a time lag. Very often it is only after the session that the child analyst becomes more clearly aware of what was going on during the session. This time lag which the child analyst must tolerate is trying and is one of the many special strains which are connected with child analysis. These difficulties are far too infrequently discussed.

The differences between the analysis of adults and children, especially in relation to the appearance of visual images with adults and emotional states with children, can be summarized in three points.

1. *The adult's structure versus the child's emotionality and lack of perspective.* The adult has been a child and although the "child within" may be dominant, the adult has "made it." The adult has managed to form all those defenses, compromises, and symptoms which enabled him to lay aside those conflicts, thoughts, and fantasies which were unsolvable, unmanageable, too painful, or simply not useful. In this way he acquired at least some development, structure, and stability. In development a great deal of mental content connected with unintegrated affects is left behind, but these residues are always only minor parts of the child's phase-specific mental world. Even the most regressed adult is an adult. It may have been difficult as a child to learn cycling, but it is still even more difficult as an adult to forget how to do it. One of the implications of becoming an adult is the development of a tension between conscious and unconscious. The unconscious ideas, repressed or by other means kept out of awareness, can become conscious only by the connection to memory-traces and "anything arising from within (apart from feelings) that seeks to become conscious must try to transform itself into external perceptions: this becomes possible by means of memory-traces" (Freud, 1923, p. 20). Although the memory-traces which consist of word presentations have the central role, visual elements sometimes have a part as one step in this process of transformation. The tension in the adult's psychic structure contains the driving force for the analyst's visual images.

This process is not the same in the child because the child cannot tolerate the tension inherent in the adult's structure. The child is in the process of development and, as Freud (1923) says, the feelings that seek to become conscious are not going through the same transformation as unconscious ideas to external perceptions. The driving force for the analyst's visual images is missing.

The child has never been an adult and has no possibility of knowing the end of the story. He is in the middle of an ongoing developmental phase and cannot comprehend anything beyond it. Even the identification with the adults is a part of the ongoing process and the child has no possibility of imagining what must be done to reach adulthood. This lack of perspective contributes to the urge and despair characteristic of the child's demands.

2. *The analyst receives and responds differently to the material of an adult and a child.* A central question for the countertransference in both adult and child analysis is the consequence of the "free-floating responsiveness" of the analyst (Sandler and Sandler, 1978) and "emotional availability" as discussed by Emde (1987). But there are also differences in the analysis of adult and child.

The adult in analysis tries to engage the analyst and to tune him in. The strong ego defenses increase the intensity of the derivatives of the unconscious and the repressed. The surrounding world, and especially the analyst, becomes the target for these charges, which we all are accustomed to as transference and unconscious communication. When the analysand is unable to accomplish the transformation of unconscious ideas to conscious memory and thought, different aspects of the analyst's own mental biography can reappear, reactivated by the analysand's material. In empathy the analyst makes a partial and temporary regression which involves some ego functions, but mainly the drives and object relations. The border between id and ego is unimpaired, and so are the defenses of the ego. Those parts of the analysand's material which the analyst cannot catch in words approach the analyst's ego through the mechanisms of the dream work, though they manufacture not a dream but a visual image.

The child bombards the analyst with urgent demands. The child's drive wishes and demands for managing drive objects and external reality are very powerful because the elements in the compromise are not yet integrated. When the child's unintegrated, phase-specific wishes and fears are directed with full force at the analyst, the analyst will be reminded of his own feelings and conflicts which belonged to that particular developmental phase before its integration. Empathy with the child implies a regression not only of drives and object relations but also of the ego to a more immature ego with an unclear boundary to the id. The analyst is brought by the child into an emotional state which is characterized by the child's developmental phase and the way the immature ego handles it. What is transferred by the child is not only the content but also the structure. This is of course only a temporary and partial regression in the analyst; usually it is not so evident as in the cases described above. But the analyst continuously experiences emotions of enchantment, love, boredom, sadness, anger, hate, confusion, etc., as a more or less silent emotional commentary in the session with the child. As a consequence of the urgency of the child's demands the child's efforts to create a wish-fulfilling object relationship in the analysis is very strong. He can more easily "press the right buttons" in the analyst and make him comply with the role that the child wants him to play (Sandler and Sandler, 1978). The child analyst is once again reminded of his own neurosis, even if it was successfully solved in his own analysis. "Fixation points retain their cathexis, even where regression to them is reversed" (A. Freud, 1972). This statement is relevant from the point of view that we never lose the possibility to be reminded of the emotional state, vulnerability, fears and wishes connected with the fixation points and the developmental phase in which they were established. If the child analyst dares to go along with the child in this temporary regression, he can obtain insight into the child, but it involves a greater risk in the sense that the analyst is brought in contact with such unintegrated material which is not so well analyzed, and therefore either defended against or enacted as a countertransference. The child analyst is continuously dealing with primitive emotional material, while the analyst listening to an adult is approached by visual images.

3. *Introspection is different in adult and child analysis.* While listening to an adult analysand the analyst can engage in free-floating attention and oscillate between wakefulness and a more dreamlike state. The analyst's ego is unimpaired and his introspection can catch what happens at the edge of awareness. When disturbances appear in the analyst, the analytic frame safeguards the analyst's space for self-reflection and contemplation.

It is difficult to attain this kind of freedom during the session with a child. The inwardly directed, free-floating attention is counteracted by the child demanding the analyst's attention. The analytic technique with a child implies that seeing is directed toward the outside, the analyst is looking at drawings, play, movements, etc., and the child says just that, "Look!" The frame in child analysis does not safeguard the analyst's space. The child has only a limited capacity for introspection, and the immediate contact with the child's immature ego functioning burdens the analyst and limits the access to his own introspective capacity. But sometimes the child permits the analyst to catch his own emotional state which otherwise is more vague. These moments of clear perception of the analyst's own emotional state can constitute a central element in the analyst's concept of the child.

SUMMARY

The analyst's experience is different with an adult and a child. One element that constitutes the difference is that the analyst while listening to the adult can become aware of visual images which are created as a continuous commentary to the analysand's material, while the corresponding phenomenon in the child analyst is an emotional commentary. The child can break through the analyst's defenses and catch him in a trap consisting of his own unintegrated, phase-specific emotions and at the same time inhibited ability to introspect. Case material from adult and child analysis is presented to describe these phenomena and to demonstrate how the analyst's visual images in adult analysis and emotional states in child analysis can constitute a central element in the analyst's concept of the analysand.

BIBLIOGRAPHY

BERGER, M. ET AL. (1980). Second report on problems of adopted children. *Bull. Hampstead Clin.*, 3:247–256.

BERNSTEIN, I. & GLENN, J. (1988). The child and adolescent analyst's emotional reactions to his patients and their parents. *Int. Rev. Psychoanal.*, 15:225–242.

BLUM, H. P. (1986). Countertransference and the theory of technique. *J. Amer. Psychoanal. Assn.*, 34:309–328.

EMDE, R. (1988). Development terminable and interminable. *Int. J. Psychoanal.*, 69:283–296.

FREUD, A. (1972). The widening scope of psychoanalytic child psychology, normal and abnormal. *W.*, 8:8–33.

FREUD, S. (1893–95). Studies on hysteria. *S.E.*, 2.

――――― (1900). The interpretation of dreams. *S.E.*, 4 & 5

――――― (1912). Recommendations to physicians practising psycho-analysis. *S.E.*, 12:109–120.

――――― (1929). The ego and the id. *S.E.*, 10:3 66.

GARDNER, R. M. (1983). *Self Inquiry*. Boston: Little, Brown.

GREENSON, R. R. (1967). *The Technique and Practice of Psychoanalysis*, New York: Int. Univ. Press.

LEVY, S. T. (1985). Empathy and psychoanalytic technique. *J. Amer. Psychoanal. Assn.*, 33:353–378.

LOEWALD, H. W. (1986). Transference-countertransference. *J. Amer. Psychoanal. Assn.*, 34:275–288.

PIENE, F. ET AL. (1983). Countertransference-transference seen from the point of view of child psychoanalysis. *Scand. Psychoanal. Rev.*, 6:43–57.

SANDLER, J. & FREUD, A. (1985). *The Analysis of Defense*. New York: Int. Univ. Press.

――――― & SANDLER, A.-M. (1978). The development of object relationships and affects. *Int. J. Psychoanal.*, 59:277–296.

TYSON, R. (1986). Countertransference evolution in theory and practice. *J. Amer. Psychoanal. Assn.*, 34:251–274.

WOOLF, V. (1927). *To the Lighthouse*. London: Hogarth Press.

The Psychoanalyst's Use of Tact

WILLIAM SLEDGE, M.D.

TACT IS A FUNCTION OF THE ANALYST THAT SERVES TO MAINTAIN THE collaboration between the analyst and the analysand for the task of the analysis (Loewenstein, 1982). The analyst's tact serves to minimize defensiveness while directing the patient's attention to that which has been avoided (Freud, 1910; Ferenczi, 1928). It involves considerable judgment and acumen, permitting analysis to go forward when the conditions are not entirely optimal, for example, when the patient's defensiveness or psychopathology threatens to disrupt the analysis. A more careful conceptualization of tact may make it possible for a wider range of patients to be treated with psychoanalysis without modification of the basic psychoanalytic process (Whisnant Reiser).

Poland (1975) presents the idea that tact is a technical function of the psychoanalyst's work ego that relates to how an intervention is made. He differentiates tact in the analytic situation from manners and politeness in ordinary social intercourse, and indicates that tact does not involve an avoidance of issues but is mainly a matter of timing and dosage so as to minimize unnecessary defensive reactions from the patient. Viewing the capacity for tact as stemming from the analyst's development of a sense of shame, he suggests elements in the decision to use tact as having to do with the analyst's capacity to perceive shame and defensiveness in the patients' responses. In his formulation, tact functions to keep the relationship between analyst and analysand a collaborative one.

PRELIMINARY FORMULATION

Tact refers to touching (and the sense of touch) and a sense of what is proper and fitting. In the service of the analysis of a regressive trans-

Associate professor of psychiatry, Yale University School of Medicine; director of the outpatient division at the Connecticut Mental Health Center; and a graduate of the Western New England Institute of Psychoanalysis.

ference experience the analyst's tact functions so as not to shame the patient or deal an unnecessarily traumatic blow as the analyst interprets between what the patient clearly cannot acknowledge about himself without the precipitation of considerable defensiveness (and risk to the analytic work) and what the patient already knows in his relationship to the analyst. It functions to maintain an appropriate form of connection between analyst and analysand in the face of this difficult work. The analyst's tactful functioning draws on empathic capacities but also differs in that cognitive, learned elements are also used. It is the specific application of technical principles to a particular patient, and may be considered to be a bridge between technical considerations and the empathic relatedness necessary in any effective psychoanalysis.

I will describe several dimensions of tactful interpretations.

Level. In the broadest terms "level" refers to accessibility to consciousness. Material that is not too divergent from what the analysand has previously been able to acknowledge or that can be linked to what has been or can be freely acknowledged has the best chance of being interpreted successfully (i.e., made conscious) to the analysand. The use of "level" is a topographical metaphor referring to the likelihood that warded-off material will not be admitted to consciousness. The "closer to the surface," the more likely is it that the material will be accepted by the analysand. The "deeper" the level, the more likely is it that interpretation on that level will provoke defensiveness and more resistance.

Of course, that which determines accessibility to consciousness is a function of character, the state of the transference, and other considerations. I will focus on habitual defensive structures or character. The analysis of character structure and character traits is frequently more difficult to effect than the analysis of instinct-driven material because character is likely to be syntonic to the analysand. Gray (1986) has emphasized the importance of the analysis of habitual character defenses for their role in the resistance to analysis and free association. The analysis makes these ego-syntonic operations dystonic and then analyzable. Tactful interpretations are those that are cast at the level that moves the patient toward greater awareness without provoking defensiveness that interferes with the continued development of awareness.

Sequence. Similar to level, sequence refers to the order in which material evolves and, in turn, is interpreted to the analysand. Greenson (1967) emphasizes the need for some ideas to be established before other material can be interpreted. If an interpretation entails an explanation for being angry, anger must be acknowledged by the analysand before such an intervention can be effectively made. The idea of sequence also refers to the situation of a complex interpretation or series of interpretations in which some of the elements may be more difficult for the patient to acknowledge than others. In such a circumstance the more difficult elements should follow the more readily accepted ones. Tactful interpretation is constant movement toward attaching what is unknown to what is known, moving from least highly charged to more highly charged material.

Phase of analysis. At different stages of the analysis different levels of work are possible. The idea of phase suggests that the beginning and the end of an analysis pose characteristic problems for the analysand. Furthermore, at one time or another the nature of the transference may dictate the manner in which the patient can work. A critical aspect of phase is the balance of the collaborative component relative to the defensive, resistant component of the relationship between analyst and analysand.

Neutrality A. Freud (1936) defines "neutral" as mid-point between ego, id, and superego. The tactful intervention does not take sides with or against an analysand's harsh conscience in the form of admonishing or giving permission. Neither does the analyst stimulate drive components by being seductive or implying a special relationship with the analysand. However, interpretation, the production of insight, and working through are activities of the ego so that in one sense the tactful analyst allies himself with the work-oriented ego of the patient. The analyst's interpretative activity must not side with the defenses and resistances of the ego in the form of collusion with character formations and ego defenses (Gray) that resist the analysis.

Transference vulnerability. The transference provides opportunities for interpretation and the production of insight while also creating dilemmas and blind spots for the analysand. The patient's transference may create hopes and expectations of attitudes from the analyst so that the patient is particularly vulnerable to trauma and frustration. A masochistic, guilt-ridden patient may be inclined to hear interpretations of hostile, aggressive wishes as condemnation and criticism. The tactful comment from the analyst takes the patient's transference vulnerability or disposition into consideration. Tact is, in part, the result of the analyst's ability to hear his own interventions as if they were addressed to him.

Ambiguity. There is no place in psychoanalysis for vague and incomprehensible interpretations. For the most part interpretations must be specific, concrete, focused, and repeated. There are occasions, however, when ambiguity can be useful for the patient. By ambiguity I refer to the indeterminateness of language so that multiple, specific meanings are carried by one act of speech. Vagueness (where the meanings of a particular utterance are indefinite, confusing, contradictory, or imprecise) is to be differentiated from ambiguity. The avoidance of relentless explicitness through the proper use of ambiguity allows the patient to find his own level of response to an interpretation. Metaphorical interpretations (Sledge, 1977) carry an element of ambiguity which have multiple levels of meaning that allow a choice of meaning for the patient.

CLINICAL MATERIAL

These formulations will be illustrated through clinical material from one analysis. I have chosen one case rather than isolated vignettes from several cases in an effort to demonstrate how tact is present throughout an analysis. While I have not tried to give a complete account of the analysis, I have arranged the material in chronological order so that the reader can develop a sense of the conduct of the analysis. Furthermore, the case material exemplifies how a consideration of tact may help in extending the range and applicability of psychoanalysis without giving up the basic process or aims.

Mr. A. was in his late 20s when he sought a low-fee analysis. A graduate student, he had had considerable difficulty being effective in his academic work; he was full of self-doubts and inhibitions in his relationships with friends, lovers, and family. The screening interviews revealed a young man who was suffering from faulty self-esteem, lack of vitality, and low energy. He was beset with profound doubts and depressive ideation. His assets were considerable intelligence, a strong wish to get better, and a nascent sense of relatedness that suggested he might be able to make use of an analytic experience. He was concerned about his ability to love women and wondered if he had some kind of "homosexual" problem, although he denied he had ever had an explicitly homosexual experience. He was preoccupied with his relationship with his father, whom he described as intrusive, anxious, and hard to talk with. As he began a five-times-per-week analysis, he experienced considerable trepidation. It soon became clear that he feared a profoundly regressive experience. He quickly developed a primitive, regressive stance toward his analyst that carried with it a passive, homosexual longing and a keen vulnerability to narcissistic injury.

Example 1. During a session (session 4) in the first week Mr. A. indicated that he felt he had already gained quite a bit from the analysis. He had found the courage to approach women whom he admired. In this session he reported vivid castration fantasies followed by a series of associations about homosexuality and transvestism. He remembered being the center of attention of a homosexual teacher. At this point in the session he indicated that he felt he was a woman (as opposed to being "like" a woman). This feeling was accompanied by bodily perceptual distortions in which he believed his hips and breasts were feminine. Because of what seemed to be the rapid rate of regression and the potential for an early disaster in the form of a psychotic transference, I indicated that he seemed to be saying that he wanted to be admired by me and that he sometimes got different forms of admiration mixed up. He was relieved; and he began to talk about his need to impress people and to feel admired by them, a goal which has always been elusive.

By addressing the narcissistic aspects of this situation on a relatively superficial level, I helped him check this maladaptive, regressive plunge. One tactful component of this intervention concerned the concept of level in the sense of accessibility to consciousness as well as the nearness to social reality. By choosing a level close to social reality and within the range of everyday social interactions (but still on a theme deeply meaningful to him at the moment), I helped him master his frightening, regressive wishes in a manner which did not preclude later exploration of the experience. Because the intervention was ambiguous in that there were different meanings in the idea of wanting to be admired by me, he could more easily find the level at which he was able to work.

Other aspects of this interaction are phase-related considerations. The interpretation created time for him to be more acquainted with the psychoanalytic situation and his reactions to it. This interaction was also sensitive to his vulnerability to developing a destructive, negative transference reaction without the protection of positive transference or a reality-oriented conviction that I was there to help him. It seemed he was unwittingly attempting to make the newness of the analytic situation the familiar one of his childhood relationship with his father in which his anxious, overbearing, overprotective father would come intrusively rushing in, much to his gratification and consternation. In some sense it was an early test to see if I, like his father, would be provoked to infantilize and attempt to control him. In this sense my comment was neutral. It also may be that he was relieved by the manner of the interpretation as much as by the content.

Example 2. An example of a tactless intervention might serve to highlight some ideas about tact. Tact is invisible in most cases; and its absence points to the qualities of its presence. This example illustrates another side of the issue of ambiguity as noted in the previous example.

This session was during the sixth month of the analysis. The return from the summer break was still an issue but fading. The patient had become enraged at his parents because they were planning to visit his younger brother in a nearby city without visiting him. He talked poignantly about how he felt neglected by them and that when he got to be a father, he would be more sensitive to his children's feelings and needs. That evening he called his parents and told them about a pain he was having in his abdomen. His father insisted that he come home immediately to get it looked into (home was several hours away). Mr. A. made a half-hearted attempt to get his stomach distress taken care of locally. His encounter with medical intake personnel ended in frustration and anger (it seemed this was inevitable); he was persuaded by his parents to come home immediately. He arrived in his hometown around midnight and was taken to a local emergency room where a physician with a tie to the family examined him and said that he might have had some gastritis, but that there was no cause for alarm. He missed his next-day analytic appointment.

In the next session following this episode, Mr. A. began with an account of the event. He emphasized the lack of care at the local clinic and recounted a dream in which one of his cousins had cancer of the bladder with pain in the abdomen (at the same place as his pain). In the dream his father had asked a lot of irrelevant, ineffectual questions. His associations to the dream led nowhere. I made several explicit comments to the effect that he had gone home because he felt he was not getting good care from me. This was met by distant but polite indifference. I also commented that his actions and the dream suggested that he feared there was something malignant inside of him which was driving people away, and he had to go home to reassure himself that his parents cared about him. In response to this interpretation, he changed the subject and talked about his girlfriend and how she had let him down. After he spoke of his disappointment in himself for his performance in graduate school ("I started out a ball of fire and ended up a piece of shit"), I suggested that he was concerned he might come to feel disappointed in me. Again his response was to deny and fend off the content of the comment.

These comments were tactless (as opposed to incorrect) interpretations because they did not contain an acknowledgment of the embarrassment and humiliation that the entire episode contained for him in the context of his passive, dependent, reproachful orientation toward me. In some sense they were too direct and too painful for him to acknowledge until he had reestablished a sense of connection with me. This sense of connection was a necessary condition for him to be able to acknowledge and understand some of the painful aspects of his feelings toward me which in this instance were dependent, passive longings with narcissistic overtones. I failed to recognize the extent to which the connection had been broken and how essential it was to the conduct of the analysis. Although my comments were accurate and perhaps even helpful, their usefulness to the patient was limited by the relative absence of tact. It would have been more tactful for me to address his wish to reestablish the connection between his father and himself as a prior step before addressing the transference issues explicitly. Presumably, this wish was closer to consciousness.

Example 3. Illustrating the elements of sequencing and neutrality, this example from the second year of analysis also demonstrates addressing the defense before the affect of anxiety and the warded-off material becomes manifest. Mr. A. was expressing scorn for others and trailed off into a desultory wandering when I noted, "You are lost." He was stunned but agreed and reflected on the feeling of being lost, not knowing what he wanted and not being able to love and admire people in his life. He complained bitterly about how critical and negativistic he was toward everyone. I said to him, "This sense of being lost and confused is, I believe, related to your being afraid that your scorn is going to get out of control and then you will be scorned by those people whom you care about." He responded with tears; and after gaining his composure, he talked for the remainder of the session about his negativism and how it had served him over the years by helping him with a sense of who he was in relation to others. This theme was repeated and further elaborated over the next several months.

The sequence of the interpretative activity that indicated my understanding of how he felt ("You are lost") reestablished an empathic rapport which led him to feel understood, so that he could tolerate and respond to the more narcissistically injurious comment (you are scornful) with a useful exploration of his negativism. The idea that his scorn was in response to the fear of losing people also made it possible for him to explore his scorn. These comments were neutral in that they remained midway between his overbearing superego and the infantile wish to be found.

Example 4. This session, from the last month of the analysis, began with more than the ordinary strain and anxiety. Mr. A. started by talking about his feelings about termination; he was both glad and sorry that he was stopping. He talked about how his life had taken a new sense of direction when he finally broke up with his girlfriend and started out on his own. At the same time he hinted that he feared he had become too dependent on me. He remembered a dream from the night before in which he had gone out with a revered, much older teacher; the older man was seized with a "form of attack." Mr. A. slapped him on the back, at which point the entire episode was revealed as a practical joke on Mr. A. His associations led him to a consideration of his worries about the future (his work and his love life) and how it all would turn out. He revealed that the night before he had been looking at himself in the mirror naked and became convinced that his hips were asymmetrical and that one hip was feminine and one masculine. He reported the fantasy with some anxiety as he noted that this was the kind of thing that he used to be preoccupied with before the analysis. Although he rarely thought this way anymore, he was again having these "kind of thoughts." I responded that it seemed to be "your way of trying to figure out who you are in relation to me." He readily agreed and began to consider his scheduled job interview for the next day. He reasserted his wish to become more independent, to finish his thesis, and to terminate the analysis, while at the same time considering his wish to be passive (i.e., womanly) and how this was an expression of his wish to attack me and his fear/wish that he would be attacked. Furthermore, he was able to consider how terminating was like an attack both against himself and against me.

The element of tact that is represented here is putting his experience into relatively abstract terms that permitted him to obtain some distance and mastery of a regressive experience. A prominent theme in this session was his struggle with his frightening, humiliating, and dependent longing. The symptomatic, regressive expression as well as the content seemed to suggest that he would not be able to terminate. When the problem was cast as a matter of his relationship to me, the strange and frightening aspects of his experience were turned into something familiar. As I was ambiguous, Mr. A. could find his own level of how to react to the material and proceed with his secondary process, conscious goals. If this had not been two weeks before the planned termination and if this had not been a patient who clearly had the potential for a severe regression, then an abstract comment would not have been as useful as a more direct and vivid statement. My comment aided the defense of intellectualization which under these circumstances seemed appropriate.

DISCUSSION

The psychoanalyst's tactful functions keep the analyst and analysand "in touch" by maintaining a therapeutic connection between analyst and analysand so that the work can go forward in the face of the inevitable frustrations, fears, and resistances. But this connection also allows for disruption and the momentary (or even prolonged) falling out that seems to accompany some analytic work. The reality-oriented, explicitly collaborative dimension of the relationship between the analyst and analysand and the unreality of the transference are integrated through the tactful work of the psychoanalyst. With a keen sensitivity to the transference of the analysand, the tactful analyst gauges how much pain and frustration and how much insight the analysand can tolerate without undue defensiveness, resistance, and disruption of collaboration. Tact is a feeling for what is available now and what is a potential for the future.

The principles of tactful functioning are also sound rules for interpretative activity. Guiding analytic interpretation, tact integrates and applies the details of technical intervention. Combined with empathic understanding of the patient and a knowledge of technical rules, the analyst's tact guides specific technical interventions or tactics.

The analyst's use of tact should be invisible except in extreme cases of psychopathology where the potential for disharmonious relationships is very high. The patient reported here had the capacity for fragmented and chaotic interpersonal relationships so that tact was particularly important and prominent. Tactful functioning on the part of the analyst may serve to broaden the range of psychoanalytic treatment by making it possible for some patients to begin psychoanalysis and weather a severe regressive experience and return to the material when they are better able to address it analytically. Tact also becomes apparent by its absence in the case of blunders or countertransference problems of the analyst.

While facilitating the work of analysis, the analyst's tact does not avoid difficulty at all costs. It is neither simple politeness nor the participation in deception or denial. Such an activity, appropriately labeled pseudotact by Poland (1975), is in the service of resistance. Pseudotact, the attempt to gloss over painful material, may represent a difficulty of the analyst in binding his own aggressive impulses so that the analyst has the sense of using tact to make things go well. True tact lets the patient determine the level of intensity, vividness, and insight; pseudotact involves an active participation by the analyst in the patient's disavowal.

Psychoanalytic tact differs from ordinary social tact. In everyday events tact functions to regulate situations in which there is the possibility for offense or embarrassment. Everyday social tact helps avoid offense even in the face of conveying painful messages. In the psychoanalytic situation the goal of tact is also the avoidance of unnecessary offense but for the added purpose of maintaining an appropriate therapeutic collaboration. Painful things are said in the psychoanalytic situation; but the potential for humiliation and pain is tempered through the relationship with the analyst (Freud, 1940). Tactfully given interpretations, even of painful content, are not usually experienced by analysands as humiliating or painful but are more likely to be accompanied by a feeling of relief.

Tact includes considerable empathic contact with the patient. But tactful functioning is also a product of conscious activity and effort from the analyst. It is a function of experience, training, and intelligence. Tact is blended with other functions of the analyst and is integrated with judgment, self awareness, and the wish to help others.

One has to ask if psychoanalytic clinical theory needs the concept of tact. After all, what does this idea add to the notions of empathy, technique, interpretation, therapeutic alliance, and transference? Is there anything in the psychoanalytic situation that requires tact as an explanatory construct or an addition to clinical theory? I believe a concept of tact is necessary in order to conceptualize how one applies general technical interventions with specific, particular individuals. Tact is a function that belongs to the analyst's work ego and draws on a trial identification with the patient as analysand. It is a bridging concept between the particular, discrete understanding of an individual patient and the application of more universal rules for interpretation.

BIBLIOGRAPHY

BRENNER, C. (1979). Working alliance, therapeutic alliance, and transference. *J. Amer. Psychoanal. Assn.*, 27(suppl.):137–157.
CURTIS, H. C. (1979). The concept of therapeutic alliance. *J. Amer. Psychoanal. Assn.*, 27(suppl.):159–192.
FERENCZI, S. (1928). The elasticity of psychoanalytic technique. In *The Problems and Methods of Psychoanalysis*, ed. M. Balint. New York: Basic Books, 1955, pp. 289–299.
FREUD, A. (1936). *The Ego and the Mechanism of Defense*. New York: Int. Univ. Press, 1966.
FREUD, S. (1910). "Wild" psychoanalysis. *S. E.*, 11:221–227.
——— (1912). The dynamics of transference. *S.E.*, 12:99–108.
——— (1940). An outline of psycho-analysis. *S.E.*, 23:41–207.
GILL, M. M. (1982). *Analysis of Transference*, vol. 1. New York: Int. Univ. Press.
GRAY, P. (1986). On helping analysands observe intrapsychic activity (in press).
GREENSON, R. R. (1967). *The Technique and Practice of Psychoanalysis*. New York: Int. Univ. Press.

KANZER, M. (1979). Book essay: developments in psychoanalytic technique. *J. Amer. Psychoanal. Assn.*, 27(suppl.):327–374.

LOEWALD, H. W. (1960). On the therapeutic action of psychoanalysis. In *Papers on Psychoanalysis*, New Haven: Yale Univ. Press, 1980, pp. 221–256.

LOEWENSTEIN, R. M. (1982). *Practice and Precept in Psychoanalytic Technique*, New Haven: Yale Univ. Press.

PARSON, T. (1951). Social structure and dynamic process. In *The Social System*. New York: Free Press, pp. 428–479.

POLAND, W. S. (1975). Tact as a psychoanalytic function. *Int. J. Psychoanal.*, 56:155–163.

SLEDGE, W. (1977). Therapists' use of metaphor. *Int. J. Psychoanal. Psychother.*, 6:113–130.

STEIN, M. H. (1981). The Unobjectionable part of the transference. *J. Amer. Psychoanal. Assn.*, 29:869–892.

WHISNANT REISER, L. Personal communication.

Gifts in Psychoanalysis

Theoretical and Technical Issues

KENNETH H. TALAN, M.D.

AS A SECOND YEAR RESIDENT IN PSYCHIATRY, I WAS GIVEN A GIFT BY THE grateful parents of an inpatient whom I was treating. The beautiful and obviously expensive jacket was manufactured by the family's company. I approached my ward chief with my dilemma of whether or not to accept the gift, i.e., was it "ethical" to accept the gift, would I offend the family if I didn't? He smilingly counseled me to "keep it; one day people will even pay you for what you do."

As an advanced candidate in psychoanalysis, my female analysand unexpectedly presented me with a gift at the first Christmastime of the analysis. Once again I was perplexed with how to respond; my ward chief's advice no longer sufficed; my many unaddressed concerns returned and focused this time on the question of what response would most foster the analysis. My search for specific references in the psychoanalytic literature yielded surprisingly little. My struggle with the theoretical and technical aspects of gift-giving in the analytic setting led to this paper, which is a review of the relevant literature, a presentation of my clinical experience, and a discussion of the topic using the clinical material presented.

REVIEW OF THE LITERATURE

The first psychoanalytic reference to gifts in the treatment setting was made by Freud (1917). Examining the path of the child's erotic interest from feces to money, he discusses "the gift" and counsels those who question this libidinal derivation of gifts to "study the gifts they receive as doctors from their patients" (p. 131). He states that "faeces are the infant's first gift . . . he will give [it] up only on persuasion by someone

Graduate of the Western New England Institute for Psychoanalysis.

he loves. . . . Defaecation affords the first occasion on which the child must decide between a narcissistic and an object-loving attitude" (p. 130).

The theoretical ideas embodied in this early reference center around the concept that gifts have unconscious meaning and that there is a developmental perspective to understanding that meaning. In addition, gift-giving has narcissistic and object-libidinal components. These ideas became the focus of interest by later authors who investigated the topic of gifts, both in and outside of the therapeutic setting.

Bursten (1959) developed the idea of the gift as a communication. He discussed this from three perspectives: the conscious and unconscious meaning of the gift, as well as the manner in which it is given— where, who, and what is said. He emphasized that the role of the receiver had an impact on the gift proffered, for the giver reacts to that role and may attempt to modify it through the gift given.

Stein (1965) more specifically addressed the gift in the therapeutic setting. Placing the meaning of the gift in a cultural context, she reviewed the derivation of the word "gift" in several languages, noting the linguistic connotation of a gift as "expecting a response from the receiver, or tying the giver and donor together" (p. 481). The idea that a gift can be used to bind two people together is also raised by Orgel and Shengold (1968). Stein stated that she understood a gift as a "fragment of communication . . . an intermediate role between the dream fragment and a form of acting out." Thus it is a form of "magic action" substituting for verbal recollection and may "conceal a repressed traumatic memory" (p. 486). Gifts therefore can serve a defensive function.

Silber (1969) used clinical material from a psychoanalysis and graphically demonstrated that a gift had multiple meanings, "It can represent a body part, it can be invested with both narcissistic and object libido, it can represent a libidinous or aggressive discharge, and also a defence against either or both" (p. 340).

Kritzberg (1980) gives perhaps the most comprehensive review and discussion of the multiple meanings which a gift may have in a therapeutic setting—psychoanalysis or psychoanalytic psychotherapy. He examines both the conscious aspects of gift-giving, which frequently are rationalized by taking place at acceptable occasions like holidays, vacations, and terminations, and the unconscious ones, which on examination reveal, like dreams, primary process thinking and the desire to become a "real object" to the therapist. The many meanings involved in the content of the gift include attention to the significance of the properties of the gift (form, shape, color, function) as well as the timing and manner of gift-giving. This leads into the third area under discussion: gift-giving as a form of acting out of the transference. The behavior also subserves defensive functions and therefore makes it difficult for the patient to recognize the transference qualities, especially if it seems congruent with superego and cultural values. The gift is seen as a defense against recall and is a form of acting "in" the therapeutic situation.

While the preceding clearly indicates that gifts are offered in the therapeutic setting, there is much less attention given to the response of the analyst, i.e., whether or not he accepts the gift. Freud's comments on this matter are almost incidental: (1) in the 1917 paper, there is a recommendation for doctors to observe when they give patients gifts (!) the "storms of transference" (p. 131) which arise; (2) in his comments on his dream of the open-air closet (1900), he referred to a piece of furniture "given by a grateful woman patient" (p. 470); (3) in 1933 he made a reference to receiving gifts of books from the library of his patient P. These references seem in stark contrast to his papers on technique where he advised his colleagues to be "opaque to his [the doctor's] patients and, like a mirror, should show them nothing but what is shown to him" (1912, p. 118). This confusion might have contributed to the fact that there is very little in later papers regarding the technical matter of responding to the patient when the gift is offered. Stein only says, "It is far easier to refuse a gift; but one must know how and when to accept a gift. . . . If it is an aid in the mastery of anxiety, the giving of gifts should not be interpreted or curtailed too soon" (p. 485). Her comments do not address the analytic situation in any particular manner. Kritzberg, whose clinical examples are all situations in which he has accepted the gift offered, also does not seem to be talking about the psychoanalytic setting. What he does not address is how he responds when a gift is not accepted. While he does make reference to the "countertransference feelings aroused," he does not elaborate. Silber gives the most extensive comments on this issue: "As a general rule, in the analysis of a neurotic patient, most analysts would agree that it is preferable to analyse the wish of a patient to give a gift rather than to accept the gift itself. It is conceivable that with certain types of patients this general rule would need to be modified" (p. 337). He concluded that the technical aspects of the matter warranted a review. This conclusion seems to be a reflection of the earlier findings of Glover (1955) who used a questionnaire approach to the issue of gifts in the analytic setting. He found that in regard to accepting or rejecting gifts, the responses "were much less free and voluminous than when the issue appeared to touch more obviously on [other] technical principles" (p. 320). This seems to indicate that, at least relative to other technical matters, gift-receiving needs more clarification.

The literature on gift-giving in the analytic treatment of children also covers a spectrum of perspectives. Weiss (1964), using Eissler's criteria in his discussion of child analytic parameters, calls for a careful scrutiny of all interventions commonly used in child analysis which are departures from the use of verbal intervention as the exclusive tool. Among these he includes gift-giving. He notes that action of almost any kind on the part of the analyst, e.g., playing a game with a child on request or refusing to do so, is a parameter of technique and should be thought of as one.

Levin and Wermer (1966) take a different position. The analyst's giving a gift to a patient, which is a modification of the rule of abstinence, is viewed not as a parameter but as part of standard procedure; it is a measure used to establish a secure therapeutic alliance which can endure the patient's resistances. Gifts can be used to achieve specific therapeutic goals or as a means of counteracting excessive superego pressure. They quote Issacs (1933), "The gift . . . is also a sign that the recipient is believed to be loving, not hating and hateful. . . . [The gift] brings him reassurance against his own sense of guilt and pressure of his superego" (p. 634). They also cite Melanie Klein's (1961) observation that a child's drawings are gifts to the analyst which, when accepted, may be "a means of making reparation." A conflict over accepting gifts was linked to the association of such action with repressed oral and anal impulses. They acknowledge that gifts may represent more than a simple expression of affection; this may include the wish to "deceive, obtain a gift in return, reward, control, satisfy exhibitionistic desires, evoke envy, humiliate, appease, and hide hostility" (p. 646). In summary, they propose that the giving of gifts to children is a useful means of conveying feelings of respect and liking; and that children, like borderline and psychotic adults, need a form of concrete giving to preserve their view of the positive interest of others.

While this paper was seen mainly from the perspective of the therapist as the giver of the gift, Kay (1967) wrote about the child analysand giving a gift to the analyst. Using a clinical vignette, he addressed the analyst's struggle to find a level of interaction which would gratify the patient and also foster verbal expression and the analysis of conflict. The factors to be considered in finding that level for each patient include the state of the therapeutic alliance, the transference, and the patient's ego functions. Kay maintained an analytic attitude with his child patient by delaying his acceptance of the gift and reflecting with his patient on the meaning of the event. This allowed the transference resistance involved in the gift-giving episode to be clarified, interpreted, and worked through in a manner that clearly fostered the analytic process. Kay's paper, like the preceding ones, supports the overarching theme that gift-giving is a highly symbolic act with multiple levels of meaning.

CLINICAL MATERIAL

The patient, Ms. M., was a 32-year-old divorced artist who entered analysis one year before the incident under discussion. Her main concern centered around her great anxiety when performing. She was also troubled by an intense infatuation with her married gynecologist. She was an only child and had devoted her life to her art, an area of major interest to her father, a dentist. She remained very close with her parents, although living a great distance from them during most of her adult life. At the last screening meeting, six weeks before the start of analysis, which was to be February 4, she presented me with a box of candy as a "Christmas gift and for all the garbage you will have to put up with." I accepted the gift and, making no opportunity, did not explore it further with her.

The analysis during the first year was concerned with Ms. M.'s obsessional struggle to deny and avoid intrusive "mean" thoughts. Erotic ideation was similarly experienced as intrusive, although less distressing to her. Ms. M. was preoccupied with my personal life, and her thoughts became focused on my elder daughter whom she had accidently met. She openly yearned for and unambivalently expressed a wish to know more about me and to make our relationship "more personal." She was extremely sensitive to the time element in the analysis. She focused obsessively on whether or not the session began even seconds late or whether I held her over in sufficient compensation for sessions which truly began late. During weekend breaks, she frequently experienced thoughts, accompanied by tears, about the time when analysis would end.

Ms. M. knew our holiday schedule in early November; in addition to Thanksgiving, there would be a few days off before and after Christmas and a week at the end of January. In early December, Ms. M., who paid a reduced fee, but had to pay more of the fee the preceding three months because her insurance for the year had run out, made multiple references to money. She felt that she had to pay her bill completely right away because she did not want to "have a check hanging over my head" and she did not want to "pretend the money in my account was

all mine." She talked about a "greedy Jew" and made extensive references to having given someone something and wanting to be paid back.
She spoke of being "willing to do anything to get money out of my
father" when she was a child. She presented a dream about a rich,
elderly lady being driven around in a car by her chauffeur. These
dream thoughts were discussed as representing her view of the analysis. One day when I came in a few minutes late, she fantasized that I had
been skiing. She thought that the week interruption in her analysis in
January was because of my ski vacation.

About two weeks before Christmas, she made reference to giving me
something for the holiday; she had thought of a tie, but that seemed
"too personal." She wondered if I would accept gifts as I had last
holiday. She recalled having expected a thank you note for that gift.
While it was hard, she had to admit that she felt hurt at the time when
she did not receive one from me. She thought that not giving something to me created a distance, but persons who would not accept a gift
were "acting as if they were superior and there wasn't anything good
enough for them." Her mother was "one of the most gift-giving people" that she knew. She was not sure what she wanted me to answer.
"Yes" meant, in part, that she would feel obligated to give a gift to me.
"No" meant that she would be relieved that she did not have to give a
gift. "No" also meant a missed opportunity to express the idea, "You
are special to me." She wished to make little of her very strong feelings
about this issue. While telling me of a dream in which the gynecologist
was "just talking" instead of going on with giving her novocaine, she
recalled that as a child she once gave her father "shot needles" for
Christmas. These were needles for reusable syringes with which he
gave injections to his patients. As the sessions passed, she spoke increasingly of strong feelings of wanting to give me something for the
holiday. I did not say at that time that I would not accept a gift. In
associating to a dream about following an elderly woman and having a
sense of helplessness about it, she spoke of her cousin tickling her. She
felt so helpless that all she could do was talk; she could not take action to
stop the tickling.

She recalled an early memory of walking along a wall. She was yelled
at by a doctor to get off the wall and her fun was spoiled. She reported a
series of dreams having to do with such themes as trying to climb
higher and find a secure path, having her breasts exposed while swimming, and crawling up to a doctor with her mouth open. When she was
talking about giving a gift, she did not like the idea raised in the sessions
that it might be "covering what I do not wish to expose."

On the day before Christmas, the patient handed me a gift. In it were an envelope which contained 25 dollars; a wedged-shaped package wrapped in white paper looking like a ski slope, which contained a cake; and upon the package a figurine of a skier, which actually was a Christmas tree ornament. Surprised and perplexed, I took the package and listened; Ms. M. immediately began telling her dreams from the preceding night. One involved her looking for a box to put presents in. She was in a "big open space, an attic" walking "upside down." It was a place that did not seem to have enough room for her. She was on a support beam which might not hold her because there was too much "weight" on it. Another dream involved her being concerned about being late for the session. Her associations centered on her fears of my not accepting her gifts, of exposing her feelings, or, if she did not give me the gifts, of missing "the fun, and the act of creating." The skier reminded her of me, and she hoped I too would "hang in there" with her. The cake was a gift for my family. She had tried to find something that was not personal, "because your wife would not be approving." The money "could be used by anyone, not personal." It had to do, in part, with the fact that her fee was lower than my usual one. She also told of having the fantasy, on the way to the session, of developing appendicitis and needing to have surgery.

After a day of reflecting on the implications for the analytic work of keeping or not keeping the gift, I decided that in the next session I would give her back the money, telling her that I would not accept it because we had an agreed-upon fee, but that I would keep the rest of the gift. In response to my statement, she said that she had wondered if I might give back the money. She thought that it was generous of me. She could use the money herself. She also felt, however, that by taking the money back, she was giving up something. She felt sad. She wondered how this was different from the situation with her father and his patients; he accepted gifts. How was this different from a social situation; if she cared for someone, she "would not think" of not giving them a Christmas gift?

After much more reflection on the matter of gifts and the material which arose in the preceding two sessions, I returned the remainder of the gift in the third session following the gift-giving. She was angry. Why did such an ungenerous act follow such a generous one? She felt unappreciated; it was a positive feeling and act, not a negative one. She then acknowledged having had the fear that I would "find something wrong" with her giving. She pursued several images of my daughter who was being burned, was on stage and shot, and was paralyzed. She felt that she had lost the opportunity to make me happy. She thought she had said so many things during the year that made me unhappy and worried, I was discouraged by her. The ornament was clearly the most personal item. She was most hurt by my giving it back. She acknowledged that the skier had been connected in her thought to my upcoming vacation. On leaving, she teasingly threatened to leave the gift in my car.

The following session, Ms. M. began by asking me, "Where's the candy?" a pointed reference to the preceding year's gift. She continued, in a sarcastic tone, by wondering, "If expressing oneself verbally was so important, why couldn't you have done that and kept the gifts instead of giving me a taste of my own medicine?" She puzzled over what her attitude might have been which had caused me to change my mind. She was reminded of her cousin's tickling her as a child; she had felt helpless and could not fight back, "only talk, but telling wasn't enough." She again acknowledged the ornament as most meaningful, "a symbol of you being away." She recalled that the preceding January, when I was away, she had at first feared that I would be killed, but then she had had the thought that she "hoped" I would be killed. This year she thought, in response to giving me the skier, "He might think that I'm sending him off on a ski trip to get killed; at least he will have fun." The part of the gift that was to be "consumed" was to say, "Remember me." The cake for my family reminded her of her father sharing with his family the gifts that he had received from patients. She referred again to my not having given back the candy and concluded that at that point there was "no depth to my feelings and perhaps that's why you accepted it." Reflecting on the whole experience, she was surprised at how much less "devastating" it was for her than she might have thought it would be. "Perhaps all the feelings were not just joy and affection," she said at the conclusion of the session. This ended her first full year in analysis.

DISCUSSION

If Ms. M. had simply talked about a gift which she thought about giving me, then the meaningfulness would have been confined to the content of the gift itself and the way it was brought up within the analytic hour. However, she acted; she gave me a gift and engaged in a process which itself conveyed meaning. This is especially so because of the context in which the action occurred—a psychoanalysis.

While it is not emphasized in the literature, the act of giving a gift, like the gift itself, has multiple levels of meaning. The most salient one is the communication about the analytic process. Through the act, the patient communicates a sense of the inadequacy of words and the desire to have more activity within the analysis. There is inherent in the act itself a demand for reciprocity from the analyst. It is action which is wanted. This is of course in marked contrast to the goal of the analytic process—remembering, reminiscing, and reflecting through language. The view that words are insufficient as the principal means of expression and the desire for more action-oriented communication reflect an early stage on the developmental continuum, a stage when self, object, and the relationship between the two are defined more by symbolic acts than by linguistic symbols. Either regressively reawakened on the analytic couch or simply as an expression of a characterological style, the state resembles that of a young child who has the need for concrete action, more than for words, to express and affirm the libidinal attachment to the parent. It is a stage when action is very important in defining the object. Thus Ms. M.'s giving a gift communicated her desire for me to act in order to reaffirm her tie to me, which she feared she was going to lose. As a form of acting out, giving a gift embodied what Freud (1914) identified as the "perpetual struggle" with the patient, "to keep in the psychical sphere all the impulses which the patient would like to direct into the motor sphere" (p. 153). The communication about the analytic process—that words feel inadequate, talking seems insufficient, and there should be more action—was reflected in Ms. M.'s material before she gave a gift: the dream of the physician who "only talked" rather than went ahead and gave her the "shot of novocaine"; the memory of wanting to respond to the tickling by her cousin, but she "could only talk." More specifically, words seemed inadequate to express the intensity and complexity of the affect generated by her multiple wishes and the defenses against them. My words seemed insufficient to take away the pain of her frustrated desires and her sense of helplessness. The process, giving, and the content, the gift, were of course linked. Ms. M. felt that words were inadequate; she "told" me this by her act of giving (process). She also "told" me, embodied in the gift itself (content), what it was that words were inadequate to express.

While she consciously said that she was simply giving a Christmas gift, Ms. M. was unconsciously making use of the holiday time as an acceptable occasion and means for the expression of fantasies which at another time or in another manner might not have been considered so acceptable. While objects conveying fantasies are given to the analyst, there is a wish to receive from the analyst inherent in any gift-giving. Thus Ms. M. had a desire to receive similar gifts from me.

Taking the gift as a whole, rather than regarding each component of the gift as conveying a separate and unrelated meaning, we can identify an oedipal level fantasy organization. The figurine, which seems to have been the most meaningful component, expressed her unconscious desire to give and receive a figurine (baby). This interpretation is also supported by her associations to the gift: giving was linked to "the act of creating"; the fantasy on the way down to my office was of needing to have an operation to take something out of her, consciously her appendix, unconsciously her baby; the cake was for my family because my "wife would not be approving" of the other part of the gift—the figurine. This dynamic organization also includes a positive oedipal identification with her mother, "one of the most gift-giving people I know." In this situation there are also preoedipal elements reflected in the gift of food (oral) and money (anal), which embody the wish for a closer bond with me, one that is orally more gratifying and "rewarding." The narcissistic significance of the gift is seen in the use of it as an affirmative expression: "I wouldn't think of not giving a gift to someone I liked." Her giving money also represents an unconscious, grandiose self-image of having limitless resources, more clearly expressed in her dream of being a wealthy woman driven around by her chauffeur. In the subsequent months' material, Ms. M.'s desire for a baby became a much more conscious preoccupation.

On an unconscious level, the Christmastime giving represented the upcoming vacation-time loss. Thus the gift was very closely associated with my holiday and was represented by the little skier. The "parts" quality of the gift conveyed to me her experience of the separation, i.e., feeling fragmented. The gift also served as a resistance to acknowledging the ideation and emotion associated with my leaving. Her subjective experience of the separation was graphically expressed in a dream of being in a large open space, an attic, while being "upside down" on a support beam; this was a dangerous act, she said, because there was "too much weight." The play on the word "weight" conveyed her sense of danger about the long "wait" she had to bear while I was away. Her feelings of emptiness, confusion, and being placed in storage, in response to the separation, were also embodied in the dream. Through the gifts she attempted to deny the presence of such feelings. The gift of food represented the oral supplies she was losing by my being away. The gift of money represented the sense of poverty my absence engendered. By giving what she felt she was losing, she turned a passive experience of deprivation into an active one of giving something up willingly. Her fear of not being remembered, of being seen as greedy, and of harming me by her murderous thoughts came to light when the defensive component of the gift was thwarted by my returning the objects. The murderous thoughts were expressed in fantasies of injury to my daughter—burned hands, being shot, and paralyzed, as she herself felt burned, shot down, and paralyzed. After the present was returned, she used words to convey her earlier wish and fear that I would be killed. She then went on to talk about one wish, represented by the cake. That was the part of the gift "to be consumed" and was a way of saying, "Remember me." The full impact of the loss was only acknowledged more fully a year later when she talked of thinking about me several times a day during my vacation and repeating over and over to herself, "It's only a week; it's only a week." These dynamics, embodied in the gift, and those present in the act of giving, reflect a significant degree of preverbal psychic organization. At that level, the one act of giving served defensive, restitutive, expressive, and communicative aims. It also served to evoke a response from the analyst.

The analyst's response to the gift and to gift-giving is determined, as are responses at other times, by the interplay of conscious and unconscious reactions to what the patient says or does. Highly charged libidinally and aggressively colored material, along with demands for action on the part of the analyst, are familiar components of the analytic setting. One difference between other situations and the one under discussion is that the former are largely verbal, while gift-giving expresses the unconscious material nonverbally, through action. One principal effect of this action is to put pressure upon the analyst to move from being more of a participating observer to being more of an observing participant. In other words, as Weiss (1964) noted, the analyst, in such circumstances, is put into the position of engaging in a parameter (Eissler, 1953) of psychoanalytic technique, whatever the response; i.e., either accepting or rejecting the gift involves engaging in action within the analytic setting.

This shift on the participant/observer continuum in the direction of participant increases the likelihood of countertransference responses. There are several reasons for this. Action itself is very stimulating and, more than verbal stimuli alone, may arouse impulses in the analyst which had been inadequately repressed or insufficiently resolved. Also, there is a challenge to the preferred stance of the analyst as interpreter rather than actor. This may be experienced as a threat to the analyst's identity, which, especially for the young analyst, is reaffirmed in the continued use of reflection, introspection, and interpretation within the analytic hour. The action of the patient runs counter to the use of these analytic tools. In such situations the beginning analyst is frequently more focused on what he should do or say than on what the patient is experiencing and communicating. Lastly, the unavoidableness of the demand, i.e., the analyst must, at that moment, accept or reject the proffered gift, may stimulate conflictual responses in the analyst because of the heightened sense of passivity and lessened sense of control accompanying such a position. The reactions thus evoked may result in extreme responses by the analyst, such as outright acceptance of the gift or rejection of it without sufficient attention to the multiple levels of meaning present for the patient in the gift and in the act of giving. As with other situations, if the analyst appreciates the presence of countertransference, he can more successfully evaluate the determinants of the patient's need for action, i.e., the degree of regression in the patient and the state of the transference (Kernberg, 1965). Weiss's example (1964) of responding to his young analysand's wish for action from him, with a clarification of Weiss's dilemma created by the call for action, highlights how the analyst's awareness of his reactions to such a situation can be used to keep the therapeutic interaction "on an analytic keel." The disruptive impact of countertransference reactions raised by gift-giving can be limited by anticipating their presence. This awareness is aided by appreciating the acting-out nature of gift-giving, which, by calling for action, places a demand for both gratification and treatment upon the analyst. Understanding this demand as a communication about the patient's experience of the analytic process aids the analyst in relocating the conflict within the patient. This is especially needed in the young analyst who is struggling with his own sense of competence.

Ms. M.'s first gift-giving, the Christmas before the analysis actually began, evoked feelings of perplexity in me. On the one hand, I regarded her gift as she consciously offered it—as a gesture of goodwill toward our working together. On the other hand, I experienced it as an ill-defined challenge to my analytic neutrality. Not fully cognizant of the conflict-filled dynamics represented in her behavior, I went along with Ms. M. and viewed the gift-giving as if it were "outside" the analysis because it had occurred before she actually began her analytic sessions. Thus her view that there needed to be, or there was permitted to be, some form of action to supplement our analytic work was established. In essence, a parameter went unaddressed. This condition contributed to my failure to anticipate gift-giving at the end of the first year of analysis. The second experience reopened the issue. I was initially taken aback by her presenting gifts and thought that perhaps my not accepting them would result in some profound injury or insurmountable hurt, that there would be irreparable damage to our working alliance, and that the analysis might end. At that point in my analytic career, Ms. M. was my third analytic patient. The first patient had terminated successfully after four years, and the second was at that very time of the gift-giving incident planning to terminate—prematurely. Ms. M. then was to be my only analytic patient.

In retrospect, both my unconscious feeling of vulnerability at the possibility of having my only analytic patient leave as well as my not addressing the gift-giving the year before contributed to my initial inability to see more clearly behind her gift-giving the attempt to deny any discontent with the analysis, any experience of my vacation as abandonment, and any anger associated with that event. I initially accepted her projection of our inability to tolerate her anger and disappointment. This reflected a transference resistance which, only later, was clarified as characteristic of her interaction with her father. She had experienced him as having great difficulty accepting her anger and disappointment when he insufficiently provided her with what she felt she needed. I attempted to maintain my analytic identity and perspective by reflecting on what was happening and delaying my full acceptance of the gift. I kept it in "limbo" and returned it in the manner described. In effect, my response was similar to what Kernberg (1965) noted: "The therapist may have lost his 'analytic objectivity' during that hour, but after leaving the sessions or a few hours later slowly regains his equilibrium. . . . [The] structures formed around his later and more mature ego identity act, one might say, in a supportive way toward the part of his ego in which primitive identifications, defense mechanisms, and impulses have been activated" (p. 46). This leads to the last part of the discussion: a review of perspectives which might help the analyst not become excessively caught up in the transference/countertransference storm provoked by gift-giving.

As indicated earlier, central to the technical handling of gift-giving are the analyst's appreciation that there are multiple conflicting levels of meaning in the act of giving gifts and that the act may have a powerful impact on the analyst himself. An understanding of the patient's developmental level at the time of the gift-giving is also important. The patient giving a gift is likely to be at a stage characterized by the inclination to define the relationship with the analyst through action, i.e., words are inadequate and states are "shown" rather than verbalized. It is further characterized by an impaired capacity to differentiate well between the content of the gift and the mental contents, the wish and its enactment, and the analyst and the analytic process. The analyst must respond to the patient's level of experience—cognitive and affective—if he is to remain a "meaning-giving and meaningful agent" (Loewald, 1978, p. 501). The times when these states are more likely to be present would include the early and regressive phases of analysis. Ms. M.'s first gift episode occurred at the start of analysis. The second episode occurred early within the analysis under the influence of regressive forces triggered by separation. It was an attempt to cope with a loss, the full impact of which she only acknowledged a year later. There was no gift-giving at the end of the second year, although there was reference to the gift-giving the preceding year.

With these perspectives in mind and the timidity born of the realization that specific responses to situations cannot be prescribed, I suggest a few guidelines regarding the technique of working with a patient who offers a gift to the analyst. If the act of giving can be anticipated, appropriately clarified, or interpreted before the patient actually gives a gift, the analyst addresses the material as he would at any other time in the analytic setting. Once the gift has been offered, the analyst, in order to promote the analytic process, declines the gift, with subsequent analytic work making use of the points highlighted earlier: (a) the gift contents are a nonverbal communication of the mental contents; (b) the act of giving expresses the thought that words are insufficient as a vehicle of communication; (c) there is a narcissistic injury provoked by almost any response, especially one other than outright acceptance of the gift. In some circumstances, such as very early in the analysis, at the very end of an analysis, or if the patient is quite regressed, the analyst may consider the alternative of accepting the gift. An attempt temporarily to suspend action toward the patient, by offering a third alternative to either immediately declining or accepting the gift, might be tried in some situations. Kay (1967), in getting the patient to agree to his putting the gift aside, seems to have done something like this in the situation he discussed. This alternative requires sufficient sensitivity and attention to the reactivation of narcissistic wounds which are secondary to the delay in responding immediately to the patient's desire and difficulties in making and tolerating the distinctions between the analyst and the analytic process. The temporary suspension of action may allow time for the patient to explore and clarify the meaning of the gift and gift-giving, with special attention to the impact of such action on the analysis. Whichever action is ultimately taken, the analyst should address the communication that words, at that point in time, seem inadequate to convey the patient's experience. This would begin to address the parameter introduced by the patient's behavior and foster its becoming an object of understanding and interpretation.

BIBLIOGRAPHY

Bursten, B. (1959). The expressive value of gifts. *Amer. Imago,* 16:437–446.
Eissler, K. R. (1953). The effect of the structure of the ego on psychoanalytic technique. *J. Amer. Psychoanal. Assn.,* 1:104–143.

FREUD, S. (1900). The interpretation of dreams. *S.E.*, 4 & 5.

—— (1912). Recommendations to physicians practising psycho-analysis. *S.E.*, 12:109–120.

—— (1914). Remembering, repeating and working-through. *S.E.*, 12:145–156.

—— (1917). On transformations of instinct as exemplified in anal erotism. *S.E.*, 17:125–133.

—— (1933). New introductory lectures on psycho-analysis. *S.E.*, 22:3–182.

GLOVER, E. (1955). *The Technique of Psychoanalysis*. New York: Int. Univ. Press.

ISAACS, S. (1933). *Social Development in Young Children*. London: Routledge.

KAY, P. (1967). A boy's wish to give his analyst a gift. *J. Child Psychol.*, 6:30–50.

KERNBERG, O. F. (1965). Notes on countertransference. *J. Amer. Psychoanal. Assn.*, 13:38–56.

KLEIN, M. (1961). *Narrative of a Child Analysis*. London: Hogarth Press.

KRITZBERG, N. I. (1980). On patient's gift giving. *Contemp. Psychoanal.*, 16:98–118.

LEVIN, S. & WERMER, H. (1966). The significance of giving gifts to children in therapy. *J. Child Psychol.*, 5:630–652.

LOEWALD, H. W. (1978). Instinct theory, object relations, and psychic structure formation. *J. Amer. Psychoanal. Assn.*, 26:493–506.

ORGEL, S. & SHENGOLD, L. (1968). The fatal gifts of Medea. *Int. J. Psychoanal.*, 49:379–383.

SILBER, A. (1969). A patient's gift. *Int. J. Psychoanal.*, 50:335–342.

STEIN, H. (1965). The gift in therapy. *Amer. J. Psychother.*, 19:480–486.

WEISS, S. (1964). Parameters in child analysis. *J. Amer. Psychoanal. Assn.*, 12:587–599.

Coercion

Technical Problems in the Psychoanalysis of Children

JOSE A. VALEROS, M.D.

THE CHILD PSYCHOANALYST SETS OUT TO UNDERSTAND HIS PATIENT'S behavior and to interpret its unconscious meaning in a systematic way. For this purpose, he has a special setting at his disposal which includes toys and an appropriate office where the child can play. His knowledge also enables him to understand the child's play as a special language.

The analyst sets out systematically to interpret the unconscious content of the child's behavior. This systematic interpretation is his basic therapeutic instrument and also his fundamental way of participating in the analytic relationship. However, the analyst often finds, almost consistently at the beginning of the analysis, that the child is not willing to participate in the interaction proposed by the analyst: its paradigm would be: patient's behavior → analyst's interpretation → patient's behavior → analyst's interpretation.

The analyst's interpretation affects the patient in diverse ways. One of these is to provoke some degree of psychic pain, a natural, unavoidable, and beneficial part of the interpretation. Ideally, the analyst's interpretation should not provoke greater psychic pain than the patient is able to tolerate. The analyst's interpretation is rejected when (1) the interpretation has caused a degree of psychic pain which is greater than the patient's capacity to bear it; and (2) the excessive pain has seriously disturbed the transference relation which the patient needed to establish with his analyst at that moment.

The rejection of the interpretation can be classified descriptively: (1) a classic form of resistance; (2) an interruption of play; and (3) an interruption of the contact with the analyst. This differentiation is

Buenos Aires Psychoanalytic Association.

justified, since in each situation the dynamic motives, the nature of the conflict, and the quality of affects will vary along with the structure of the patient's mental state.

The interpretation provokes resistance behavior. The child opposes the interpretation because of intrapsychic problems. The specification of unconscious content awakens anxiety related to conflicts between unconscious impulses and internal objects. This anxiety which is activated by the interpretation triggers the defense against the interpretation.

The interpretation interrupts the child's play. When the child is playing by himself in a creative way, the analysts's interpretation interrupts the child's play. This interruption is due to (1) the invasion of the field of play which at that moment must be private; (2) the failure of the psychological functions which the analyst should have provided for the continuation of the child's play: (a) to maintain the analytic setting; (b) to tolerate the greater degree of differentiation between himself and his patient when the latter is concentrating on his play; and (3) to keep up constant contact with the child's play without intruding.

The dynamic causes that lead the analyst to intrude into the child's play are generally related to his difficulties in tolerating the differentiation between himself and his patient. This difficulty, which is perceived by the patient, is largely responsible for the child's response to the analyst's intrusion. Of course, the ways in which the child responds will vary. Some children are able to explain to the analyst that he should not interrupt their play with interpretations. Other children are directly harmed, not having any possibility of directly opposing this disruptive intrusion. It will be more difficult for the analyst to recognize the origin of this damaged clinical situation, since he will tend to attribute the disturbance of the process to the patient.

The problem described forces the analyst to review his theory of play. At least, it will require that he (a) expand the view that play is "merely" a form of communication; (b) investigate the possibilities of working through in play; (c) differentiate between different forms of play; (d) think in terms of important therapeutic contributions of the analyst as related "to the child who plays by himself in the session," which differs from interpreting the unconscious content of play; (e) integrate the interpretative function with the functions of supporting play.

This point summarizes the situation of the child who plays creatively by himself in the session. This special psychological situation is rare at the beginning of the analysis; when it does come up, it tends to be very brief. However, toward the end of the analytic process, it becomes more frequent and lasts longer. Another characteristic of the last stages of the analysis is that the child plays the same game nearly all the time; this game is obviously personal and highly meaningful for the child's whole personality.

The interpretation interrupts contact with the child. This situation is by far the most frequent one during the initial stages of child analysis. *The child is opposed to the analyst's systematic interpretation because the analyst's interpretation implies a degree of differentiation and a type of object bond which are incompatible with the degrees of undifferentiation and types of object bond which the patient offers in his transference reaction.* This psychological situation will force the analyst to review some aspects of the theory of transference that he uses. Although the patient's transference arises from his internal world, the analyst will admit that the transference is not just an instantaneous projection by the patient or simply a distortion; it has a quality of necessity: that of extending itself into the here-and-now of the psychological reality of the patient's interpersonal relationship with the analyst.

In descriptive terms, this means that the patient asks, requires, and demands that the analyst do certain things and play certain roles, all of which differ from the role mentioned for the analyst in the first definition: interpret the unconscious content. If the analyst does not accept the roles transferred by the patient, in the manner and for the time the latter needs it, the natural evolvement of the analytic process is arrested. I believe this to be a universal observation. The conceptual explanation of the course taken by events in the analytic process will vary depending on the theoretical instruments used by each analyst. But from the immediate psychological point of view of the analytic process, all analysts will frequently and dramatically be faced with the problem of whether or not to consent, to what extent, and in what way, to what the patient asks him to do.

At these moments in the analytic process, the analyst may be faced with a possibility for conflicts. His theory and technique, on the one hand, and his personal factors, on the other, will be sources of impediment for the very difficult psychological process which his patient's particular need to transfer imposes on him. Essentially, *the acceptance of the patient's transference requires a process of depersonalization in the analyst.* This is the source of the greatest emotional difficulties in the task of psychoanalyzing and also the origin of a possibility for greater personal integration for the analyst; this can be said for each analytic process that he is able to lead to its termination.

A Type of Object Relation

I will now discuss a type of transference which I name "coercion." When I took on my first child patient, a 9-year-old girl, I had relatively

extensive theoretical training for a beginner. I had had the opportunity to study considerable portions of the works of S. Freud and M.
Klein. Those readings and many personal reasons came together in me
in a way that led me to confront that first psychoanalytic experience by
clinging closely to what I then understood analytic technique to be,
including the *task of interpreting the unconscious.*

Mary took it upon herself to challenge, with violent blows, kicks,
bites, and spitting, all my attempts to establish the analytic setting,
especially my efforts to interpret the unconscious content of her behavior. Among my limited resources I had the ability to attribute Mary's
response to some kind of resistance on her part, which it undoubtedly
was, or to some kind of functional or structural conflict in her personality, which also undoubtedly existed. On a parallel, I blamed many
shortcomings of mine for this sort of ruthless all-out battle which we
fought daily throughout the time that should have been an analytic
session.

At the same time, it did not seem to me that the theoretical resources
at hand were enough to understand, to solve, or to put a stop to the
clinical situation I was faced with. My opinion that the available theoretical concepts were insufficient had no more value than an intuition. I suffered, and still do, from the problem that intuitions typically
pose the danger of giving them an objective conceptual value that they
do not in themselves possess, the temptation to leave them aside and
cling to other certainties, and the vexation because of the tremendous
effort which the challenge of the intuition requires to give it conceptual
form.

Since that experience, 20 years of analytic work have passed, most of
them devoted to the analysis of children. On the basis of this clinical
experience, I consider Mary's behavior—attacking me physically in a
violent and continual way—a type of opposition to analytic work
which, although extremely spectacular, is neither infrequent nor the
most serious form of it. More importantly, I have found that coercive
behavior is nearly universal in all patients, though its form, persistence,
and intensity may vary.

I have chosen "coercion" for the type of object relation which I will
discuss in this paper. This kind of bond has been identified in the
beginnings of psychoanalysis and also has been a subject of special
interest for many authors. Adler (1929) devoted the greater part of his
extensive work to this kind of human relationship. He gave coercive
behavior a conceptual category that is nearly the same as instinctive
disposition; he named it the tendency for mastery, which he considered to be independent of the sexual instinct. Mahler (1968) discussed

this type of relation in her studies on pathological symbiosis, since this is precisely the type of relation which occurs in that clinical condition. M. Klein (1932) mentions it throughout her work, calling it "hostile dependency." While she contributed widely and quite significantly to our knowledge, she did not treat it as a systematic way of relating. Meltzer (1972) concerned himself extensively with this type of bond in his studies of the "addictive bond." He investigated it within the intrapsychic field of the patient. Searles (1965) has made a detailed study of the coercive aspects of transference in psychotic patients and within the field of the interpersonal relationship with the analyst, placing special emphasis on its place and meaning within the analytic process. In his writings, he names the coercive relation "ambivalent symbiosis." Winnicott (1971) made important contributions to the understanding of the genetic and developmental aspects of this type of bond, especially in his studies on submission, which is the unfailing complement to coercion. Bowlby (1979) studied this form of human relation, especially in the field of development, calling it "anxious clinging."

THE COERCIVE BOND

From the observer's point of view, coercion may be defined as the conscious and/or unconscious intention which a subject has forcibly to control the behavior of an object.

Depending on the level of behavior which the observer focuses on, he may say that coercion is aimed at limiting the object's autonomy, at tyrannizing it, at eliminating differentiation from the other, at restricting the other's liberty. If the observer makes a detailed examination of the nature of the coercive behavior, he will see that it is aimed at specific aspects of the analyst's person. He will also find that the specific aim of coercive behavior varies from patient to patient and at different moments in the same patient. It can include all the functions of the analyst's personality; the spatial limits (doors, windows, walls, the body of the analyst, and especially his clothing, his skin, and his movements) and temporal limits (the beginning and end of the sessions, their placement in the week, their frequence). Other patients direct their coercion to more central aspects of the other's mind: the affects, thinking, judgment, attention, language, the gaze, understanding, memory.

Essential components which are common to all coercive behavior, again from the observer's viewpoint, are the aim of mastering the other and the anxiety which motivates it. *This anxiety is a type of separation anxiety the deep content of which is not having the object, even when it is physically present and nearby.* Coercion is precisely a vehement effort to

take concrete, material, immediate, and constant possession of the
object. The observer will notice that all attempts by the subject to coerce
the object are simultaneously bidirectional. The subject not only requires the other's submission but also offers his submission for the
object's coercion. This offer may be explicit, in which case its apparent
form is a negotiation, or it may be implicit. What is sought is not simply
coercion of the other, but the establishment of a bond of mutual coercion with this paradigm:

order—submission

submission—order

From the observer's point of view, there is a remarkable correlation,
both structural and dynamic, between the bonds of coercion and the
defects in the differentiation between subject and object: the subject-
object undifferentiation is the cause and also the effect of coercive
bonds. In the same way, defective individuation is the cause of the form
which separation anxieties assume. The subject seeks to establish unity
with the object, moved by the illusory conviction that this fusion will
provide all he needs and calm all his anxieties. The failure to bring
about the fusion is felt to be the fragmentation of the subject's illusory
identity.

The subject who exerts the coercion sees obstacles to his demand to
have the object. The way in which the obstacle is experienced will vary
widely, but its meaning is always that of colliding with a barrier or a
wall. This barrier which actively prevents the literal possession of the
object may be placed by the subject in the office door, the walls, the
windows, the analyst's skin, the temporal limits of the session, or in
more directly mental aspects of the object: barriers of lack of interest,
lack of attention, lack of affect. In his fantasy, the subject attributes
these obstacles to the object's hostile intentions: the desire to abandon
him actually, violently, and everlastingly.

The failure of his attempt to possess the object provokes severe
separation anxieties and intense hate in the subject, as a response to the
hostility which he attributes to the object. These separation anxieties
take the form of an experience of dismemberment and frequently
appear in the conviction that death is imminent, either his own or the
object's.

Physical Attack on the Analyst

When the analyst resists the patient's physical attacks in a systematic
way without abandoning the analytic process, the attacks finally disappear and the analytic process continues its course. This repeated expe-

rience naturally led me to make the technical recommendations "systematically to resist any attempt at coercion as the first step in the approach to coercive behavior" (Valeros, 1979). I noticed some events which tend to develop along with the physical attacks on the analyst and which seemed to be pertinent to the theory of this technique. The patient's physical attacks tend to persevere for a long time. When the analyst, firmly, rapidly, and simply, manages to limit the patient's aggression so as to reestablish the setting, the patient will change his mode of aggression in a renewed attempt to break the limit. If he was using his hands to throw punches, he will now use his feet to kick and then will spit or resort to the nearest object to throw at the analyst from afar. The analyst will necessarily have to change his technique of restraint in order to adjust it at each moment to the patient's type of aggression.

Throughout this battle, two significant processes arise. The patient, because of his transference, has seen the analyst, his setting and his body, in a negative and persecutory light. The patient attacks anything about the analyst that interferes with the type of bond which he tries to establish. From this perspective, the limits imposed by the setting, the personality functions of the analyst, and even his body, are material and active enemies of the patient's attempts to establish an undifferentiated bond. Over long periods of time, no other transference appears than this negative, persecutory form. But at the same time, the patient discovers a coherence that connects the different kinds of restraining behavior that the analyst used against the different kinds of attack. When the patient discovers that coherence, he can see a meaning in the analyst's behavior that is different from the former one which was persecutory. What usually follows is an evolvement of the patient's fascinated interest in widening his knowledge of the meanings of his analyst's behavior.

This description applies only to the analyst or observer. The patient, from his point of view, does not attack limits which he does not yet recognize as such and much less accept. He is attacking "things" which prevent him, "actively" and for "evil reasons," from getting what he demands, the material and immediate achievement of an undifferentiated relationship. For this reason, the patient feels that the analyst is a thief, a wizard, a killer. The discovery of coherence in the different kinds of opposition behavior used by the analyst makes for a decisive change in the patient's mental state and in the interpersonal relationship with the analyst. The patient's mode of functioning is magic: he is fighting against the analyst's demonic forces which he endeavors to destroy with action. The appearance of another meaning for the analyst's behavior ushers in a nonmagic type of functioning, one of understanding communication, even though the patient's level of understanding is initially purely intuitive. The meaning which the patient discovers in the coherence of the analyst's behavior psychologically establishes the limit for the patient, although it has not yet been accepted.

Once the limit has been established, the battle will take place *around* the limit. The patient will try to move it a little, to go over it a little, to break it a little. The patient's behavior and his unconscious motivations for these transgressions will be similar to the former ones, but they now appear limited by the recognition of the same limit which he challenged. However, in spite of the similarity in the style of the attack and of the unconscious motivations, the limited attack on the limit is now symbolic behavior, unlike the former magic-manic attack. The attacks on the limit gradually become more subtle and less pressured by anxiety; and finally, we come to a typical moment, both precious and estimable, in the analytic work. A moment arrives, unpredicted by patient and analyst, in which neither of the two can tell whether or not the limit was literally transgressed. In this very special situation, the interaction between patient and analyst with regard to the limit becomes restricted, because of its structure, limited to the intentions, to the virtuality of the transgression. This is the moment of the passage from the act of magic to the behavior of knowledge. These moments are brief and rare at the beginning of the analysis, but they tend to become longer and more frequent. In them, patient and analyst exchange their understanding of their private and unconscious intentions.

It is creative play, *in sensu stricto,* and is essentially the same model of interaction which shapes the classic psychoanalysis for adults. It is relevant to remember that this same type of interaction underlies a particular game which appears at around 26 to 30 months in the development of the human infant. At that age, in normal development, the child greatly broadens the semantic meaning of language. This development is directly correlated to a remarkable development in the integration of his personality, since the semantic meaning of language is both instrument and consequence of greater differentiation and individuation for the child, especially in relation to the mothering object. These advances lead to and are furthered by the game that mother and child now play: intuiting and explaining the other's private intentions, especially the hostile ones. This possibility for explanation which language has when it is used semantically, to refer to what is potential or hidden, leads to the other possibility of hiding in play. And thus we can daily observe in the clinical setting the same type of mutually determined correlation between limit and meaning, the placing of limits and the giving of meaning, that may be found in the historical development of culture and in the individual evolution of the symbolic behavior of man: magic, myth, gesture, art, language.

By focusing on the patient's coercive behavior, I have artificially simplified the analyst's participation and included only his response of opposing or not opposing the patient's physical attack. This illusory impression must be corrected by a reference to the analyst's active and complex situation.

COUNTERTRANSFERENCE PROBLEMS

The coercive behavior of the patient tends to provoke intense countertransference reactions in the analyst. Within the wide range of the analyst's emotional reactions, outstanding feelings will be hostility, indignation, hate, rejection, which will provoke his desire to hurt, to attack, to insult, and to throw out the patient. Less noticeable than the reactions of rejection are those of submission to the coercion imposed by the patient. Although this type of response is more silent than that of hostile rejection, it can seriously complicate the course of the analytic process. The more conscious the analyst can be of his countertransference, even though it may be hostile and he can tolerate it, the better able he is to continue to direct the development of the analytic process. But the more his countertransference responses are unconscious, the more he will tend to act upon them. The decisive factor in this case is the analyst's unconscious tendency to coerce the patient as a response to the patient's attempt to coerce him. Here, the apparent form the analyst's behavior assumes is unimportant. This may be interpreting, placing verbal or physical limits on the patient, terminating the session or the treatment, being silent, etc. If the unconscious motivation for his behavior is to coerce the patient, this will be perceived by the patient and confirm his conviction that the analyst has malignant intentions. In this case, the patient will remain in the vicious circle of tyrannical behavior on his part and counterattacks from others. The other alternative, the occasional submission of someone, including the analyst, does not break this vicious circle; it only serves to perpetuate a bond of mutual coercion which is unstable, anxiety-ridden, and inappropriate for both members of the couple.

Thus, the analyst is faced with the very difficult task of tolerating the patient's attack, working through his conscious hostile reactions, and at the same time establishing precise limits without unconsciously intending to subdue the patient. The possibility for limiting coercion can be achieved only through deep understanding of the patient's behavior. In my experience, the kind of understanding which makes it possible to break the vicious circle is the recognition that *all coercive psychological and physical behavior results from a dependency bond the early development of which has been disturbed; yet all coercive behavior contains the potential for a search and the possibility for satisfying dependency needs.*

From the experience with Mary and with other children who in the course of their analyses demonstrated similar needs for physical restraint, I have gathered the impression of a series of characteristics which are common in this situation and which could be called a *restraint syndrome.*

TYPES OF ATTACK

Violent physical attack. When the vital need to be held and subdued physically by the analyst arrives, a violent attack on this restraint takes place. I believe that one can see in this, perhaps in its purest and most direct form, what psychology refers to as *pathological omnipotence.* There is an urgent and desperate impulse in the child to "break out of" the restraint and to show that his strength surpasses all the limits "in the world." The first episodes of this reaction motivated by desires of omnipotence typically occupy the entire session; the end of the hour terminates this reaction which the child seems determined to keep up until the last breath. The nature of the reaction seems to be basically physical; its rough translation into words would be: "nothing in the world is strong enough to subdue me, and this proves that there is no limit at all."

While physically fighting, the children generally do not converse, but usually shout, insult, threaten, or cry. The content of the shouts and threats refers to "winning," that nobody will be able to restrain them, but more important, that they will kill the analyst. I believe that the child's omnipotent feelings awaken the therapist's own feelings of omnipotence and that this is the source of the specific countertransference difficulty in this situation. For the psychoanalytic process, the most dangerous is the analyst's countertransference identification with the child's omnipotent desires. This difficulty in the analyst may surface in various ways; from direct action in a physical attack on the patient to the termination of the treatment. Sometimes the termination of the treatment is correctly attributed to the analyst's limitations in handling the problems which arise in such a difficult transference-countertransference relation. Other times, technical terms are frequently used, e.g., "poor control of the impulses" or "psychosis," to cover up what is actually happening when an analysis is broken off in this way and for these reasons. On the one hand, the patient is blamed for his "lack of analyzability," while at the same time the termination of the treatment is a message to the patient that he is in fact omnipotent and that nothing can subdue him. When an analysis is broken off because of this kind of countertransference difficulty, the deep psychological truth is that the analyst is not willing to restrain and eventually to dissipate his own childish omnipotence, counteridentified with the patient's. It is important to bear in mind that those cases in which the analyst is literally unable physically to restrain the patient are not included, but only those in which he can but does not do so because of the above-mentioned motivations. In my experience, the difficulty I describe occurs frequently and is the cause of the abrupt termination of many treatments of children and of adults. A similar conflictual configuration can frequently be observed in families. The parents send their pubertal or adolescent children to the analyst when they "cannot physically restrain them." Previously, when they could have done so, they did not; nor did they allow others to do it for them.

In these cases, the child analyst knows that the omnipotence which the child attempts in his office is genetically and dynamically interrelated with the parents' omnipotence, and that he must expect an attack on the restraint from them no less than from his patient.

The subtle attack. The violent attack as a reaction to the physical restraint is usually followed by covert attacks. The clinical diversity is great, depending on the style of the patient's personality. He may pretend to control his aggression or attempt to bribe the analyst. At these moments, the source of the main difficulties for the therapeutic process is the analyst's counteridentification with the patient's omnipotence, the in-depth situation already described varying only slightly. These slight variations depend on the styles of the patient's and the analyst's personalities and on the way in which these styles complement each other or resist the perpetuation of the identification.

When the patient is let loose before his need to be held is satisfied, this will only lead to a renewal of the physical attack on the therapist. There may be a lapse of time before the renewed attack, but the study of the patient's behavior during that interval shows that this is only a more or less elaborate planning for the new onslaught and that no therapeutic work can be accomplished during these periods.

Sleep. When the therapist, after repeated errors, finally holds the child enough, signs appear in the child indicating that his omnipotent impulses are calming down because of the satisfaction of his need for restraint. Real muscular relaxation can be seen then: sorrowful crying, the decrease and disappearance of anxiety, and eventually the child may slowly fall asleep in the analyst's arms. This phenomenon generally announces that interaction on the physical plane will soon disappear. This way of gradually falling asleep in the analyst's arms can be differentiated from the abrupt falling asleep in the session, which is diametrically opposed to this phenomenon. In fact, patients with marked schizoid personality traits are frequently able to resort to the magic behavior of eliminating external reality by falling spasmodically asleep as a defense against tremendous persecutory anxieties. When this sudden falling asleep occurs as a response to restraint, it warns that a long process may follow in which physical attack and restraint will remain at the center of events.

Erotization. One variety of this syndrome, though not a frequent one in my experience, is the patient's intense erotization of physical restraint. When this occurs, verbal interpretation is usually enough to resolve the erotization, and the physical attacks disappear for the moment. I consider erotization to be a complex and overall defensive maneuver which could be included in subtle attacks. Later in the analysis, the physical attack will almost surely return, this time in the usual, nonerotic way. If erotization tends to drag on, it is advisable to see whether the analyst's ambivalence toward the need to restrain the patient may not be stimulating this defense.

Variations on the direct physical attack. Another variation deserves a special reference. Instead of physically attacking the analyst's body or his office, the patient displays behaviors of touching the analyst or spitting at him. These are often true attacks on the analyst's person, which the patient effects with a thin veil of "erotic problems." This kind of attack on the analyst's individuality generally occurs before the outright physical attack on his body. The structure of the conflict is essentially the same as that which provokes direct physical attack, but in a personality whose resources allow the patient to give it this form. Again, it is advisable to warn against the possibility of the analyst's countertransference identification with the patient. This is often revealed in the analyst's verbal interpretation over long periods of time, interpreting these attacks as erotic and/or aggressive problems, while also allowing the patient to go on literally attacking his person. I said "allow" because I believe that it is basically through the setting, in this case restraint, that the analyst can provide the necessary conditions for the work of separation and mourning underlying this behavior.

Insight. Finally, I want to discuss the evaluation which the patient himself makes of his physical attack and of the restraint that he has received, once he is in a position to see that experience from a certain distance and to develop his own insight. This happens naturally in the final stage of the analysis. Although there are individual variations, patients generally feel that the violent attack on the analyst and the restraint received were vital for changing the course of their development and the quality of their personality. Generally patients feel most grateful for the analyst's restraining behavior which alleviates their guilt for the physical attack.

Unlike the behavior in which the patient attacked basic limits of the analytic situation, the analyst's body, the space and time of the session, children frequently demand the analyst's participation which removes him from his classic role of observing, understanding, and interpreting the patient's behavior, but *within* the basic analytic framework. The patient will ask the analyst to play all kind of games, imposing game rules or roles on the analyst that exclude not only the classic analytic role but also any sign of the analyst's personal autonomy. The behavior required of the analyst often lacks even the appearance of being a game; it is material slavery to the patient's tyrannical demands, be they cryptic or obvious.

One child might demand that the analyst run, jump, count numbers, walk steps, squat down, remain standing, raise his arms, draw, clean messes, floods, disarrays, make some musical accompaniment, search, hold some object in his hand, not look, not speak, not gesture. All these activities must be in the way, at the rhythm, velocity, and duration which the patient imposes. These characteristics have been widely discussed in the literature. They are generally called "inconsiderate use" or "the use of the analyst as an extension of the patient." They are generally considered to be a "narcissistic" use of the object by the patient. However, it is obvious that the patient is motivated by an extreme need for the object; this need is ruled by an urgent search for absolute identity between the external object and the subjective conception which the patient has of the object; and subjacent to this pathological type of fusion is the search for a normal symbiotic relation.

CLINICAL COMMENTS

Each attempt at coercion within the basic analytic setting places the analyst at a crossroad. To simplify, the two main roads are opposition to or acceptance of the patient's demand. The first alternative, the analyst's opposition, may assume various forms; one of these is systematically to interpret the patient's behavior without doing anything else. The second alternative also includes formal variations in the patient's and the analyst's behaviors, but what is relevant to the present discussion are the psychological processes and specifically the vicissitudes of the patient's transference and of the analyst's countertransference in each of these two main alternatives.

If the analyst does not accept what the patient asks of him, what is achieved is a complex reaction from the patient: (a) to an object which he cannot control; (b) to the break in the contact that this implies: (c) to the real impediment to the development of his transferences; (d) to the analyst's unconscious motivation for rejecting the role transferred. The patient's reaction is also of a transferential nature; he reacts to the analyst's opposition on the basis of his internal object bonds. The reaction of each patient has its own emotional content and style, but the patient's reactions will also have elements in common that are identifiable. The affect is rage because of the rejection and intense separation anxieties. These can be grouped into three types: (a) the patient insists that his transference be accepted, with great urgency and with threats of physical attack on the basic setting; (b) the patient tries to leave the analytic situation in search of an object that will accept his transference; and (c) the patient isolates himself from the analyst. Detailed study of children who isolate themselves from the analyst shows that they have replaced the analyst, as a possible receptor of their transferred bonds, with a nonhuman object: a part of physical space, an inanimate object, or body movements. All of these are clinical varieties of the autistic syndrome. Within this group, it is important to emphasize the intense and persistent manic state. In these states, the human object has been replaced by manic "achievements" that generally take the form of "brilliant" movements and actions. Their clinical form tends to provoke countertransference reactions of humiliation, hate, defiance, and irritation in the analyst, which makes it difficult to recognize the reactive nature of the manic state.

Essentially the drastic defense mechanisms used, which put the patient in contact with a nonhuman object and unnatural feelings, place him in a dramatic situation; though it will be difficult, he must be rescued. These reactions to the rejected transference are, in my opinion, reactions of pathological mourning. They show the puzzlement, protest, rage, separation anxieties, renewed search for the object, despair, abandonment, and isolation found in reactions of mourning. I have described these reactions as the patient's responses to the analyst's rejection of his transference. However, the analyst will often receive these reactions without having participated in their triggering. Particularly at the beginning of the analysis or even in the first interview, the patient has this reaction; the rejection of his transference has taken place in his mind.

Up to this point, the patient's attempt at coercion and his reaction to the analyst's opposition can be understood within the analytic setting and with the conceptual tools of analytic theory. Therefore, up to this point the analyst could maintain his technical attitude of limiting himself to the interpretation of the events observed in a systematic way. But in my experience, the situation becomes complicated because the analyst will find that, in spite of being able to cover all of these events with his understanding, *the analytic process is arrested.*

The essence of the definition which I use for "analytic process" is the natural, gradual, and constant evolvement of the potential transferences provided by the patient. In this definition, the key words are "evolvement," "natural," and "potential." When the analytic process is arrested, the nature of the patient's behavior is just as transferential; but he reacts to the impediment of its spontaneous evolution. I have repeatedly observed that if the analyst accepts doing what the patient asks him to do, this permits the analytic process to take a different course, which I believe to be the natural development of the patient's transferences. These observations led me to make the technical recommendation that the analyst accept any kind of transference which the patient spontaneously brings into the analytic relation, that is, accepting in the sense of consciously and willingly carrying out the behavior that the patient determines for as long as he demands it. This recommendation may seem to contradict what I discussed above: "the analyst must systematically oppose the patient's attempts at coercion." I now turn to the most important phenomena and concepts which I have used in my attempt to resolve this contradiction.

EVOLUTION OF THE COERCIVE TRANSFERENCE

Among the kinds of transference that the patient might bring in, I observed that the active forms of coercive behavior—tyranny and control—are the most frequent. If the analyst resists being tyrannized, controlled, coerced, the patient will persist in the same form of coercion or in equivalent varieties, or will isolate himself from the analyst in some way. In either case, the natural development of the patient's transferences is arrested. The reason for this arrest is related to one of the psychological characteristics of transference which takes the form of a need: that of being fully externalized in the interpersonal relationship with the analyst. In this, the transferences within the analytic process need the same conditions for their development as does man's subjective behavior in other contexts: their full and sustained realization as a necessary process for the acquisition of new forms; this is equivalent to symbolizing, to acquiring knowledge. If the analyst accepts the role which the patient's tyrannical transference has assigned to him, the moment will arrive when that tyranny will cease.

I observed time and again that the patient's coercive behavior breaks off suddenly and it does so at the precise moment when I finally unconsciously stopped resisting the coercion. I realized this because when I set about playing the role, for example, of slave with interest and pleasure, just then the patient changed the game. I related this phenomenon to another which is seen at the beginning of the game. The patient unconsciously selects a form of coercion which, besides responding to the structure of his internal world, also fits in with a resistance on the analyst's part which is specifically meaningful for the patient. These two phenomena suggest the hypothesis that the patient needs the analyst to work through his own resistance toward playing the role of tyrannized object. The resistances of the analyst which the patient will focus on with great precision are used for externalizing the resistances of the patient's internal object which resist being coerced and the original mothering object which demonstrated a similar resistance. The patient's imperiousness arises from his incapacity to work through the conflict on his own, intrapsychically.

Although it is valid to say descriptively that the acceptance by the analyst of the patient's transference imposes a task on the analyst that he experiences as depersonalization, it is important to see some of the deep aspects of that process. I said that the patient unconsciously selects an area and a form of coercion which provoke resistances against its acceptance in the analyst. The analyst's resistance reveals a zone of defective individuation in his person. Any aspect of the personality which achieves sufficient differentiation from the mothering object and from the external world achieves the double functional capacity for separation and fusion.

Creative play, creative and recreational moments in everyday life, normal falling in love, and all types of symbolic behavior in general are based on interwoven, undifferentiated bonds between subjective aspects and the human and nonhuman objects of the external world. These moments of real fusion—of the normal symbiotic kind—are characterized by: (a) their clear spatiotemporal limits; (b) the internal psychological context, the only one in which they take place—the satisfied dependency bond with the mothering object; (c) their recognition of the objective qualities of the external object; (d) the objective quality of the events of this special area. Only differentiation permits the tentative, sharp, specialized suspension of differentiation itself, motivated by the search for new forms in object relations.

When faced with the patient's coercive transference, the analyst must offer his real and objective but virtual acceptance of his submission. For that reason, where his personality has defects in individuation, he will feel the demands of his patient to be concrete threats to the integrity of his person. The analyst's defective individuation is dynamically meaningful for the patient who needs similarity in the external object for the transference externalization of the defects of individuation of his internal object. It seems that there are several factors which come together in this kind of unconscious search by the patient to transfer in this way. One of these is the need for externalizing subjective contents as a way of working through, symbolizing, and learning. Another is the need for the analyst to resolve the defective personification. The third and perhaps most basic one could be described as the persistence of the subject's tendency to search for types of contact that satisfy his dependency needs. Of course, this tendency appears in the analytic process in a deformed version in coercive relations. The repeated clinical finding that when the analyst resolves his defective individuation, this leads to the development of the patient's dependency bonds. This suggests the genetic hypothesis that coercive bonds are pathological developments of failed dependency bonds. This hypothesis necessarily includes the fundamental participation of the mothering object in the development of this pathology, particularly of defective individuation. If we judge from the psychological vicissitudes of the analyst in the course of the analytic process, it may be that the mothering object resisted real fusion, satisfactory contact with the infant's dependency needs, and instead set up mutual coercion as a pathological form of contact. In my opinion, three sources of data tend to support this hypothesis: (a) the clinical histories of patients who suffer greatly from coercive bonds; (b) the psychological data from direct acquaintance with the mothering object; (c) data from investigations of mother-baby interactions.

I turn once again to the contradiction between the two recommendations: "the analyst must systematically oppose the patient's attempts to coerce until they cease," and "the analyst must accept any kind of transference which the patient brings in, for as long as necessary." I realize that the model for the first group of situations is the clinical situation of the patient's physical attack on the analyst, the office, and the time of the session. I also realize that the model for the second group of observations is the analyst's submission to the patient's tyrannical transference *within certain limits.* The key to the resolution of the contradiction seems to lie in the placement of limits. The element which all kinds of coercive behavior have in common would seem to be the attack aimed at eliminating the limit or differentiation between the patient and his analyst. When the analyst is able to reestablish and maintain the basic setting, his physical integrity, the space of his office, and the time of the session, then a special field, the analytic situation, is defined in which the patient's transferences can be brought into the present. The analyst's acceptance of these transferences transforms the patient's subjective states into real situations in his interpersonal relationship with the analyst; the boundary within which they are brought into the present makes them virtual. In conceptual terms, we could say that the patient's coercive behavior attempts to transform the analytic situation into a concrete, actual, and literal fulfillment of his internal world; and the analyst accepts his objective, real externaliza-tion, but establishes its virtuality through the limits of the setting.

This is essentially the same process that is implicit in the classic psychoanalytic model. The difference lies in the nature of the patient's behavior. The classic model presupposes that the patient's behavior is discursive and conceptual-linguistic; the situations which I study in this paper deal with magic behavior. In my opinion, technical matters re-ferring to this type of behavior cannot be discussed from the perspec-tive of theoretical ideals or of personal preferences of analysts, but instead should be approached from the viewpoint of the possibilities for the natural development of the patient's behavior. Further, from this last perspective, clinical experience suggests that it is not possible to advance from magic thinking to conceptual-linguistic thinking only by means of introspection. On the contrary, gradual development is nec-essary through different ways of thinking, without skipping categories, each one of which is fundamental to the following ones. Above, I say "forms of thinking" for reasons of composition. In reality, these are overall forms of mental functioning. Magic thought is not only a way of thinking but is at the same time a way of perceiving, of feeling, of doing, of living. The same is true for intuitive and conceptual thinking. When I propose accepting the patient's transferences at all times and when I say that this is, psychologically, the objective and real, though virtual fulfillment of the transferences, this means that the analyst establishes the necessary conditions for the development of play itself. Structurally, creative play is a way of thinking and acting, of feeling, of learning, which consists of the objective, concrete, and virtual fulfill-ment of a subjective state.

I deliberately say that the analyst "establishes" the necessary condi-tions for play. "Establishes" implies that this is a contribution by the analyst and not an initiative of the patient; further, it is a *de facto* imposition by the analyst. The model underlying the limit is the line which divides two fields: the sacred and the profane; the office and what is not the office. The boundary line has forces: signifying force which gives definite values to what is on each side and another type of force which is more akin to physical force. The latter one can be described as immobility, firmness, stability, regularity, strength, depending on the point of view from which it is seen or the kind of challenges with which the boundary is confronted. It seems to me that the setting established by the analyst always has these two meanings and that both are vitally necessary for the development of the analytic process. From this perspective, I propose that the analyst establish and maintain the limits with full rigor and that inside them he give free rein to the fulfillment of the patient's transferences. "Establishes" also means that this is an act by the analyst that does not imply the patient's acceptance. The patient will continue to try to fulfill his transferences, objectively, really, and also literally. But if the analytic process takes a favorable course, the *site* of the battle against the boundary becomes placed more and more "within" the analytic situation. The patient who physically attacked the analyst or tried to escape from the session or to stay in the office after his hour will now try to dirty the analyst, to remove an object from the office, and then will try to stretch a 10-point game to 15 points and later, obeying the 10-point limit, will try to change the rules of the game. This transference may be, and often is, precisely that of breaking the rules of the game. In a well-defined game setting, the transgression—the cheating—is accepted by the analyst. It is objective, concrete, but virtual cheating, since the setting defines the transgression as cheating. Eventually, the patient's transferences will have essential meanings other than the attack on the placement of limits.

The favorable evolution of coercive behavior is important, because it leads to true play. Creative play is a form of behavior which is necessary and irreplaceable for the development, structuring, and differentiation of the personality. Play lies between magic-mythologic behavior and conceptual-linguistic behavior. Like other behavior, play is a type of mental state which lends special qualities to the processes involved in it. This could be described by saying that each type of behavior has a specific way of perceiving, expressing, communicating, elaborating, remembering, thinking, feeling, contacting, experiencing.

What I say is true for both patient and analyst. If the analyst compares what he can learn about his patient and the psychological processes that take place in analysis, if he restricts himself to understanding a request, for example, that he play teacher, or if he plays as the patient demands, the analyst will find significant differences. He will find that, for him, play is a way of getting to know his patient whose breadth, detail, precision, and privacy are not to be found in other kinds of contact. Play will also provide him with surprising opportunities to interpret because the patient only demonstrates his full capacity for insight within play. However, the interpretation must be intimately connected in form, content, and timing with the characteristics of the game. If the interpretation fails to conform to the game's form, it is an interruption just as much as is any other behavior in which patient or analyst leaves the game. Play is an extremely fragile activity. When play has been broken off or when it cannot be begun, then the interpretation of the anxieties that caused its disruption, in the classic way, is indicated. At those moments, the interpretation must provide a high degree of differentiation between fantasy and reality, analyst and patient, the conscious and the unconscious. The loss of that differentiation is precisely the dynamic cause of the interruption of a game which stopped being a game and became the literal fulfillment of an unconscious situation. But once play has begun again, the task of interpretation will change its form and will return to the game.

The analyst who forcefully restrains the patient or does what the patient tyrannically orders him to do suggests a kind of interaction which could hardly be further removed from the attitude offered by the classic figure of the analyst who observes his patient's behavior and interprets its unconscious meaning. However, this antithesis is only apparent. All of the analyst's behavior has meanings which are communicated to the patient. Of course, the form and content of communication vary according to the analyst's behavior. It can be seen that the classic interpretation, formulated in conceptual language from the position of an observer, provides maximum differentiation between subject and object, internal and external world, the conscious and the unconscious psychic reality and factual reality. Consequently, it is logical that one of the ideal goals of analysis should be to lead the patient to this highly differentiated level of insight. It is not true, however, that this is the only way of communicating the content of his unconscious to the patient. On the contrary, clinical experience suggests that for those of the patient's mental states which are related to less differentiated forms than those of conceptual-linguistic thinking, the appropriate and feasible forms of contact and communication are action, gesture, dramatization, intuitive thought, verbalization, carried out from within the game itself. And so we see that from physical restraint of the patient to conceptual-linguistic interpretation, there is a progressive range of forms of behavior which make up a logical, structural continuum with respect to the essential aspects of the analytic attitude: (a) the conscious and unconscious intentionality of establishing and maintaining contact with the patient; (b) to provide information on the patient's unconscious which tends to differentiate subject from object, the literal from the virtual, internal from external, conscious from unconscious, psychic reality from factual reality.

CONCLUSIONS

1. This essay focuses on dynamic, structural, and genetic aspects of the patient's coercive behavior, placing special emphasis on the technique of approach.

2. From an observer's point of view, coercion is defined as the behavior of a subject whose main conscious and/or unconscious intention is forcefully to control an object.

3. The analyst's conscious and unconscious intention of establishing and maintaining contact with the patient and of systematically understanding his behavior is the basic psychoanalytic function.

4. The antithesis of the basic psychoanalytic function, the intention to coerce the patient's behavior, must never by adopted by the analyst.

5. Although there is a basic, systematic, psychoanalytic function, there cannot be systematic therapeutic behavior or a systematic therapeutic factor, since patients' behavior varies tremendously and the analyst's response must articulate with the nature of the patient's behavior.

6. The key to articulating the analyst's response with the patient's behavior must be found in the understanding of the psychology of transference.

7. Constant contact with the patient is possible only on the basis of the transference relation which the patient proposes. Therefore, the analyst must consciously accept all the transferences that the patient brings in, whatever their form, mode, and duration may be.

8. Accepting implies consciously playing the roles and actions the patient demands and essentially not resisting in any way, especially not unconsciously resisting, the role transferred by the patient. Accepting also implies unconsciously not to identify with the role transferred. Rejection and unconscious identification by the analyst with the patient's transference divert the natural course of the analytic process.

9. The analyst must play the roles transferred, even when the patient does not play his own transferred roles for long periods of time. On the contrary, the patient will consciously and unconsciously try to

materialize the transferred situation in his attempt to eliminate any evidence of play.

10. This battle for the material meaning versus the symbolic meaning of the event of transference is fought within the boundaries of the analytic situation, that is, the setting.

11. The analyst must always remain in contact with the patient, observing the patient's indications as to zone and type of contact, avoiding becoming isolated from the patient, or invading the zone of contact.

12. The analyst must know about the different kinds of symbolic behavior: myth, magic, play, language, gesture, art. Each kind of behavior has a particular structure which implies certain forms of thinking, feeling, doing, learning, perceiving, relating, and resolving.

13. The analyst's understanding and the form of his response must be in accordance with the perspective of the patient's transference and of the type of behavior of that transference.

14. To all the items mentioned up to this point, the expression "within certain limits" must be added.

15. These limits must be the minimum necessary, simply, precisely, and rigorously enforced.

16. The minimum necessary limits or boundaries are: the physical space in which the analytic relation will take place, the office; the time: the appointment time, frequence, and duration of the sessions; the physical integrity of the office, the analyst, and the patient.

17. At the beginning, the battle against the placement of limits will be aimed at the basic limits. Then, in the course of the analytic process, each transference situation will have its own type of limit *within* the basic setting.

18. For each configuration of the psychological field in the session, the two principles mentioned apply: (a) full rigor in limiting and maintaining the setting of the situation; and (b) full liberty for the evolvement of the transference within the established field.

19. The analyst must be aware of the significance of and need for placing limits as the necessary condition for the progressive development of symbolic behavior.

20. The evolvement of coercive behavior within the analytic process is significant since each coercive behavior, from its genesis, involves a dependency need which may come to be expressed as such if the optimal conditions are provided.

21. Nonacceptance of coercive transferences provokes: (a) the interruption of the patient's contact with his analyst; (b) violent separation anxieties; (c) repetition of pathological mourning processes due to the

loss of the relation sought in the transference; and (d) deviation from the potentially natural course of the analytic process.

22. All of the analyst's behavior has meanings which are communicated to the patient, including of course the meanings of his unconscious. The form and content of what is communicated will vary according to the analyst's behavior. The classic interpretation formulated in discursive conceptual language provides the maximum differentiation between subject and object, internal and external world, conscious and unconscious, psychic reality and factual reality. Logically, one of the objectives of analysis is to lead the patient to this highly differentiated level of insight. Clinical experience shows that the analyst's communication must articulate with the patient's. From the physical restraint of the patient to the discursive, conceptual-linguistic interpretation there is a progressive range of types of behavior for the analyst which form a logical continuum with the essential aspects of basic analytic activity as defined in point 3. Each level of the analyst's behavior has a corresponding level of information which will be given to the patient regarding the conscious/unconscious, subject/object, psychic reality/factual reality, external world/internal world, the literal/the virtual.

BIBLIOGRAPHY

ADLER, A. (1929). *Problems of Neurosis*. London: Kegan Paul.

BOWLBY, J. (1979). *The Making and Breaking of Affective Bonds*. London: Tavistock Publications.

KLEIN, M. (1932). *The Psychoanalysis of Children*. New York: Grove Press, 1968.

MAHLER, M. S. (1968). *On Human Symbiosis and the Vicissitudes of Individuation*. New York: Int. Univ. Press.

MELTZER, D. (1972). *Sexual States of Mind*. London: Clunie Press.

SEARLES, H. F. (1965). *Collected Papers on Schizophrenia and Related Subjects*. New York: Int. Univ. Press.

VALEROS, J. A. (1979). *Experiencias con una Bruja Buena*. Buenos Aires: Kargieman.

WINNICOTT, D. W. (1971). *Playing and Reality*. New York: Basic Books.

IN HONOR OF
HANS W. LOEWALD

Styles of Connection in Analysis

Clinical Instances

ROSEMARY H. BALSAM, M.R.C.P.
(Edinburgh), M.R.C. Psych. (London)

THE STYLE OF CONNECTION BETWEEN THERAPIST AND PATIENT, BETWEEN analyst and analysand, is as unique as the way one person's face registers with another person. Therapists of the same school share theoretical assumptions which guide and influence the forms of therapy into recognizably similar shapes. For example, there is a beginning, middle phase, and termination; or there are shared ideas about the frequency of appointments and the use of the couch; or, closer to the intimacy of the interaction, there is the deemphasis of the therapist's social contact with the patient, or the invitation to the patient to lead off the session with his or her associations. Within these like frameworks, each therapy couple develops, in addition, emotional idioms particular to that couple. The ways of mutual engagement in a therapeutic dialogue are probably myriad. There will be patterns in speed or production of association, color, and particularity of imagery, characteristic hesitancies in addressing the analyst, and differing styles of distant displaced or blunt intimate reference to the analyst. The analyst in turn will develop, say, patterns of personal and reactive fantasies during a silence, or patterns of verbal or nonverbal response to certain chains of association. The precise individuality of these connections is both a fascinating and an immense study.

One avenue to the topic is to try to capture some of the overt and underlying attitudes mutually present in both therapist and patient, which, when they combine, may yield elements of an engagement discernibly unique to a given couple. The topic brings together searches for the essence of individuality, the point and counterpoint of ways of

Associate clinical professor of psychiatry, Department of Student Mental Health, Yale University; member, Western New England Institute for Psychoanalysis.

connecting, the joint task set before analyst and analysand, and the final yield of the work.

Loewald (1960) offers a passage central to this issue: "In analysis, we bring out the true form by taking away the neurotic distortions. However, as in sculpture, we must have, if only in rudiments, an image of that which needs to be brought into its own. The patient, by revealing himself to the analyst, provides rudiments of such an image through all the distortions—an image that the analyst has to focus in his mind, thus holding it in safe keeping for the patient to whom it is mainly lost. It is this tenuous reciprocal tie which represents the germ of a new object-relationship" (p. 226).

In order to illuminate the task of the analysis, then, Loewald uses an evocative metaphor. It is one used by Freud (1905) who borrows from Leonardo da Vinci's formula for the antithesis between painting and sculpture: i.e., in painting something is added, whereas in sculpture something is taken away. Therapies involving suggestion, Freud explains, seek to superimpose and thus "restrain the pathogenic idea from coming to expression. Analytic therapy . . . [seeks] to take away something, to bring out something" (p. 260f.). The metaphor celebrates at once the individuality and uniqueness of connection between analyst and analysand. No two sculptures are identical. No two artists and no two basic materials are ever identical, yet, like individual analyses, the works emanate from a recognizable discipline and art form. It seems to me that the use of this image is a good example of Loewald's own hallmark in engaging the imagination while appreciating the work of transformation, creation, and recreation in analysis. However such therapeutic connections are conceived or described in our literature, here is an image which invites contemplation upon what may be individual in both participants and how this may bear on the work.

In 1986, when Loewald sprained his ankle, having tripped off the platform at a scientific function, he explained to concerned enquirers that he had fallen. "Where did you fall?" they asked. With a twinkle he replied, "I think I fell in the gap between ego psychology and self psychology, or was it between hermeneutics and natural science?" It is clear how much we owe to Loewald for his explorations and adventures into these so-called gaps where he is, as you know, actually a bold traveler. He is not known for either *faux pas* or leaps of faith! He guides and illuminates from the foothold of experience. Closely allied with Loewald's theoretical ideas are always images of an embodied human being developing and existing within a living world. His work is not readily categorized or claimed by any specific theoretical territory. One could say that he nimbly traverses the gap between the high podium of theoretical abstraction and the basic floor of human experience. If he is influenced and gleans the wisdom of ego and self psychology, hermeneutics, natural science, object relations, structural and prestructural theory and id psychology—if he works in the substance and negative spaces of these areas, it is in the interest of eliminating false boundaries.

These areas include the space for transference and countertransference. This is the space of analytic process, of the meaning and impact of one person upon another. This is the space for the growth of individuality from the cocoon of babyhood to the formation of character and selfhood in the world. This is time as fluid, history within the present and the future already reverberating with the forms of the past.

Following the Loewald metaphor of the sculptor and his raw material, one may ask: How do analyst and analysand work together? How does the patient fire the imagination of the analyst so that he or she develops the interest and courage to "hold in safekeeping" an image of the patient at his articulated best? How may an analyst register "rudiments [of] an image of that which needs to be brought into its own" or how may he register a distortion?

THE ANALYST AND THE PATIENT

The analyst's connection with the analysand is highly specialized. Loewald (and others) have helped free the positivist scientific self image of the analyst from the studied ideal solely to become an objective mirror to the patient's neurosis. This notion risked becoming a stultifying aspiration. While it may be partially useful, the concept is incomplete because it lacks the quality of mutual engagement which also plays a part in the potential for restructuring the psyche. Loewald (1960) points out, for example, that the necessary quality of objectivity which one brings to the analytic work "cannot mean the avoidance of being available to the patient as an object" (p. 225). It is within this very availability, with all its particularity and ramifications, that Loewald sees developing the fruit of the work, which is the potential for the analyst to develop as a new object. The patient's experience becomes the "new discovery of objects." Loewald elaborates, "I say new discovery of objects, and not discovery of new objects, because the essence of such new object-relationships is the opportunity they offer for rediscovery of the early paths of the development of object-relations, leading to a new way of relating to objects as well as of being and relating to oneself" (p. 225).

One of the catalysts linking the analytic couple is the individual response to cues in the dialogue, which opens up the capacity for controlled regression and reconstitution in both parties. It is through an experience of and fascination with emotional origins that such connections can be potentiated. And it is in working through an appreciation of the past interacting and being reenacted in the present, that insight comes about. A vehicle and byproduct of insight is the help gained to express in words the heretofore inexpressible. The hope of new object relatedness can thus emerge in relief.

At play in the analyst's mind as he or she listens and responds to the patient are, together with scenes of the present, personal memories, experiences with patients sitting up in therapy, or lying on the couch. In fantasy the analyst tests the borders of outcome, scanning the similarities and differences, remembering the evolutions and rhythms of similar-enough emotional scenarios. As part of his or her skill, the analyst at work develops marked abilities to follow, tune into, and keep fluidly interactive multiple levels of thoughts, feelings, and a dialogue within mind and body as he responds to the patient's unfolding stories and attitudes. He or she pursues several different levels of object relatedness simultaneously with the patient. This requires an ongoing ready alertness for regression and recovery. Thus, can the analyst offer himself or herself as new object for potential discovery, side by side or in parallel with the transferentially imagined answering image, say, of the one who does not listen, or the one who hates women, or the one who is so self-enclosed he is incapable of appreciating separateness.

The patient offers the material for joint endeavor by communicating consciously or unconsciously an invitation to engage differing levels of his own psychic structure. This capacity resembles that of a child who is able to be deeply involved in playing dollhouse but who, when called by mother, can come downstairs and have tea with the family. A potential for psychic fluidity is nurtured in the analytic atmosphere. Ultimately, this quality can participate in "regression in the service of the ego," a state which Kris (1952) first described and Loewald elaborates as an important element of the therapeutic action in the ability to restructure the psyche.

Clinical Examples

In the clinical examples that follow, I especially try to show the analyst as sculptor. The style of connection is informed by the fantasy of the approach of the artist to his basic material. I wish to underline that the aspect of the analytic work which I present can be no more than a fragment. The process of the ongoing work is much more mutual. The analysand too is daily scanning the raw material offered by the analyst. He or she too engages in a fluid mirror-image process so that finally, as a result of the working through of the analyst's fantasies, images, and communications, the patient will become the master sculptor of his own psychic material. To the artist, his material is not mere concrete stone or wood. The substance generates excitement and energy, akin to the analyst's challenge which is the imaginative, living self-conscious and unconscious psychic material. The jar of misalignment between the psychological distortion and the limit of the original pattern is expressed here in the notion of a patient's presentation of emotional paradoxes or puzzles, which trigger the analyst's interest. For brevity's sake, and also for the sake of confidentiality, the pictures of these patients will be foreshortened. Time will be eclipsed. I will focus only on a few striking features. As the task of working through is not presented, the underlying dynamics are only hinted at.

1. A 25-year-old male doctoral candidate in a hard science walked with a swagger, yet with eyes averted. He boasted throughout the sessions, yet with no ongoing acknowledgment of the presenting complaint of his failed comprehensive examination. He visibly shook as he inquired if I would be certain to see him. Yet he said he loved my approach. In what ways was I so important? He did not know. Actually, he waited a year with my name in his pocket before acting on his need for consultation. Within these paradoxes he floated elements that would be kept in trust and appreciated through the veil of urgent anxiety. Somewhere between the false swagger and his eyes that avoided gaze, there was a sense of body importance and awareness, a wish to be registered as noticeable, confident, and attractive. The swagger and the avoidance of looking betrayed the fantasy of exaggerated power, beauty, and grandiosity, and the simultaneous shame or fear of looking at me or being looked at. Somewhere between the boasting and the failed examination lay ambition, a wish to succeed, energy, and the potential to bring enough of himself to the work to care. Yet the boasting betrayed a powerful wish to deceive me and/or himself, perhaps in pursuit of the love of a parent? He was primed to fall in love with me. Within this helplessly fast but ambivalent blind surrender was surely a core of avid romanticism—a willingness to yield himself up to passion. This capacity of his for live fantasy possibly matched the fluidity of the psyche of the analyst so that together they would enter into what Coleridge described as a "willing suspension of disbelief." There was promise of the ability to become co-actors probably on an oedipal stage. The

analytic task could possibly be to chip away at the temptation to radical abandonment of judgment and the reckless lack of assessment of the other in the service of inchoate desire which would be a liability in choosing a potential life partner. The task would expose or transmute his counterphobic approach which in elaboration revealed unknown inner dangers. The false assurance of this present masculinity could over time become more secure, and more organically connected to the romantic passionate spirit. His sense of burgeoning manhood might be held for him in safekeeping.

2. A stiff-faced 18-year-old female undergraduate talked in a high childlike monotone. Her posture was immobile but her eyes flowed with tears. She spoke very quietly of world class athletics, a safari, a glacier, a volcano, and an earthquake.

Her thin but square figure was draped unflatteringly in dark, ill-fitting denim. Yet she wore sapphire-blue sparkling ear studs which exactly matched her glistening tearful eyes. She was watchful and straight, waiting to be told where to sit, yet her eyes were often drawn to and lingered over the couch. With her, where were the gaps, the space, the paradoxes for this analyst to engage imaginatively with her dilemma? She was stiff and rigid, like a still photograph, but the content within the tight frame was brilliant, exotic. Here in the room was a cautious waif, but there outside was a fearless adventurer, a sturdy explorer. In the dull dress she was like a chameleon—perhaps aggressively protected against marauders in the environment, yet the camouflage was incomplete considering the lovingly chosen and enhancing earrings. The affect was bleak and sterile, but the freely flowing unacknowledged tears surely tapped a hidden but fervent source of feeling.

The invitation that she offered, and the one that the analyst might hold in safekeeping, could be this strong energetic pioneer spirit. Here was a thwarted capacity for enhancing herself, a held-back energy in her emotional expression, and a possible yearning to trust and to depend on another in vulnerability while fearing the adventure into intimacy. The analysis of such paradoxes could some day coalesce in a powerful, capable, but tender woman. One may intuit that the effort to camouflage, to dull, may only increase with the threat of such personal attention and scrutiny as analysis offers. Yet, like an explorer who leads the way, this young woman beckoned on the follower with enough hints of the curiosity, richness, and color that might be discovered to engage and keep hope in a possibly wearing journey where these stalwart qualities become lost, not only to the analysand, but at times to the analyst.

Thus did the analyst begin the work which would proceed reciprocally. Each tone, each fantasy was carefully brought to the fore from the realm of hints, gaps in the process, from sudden switches in affect, toward free-flowing inner revelations, from the arena of resistance and hesitancy or filibustering. The analysand lived out her inner world. She subjected each communication of the analyst to the borders of her own knowledge of the analyst and the ritual of the process: Will she be present? Listen? How will she respond? What does it mean that she does or does not comment? Will she be withdrawn, or will she be overenthusiastic? Always the focus was upon the meaning of bilateral communication and always inner comparisons with the familiar objects emerged to reignite the analysand's memories, old pains, and ancient pleasures. Confidence grew as the analysand as apprentice sculptor took on the interest and curiosity of the analyst sculptor to her own material. She rendered her dilemmas in words—words chosen from her own meanings to capture what ultimately she, the analysand, wished to retain and what she wished to discard and recognize as obsolete, but as ever-present informing centers of the possibility for new connectedness gradually experienced with the analyst.

There is of course a limit to this analogy of the sculpting process, even in its bilateral dimension. Loewald would be the first person to recognize the limit of any given analogy applied to the variousness of the analytic process, which, as in life, can never be finalized as the form of a sculpture might be. I end with a quotation from the essay "Man as Moral Agent" which Loewald included in the Freud lectures at Yale in 1978. The notion of the continuous dynamic involvement of psychic life is here brought forward.

> To own up to our own history, to be responsible for our unconscious, in an important sense means to bring unconscious forms of experiencing into the context and onto the level of the more mature, more lucid life of the adult mind. . . . What is possible is to engage in the task of actively reorganizing, reworking, creatively transforming those early experiences which, painful as many of them have been, first gave meaning to our lives. The more we know what it is that we are working with, the better we are able to weave our history which, when all is said and done, is re-creating, in ever-changing modes and transformations, our childhood. To be an adult means that; it does not mean leaving the child in us behind [p. 21].

The analyst and analysand will therefore painstakingly work toward these final forms.

SUMMARY

This paper elaborates on the meaning of Loewald's metaphor of the analyst as sculptor as it relates to the transformation toward new object relatedness. The mutuality of the process is stressed and clinical vignettes are offered.

BIBLIOGRAPHY

FREUD, S. (1905). On psychotherapy. *S.E.*, 7:257–268.
KRIS, E. (1952). *Psychoanalytic Explorations in Art.* New York: Int. Univ. Press.
LOEWALD, H. W. (1960). On the therapeutic action of psychoanalysis. In *Papers on Psychoanalysis.* New Haven: Yale Univ. Press, 1960, pp. 221–256.
——— (1978). *Psychoanalysis and the History of the Individual.* New Haven: Yale Univ. Press.

Id or Subego?

Some Theoretical Questions for Clinicians

T. WAYNE DOWNEY, M.D.

THIS PAPER IS MOST MANIFESTLY STIMULATED BY THREE OF HANS
Loewald's works: his papers "Psychoanalytic Theory and the Psychoanalytic Process" (1970), "Instinct Theory, Object Relations, and Psychic Structure Formation" (1978a), and his monograph *Psychoanalysis
and the History of the Individual* (1978b). In each he presents intricate and
yet straightforward and ingenuous reinterpretations of psychoanalytic
theory. His mode of theoretical application is a model in these post-
modern, ego, psychoanalytic times. As he presents it in a characteristically succinct and understated manner at the end of his paper
(1970) on analytic theory and process:

> ... I *reformulated* the concept of instinctual drives and suggested a
> somewhat novel interpretation of the concept of hypercathexis.
>
> It seems to me that most of the views I have advanced are at least
> implicit in Freud's work and that of many other psychoanalysts. Perhaps
> my contribution consists mainly in making things explicit and drawing
> some unfamiliar conclusions [p. 299; my italics].

Loewald's mode in writing and treatment, theory and practice, is one
of "reformulation." This term captures an essence of psychoanalysis. It
can then be understood as an attempt at a reformulation, as a revision
of the individual's understanding of himself and of his meaning to
himself and others. Loewald's model enhances standard analytic conceptualization by emphasizing circuital in addition to linear dynamics.
It stresses reciprocity as a principle in psychic functioning. Areas of the
mind and functions of the mind interact with each other rather than
relating only in relatively straight-line, unidirectional Cartesian fash-

Training and supervising analyst at the Western New England Institute for Psychoanalysis; associate clinical professor of psychiatry, Child Study Center, Yale University,
New Haven, Connecticut.

ion. Loewald nevertheless maintains a hierarchy of levels of development. He insists on the individuals' attempts to master their destiny and optimize their growth at all levels of development; a continuing process of reformulation; that is, psychic structure-building and de-emphasis in its most basic psychological sense.

This paper attempts to use Loewald's concept of reformulation in relation to structural theory. It will concentrate on the concept of the id and the problem of reconceptualizing it *in the interest of clinical gain.* It poses the question as to whether the id in its depths needs to be viewed as so caliginous and inaccessible as conventionally presented. This exercise is intended to underline and complement several of the reigning themes in Hans Loewald's continuously evolving work: (1) the necessity of dynamic exchange between all areas of the *mature* mind; and (2) the corollary *reciprocity* between psychoanalytic theoretical models of the mind and clinical practice. Is the id always malevolent? Is it potentially at times beneficent? And following these themes, since the theoretical elements of id, ego, and superego are inextricably linked in the psychoanalytic model of mind, changing one definition implies change for all. This brief presentation will be no more than an introduction to a way of thinking about psychoanalytic theory and practice which I hope is only tendentious in its emphasis on evolving change through evolving meanings.

Superego, ego, id. Let us continue this experiment in reconceptualization with some commonly accepted definitions of these terms from Webster's *Third New International Dictionary.*

Superego: "a major sector of the psyche that is mostly unconscious but partly conscious, that develops *out of the* ego by internalization or introjection in response to advice, threats, warnings, and punishment esp. by parents . . . that reflects parental conscience and the rules of society, and that serves as an aid in character formation *and as a protector for the ego against overwhelming id impulses*" (my italics).

Ego: "the largely conscious part of the personality *that is derived from the id* through contacts with reality and that mediates the demands of the id, of the superego, and of everyday reality in the interests of preserving the organism."

Id: "the primitive undifferentiated part of the psychic apparatus that reacts *blindly* on a pleasure-pain level, is the seat of psychic energy, and is the ultimate source of higher psychic components (as ego and superego)."

Let me add a fourth definition that you may be thinking about as this essay unfolds:

Subego (a postulate): The realm of the mind derived from the infant-mother experience culminating in the development or mal-development of a partial sense of self as sensate, effective, and autonomous. A structure in the psychological sense for driving experience and simultaneously interpreting it through unconscious visual imagery which later becomes overlaid by verbal symbolism. It is a functional structure in a state of constant communication and overlap with the ego and superego. In nonneurotic terms, it wakes us up "on time." It asserts through parapraxis our individual rights in the midst of profoundly social, mainly conscious ego and superego emphases. That is, wish and self-assertion may strike a better balance with accommodation and guilt. Though obviously given our conflicting goals and interests, there can never be harmony in the mind; at best there can be only the potential for resonance and conflict avowal or resolution.[1] For purposes of this paper, the "infant-mother" experience is a shorthand term for the sum of all the child's potentially nurturing experiences, including those derived from father, siblings, and significant others.

My question is: Has the term "id" outlived its usefulness? After originally dominating psychoanalytic theory for more than three decades, is it merely out of fashion, merely overshadowed by ego defensive and object relations theoretical developments? Or is the contemporary lack of interest in the id (in theory, for we see abundant manifestations of drive activity in everyday life, in the movies, and on TV) a measure of the inutility of the term; the silent assertion of a widening discrepancy between its meaning and clinical experience?

Freud's particular conceptualization of the id in relation to ego and superego served to consolidate and clarify structural theory and facilitate a clearer conceptualization of the ego and its functions. This prepared the way for ego psychology. Ego psychological assumptions eased a shift in technique from symptom analysis to character analysis. It also threw a more balanced light on the functioning of the mind. But the question arises as to whether a side effect of Freud's own reformulation of his theory was that ego psychology was institutionalized in such a manner as ultimately to render the concept of the id clinically inaccessible? Did it become "off limits"? Did it in more particular ways engender a "fear of the id" (A. Freud, 1965) in analysts and other clinicians similar to that which Anna Freud (1936) described as particular to adolescents? For here was an id conceptualized as cut off from direct contact and direct interaction with the environment and with the

---

1. In a reaction to this paper Hans Loewald wryly suggested that in keeping with its syntax and the unending struggle for harmony, if the id is to be termed "subego," the ego might be termed "superid"!

superego, as the definitions I presented initially indicated. Here was an agency of the mind cut off from direct communication with other parts of the mind. It could only be approached and influenced indirectly through the mediating influence of the ego. As an aspect of mental functioning, the id was depicted as a quite basic precursor of ego and superego and yet quite apart from these so-called higher levels of psychic functioning. Freud's conceptualization of the id may also have served to create a degree of mistrust in the psyche's capacities for healing, growth, and investment in completing psychological development. And this even though we see evidences of positive growth and development all around us!

While analysis obviously requires the presence and assistance of another person, the characterization of the id and its aims brought into constant question the degree of cooperation, collaboration, or alliance which the analyst could expect of the analysand. A view emerged of a patient on manifest and latent levels who has many qualities of a recalcitrant child; one who must be pressed and prodded through interpretation and defense analysis to arrive reluctantly in the end of an analysis at something approaching full personality development. The implication is that left to their own devices (which of course cannot be the case in the lively interchange that is analysis), patients would opt for a lollygagging sort of evasion. This is a condition of some analyses and a portion of all analyses, but it is not necessarily the most salient quality of an analysand or of the id! The phenomenon of resistance is certainly ubiquitous, paradoxical, and in need of further clarification. The id was characterized as forever immutably sealed off from the reach and influence of social experience and conscience. This functional unit of the mind partook more of biological givens. While a psychological entity, it was conceived of as much closer to physiology than to mental life. It operated solely for pleasure at any cost without regard for external influences from executive ego, critical superego, or the external world.

Id, ego, superego. This nineteenth-century conceptualization of the trifurcated mind containing fixed psychic entities in almost perpetual dysharmony may have served to add weight to clinical premises charging the analyst with a "meta-mission." The task by implication may have become the sealing off of the id in the interest of extending the ego's, and perhaps the superego's, sphere of influence by increasing rational, conscious, executive functions such as memory, motility, and conscious thought as well as increasing moral suasion. In putting this forth, I am keenly aware that we are struggling here with a common phenomenon of analysis. We might say that with every advance, theoretical or clinical, come certain trade-offs. Latent vulnerabilities are exposed which then become the object of subsequent work. So there is a certain irony in the manner in which the statement of structural theory in *The Ego and the Id* prepared the way for the increased rationalism of ego psychology.

As Loewald (1978) and others have noted, psychoanalysis, which had been born in the joy and exultation of newly discovered libidinal springs beneath the crust of Victorian pragmatism and its closeted morality (or immorality!), experienced a return of the repressed in the course of its inevitable theoretical growth. To a certain extent the ferreting out of defenses and the rational analysis of mechanisms of defense became the order of the day as the id-dominated period of psychoanalytic theory was superseded by ego psychology.

I could carry this review further by stating that it was Freud's formulization of an object relations theory in *The Ego and the Id* centered around the oedipus complex that permitted this line of development from id to ego psychology and structural theory. Again by implication we come to the notion that drives cannot exist without object relationships. Otherwise neglected, understimulated infants would grow to be savages rather than succumbing to the nonobject, nondrive states of marasmus and physical illness!

To sum up what has been said so far, in this 65-year-old structural model, the embattled ego was perenially caught between the boat of the id and the dock of the superego. A mind divided was presented: one struggling to avoid the chasm of hedonism or psychosis should the id predominate; or struggling to avoid a mind obsessionally imprisoned by the equally obdurate and paradoxically passionate energies of the superego. Not a happy prospect for achieving lasting psychological peace! And yet perhaps therapists and clinicians have been overly sensitive to the negative implications of this structural model (which, by the way, most clinicians seem to use, though they may label it differently or bury any acknowledgment beneath many layers of new terminology). We may have shied away from a closer communication through words with the realm of the id, using our theoretical model to rationalize this movement on the grounds of unanalyzability or untreatability.

Loewald (1970) proferred a solution to this theoretical logjam. His solution rested on the premise that the id is accessible to some degree or other due to the fact that it is by and large a psychological entity whose shape and meaning are taken from the object relation of child and mother from infancy on. In contrast with the 1923 model, the id is not conceived of as a fixed entity, the blind messenger of temperament, instinct, and neurophysiology. In Loewald's reformulation the id is characterized as socially available and socially amenable. The id is then depicted as the psychological resultant, a mass of mental representations, if you will, arising out of the interactions around need satisfaction and object-seeking which occurs within the "mother-infant dual unit" (Loewald, 1970).

This model, as I understand it, is an id grounded in emotions and the haptic experiences of vision, touch, and kinesthetic sensations as they are felt interpersonally. To put it in other words, in Loewald's conceptualization of the id, it along with the ego and superego is psychologized. In a certain sense it is socialized having been formed in a social matrix. As Loewald described it in 1978, the walls of its physiologically defined cell are all broken down and replaced by an active dynamic interchange with the rest of the mind and with the outside world. The id then becomes defined as somewhat mutable rather than immutable. The clinical potential for communicating more directly with the psychotic cores of schizophrenic, borderline, and any other individuals may be significantly supported by this reconceptualization. It remains to be seen how influenceable this area of mind will be. We are given the theoretical will to explore this clinical region if id is not viewed as eternally and intransigently fixed. It is as though a world once thought to be flat is now pronounced to be round! A universe thought to be infinite is, and yet looks back on us with finitude!

THE SUBEGO

I hope that in the preceding brief I have been able to do some justice to one aspect of Loewald's many contributions. Given the reformulations I have outlined, can and should the concept of id be expanded or contracted? Does subjecting the id to object relations theory make its similarities with the ego more important than its obvious affiliations with the body and the drives? Yet should it be positioned even closer to physiology? Should its commonly conceived creative and true self-messenger functions be ascribed to a significantly larger area of unconscious ego function, the subego? These questions asked and arguments presented have provided a reasonable base for considering whether the idea of a subego is clinically meaningful and additive or just "old wine in a new bottle."

I refer once again to *The Ego and the Id* and to another fruitful concept which may support proposals for such a new conceptualization. In this work, Freud also introduced the notion of a differentiating grade in the ego to highlight a particular object-related area of ego functioning. He used this concept to set apart the socially identificatory and critical aspects of the superego and conscience from the management functions such as memory, motility, and finding meaning in mental activity of the ego proper. If then the superego represents the taking in of social development and social control resulting in the formation of a conscience; if it represents our moral debt to others; if the superego is the dominion of guilt psychology: then perhaps in a similar manner we can look for a province of the mind along this differentiating grade in the ego counterbalancing this domain of conscience. Can we conceptualize a polar opposite domain where the social experience of infant with mother has ideally served to enhance, temper, and give meaning to the wish psychology of the id/subego? I suggest subego as an alternative to underline the presence of an object relations and object-related element even in this primal area of the mind and self-identity. All of our mental activities require the actual preserve of another person initially and at least the fantasied presence (or fantasied absence) of another person later on in development. Given a differentiating grade throughout the ego grounded from earliest experience in object relations, the concept subego may escape the conventional *nonobject* meanings attributed to the id. One thing is certainly clear which may support such an argument. For all his difficulties and conflicts around coexistence and for all his hostility and destructiveness, man is basically a social and, in the broadest sense, a cohabiting creature.

The infant developmentalists add positivistic weight to these arguments. Many infant observers, including Brazelton and Als (1979) and Stern (1985), have reported on the active, vigorous, object-seeking and object-stimulating behaviors of babies right from birth. They describe perceiving infants "prewired" with the physiological preparedness for sizing up their worlds and immediately entering into the object relations exchanges which will give psychological meaning to early, near-physiological ego states.

In 1923 Freud also remarked on the strange similarity in the powerful energies that fuel the superego and the id, even though their functions seem so diametrically opposed. Day-to-day clinical and analytic experience confronts us with an unconscious psychological landscape where the scenarios (object relations fantasies) of self-interest, self-assertiveness, and drive gratification are constantly in contact and conflict with superego scenarios of self-sacrifice and guilt. As we see at times in individuals with obsessional dispositions, there can be a rapid, almost instantaneous shift from self-hateful, self-defeating superego condemnation to states of angry, vicious, drive-dominated expressions of hate directed at those who have blocked various self-assertions and self-gratifications. Indeed the conscience of such individuals often seems partially characterized by a brittle, unstable quality of reaction formation. Self-assertion is hidden right under its opposite pole of self-sacrifice and conscientiousness. A socially overcompliant self-image is often supported by interpersonal scenarios of revenge and triumph fostered by lost opportunities for genuine and true libidinal and aggressive drive expression.

We also see general styles of relating in adulthood; these seem to reflect this self-sensate area of the ego which was originally defined with the aid of mother's ministrations during infancy. Somewhat arbitrarily I am thinking of the period up to age 3 as the possible period of basic subego development; for instance, overly possessive persons who are unable to share their loved one's attentions with anyone or anything else, be it friends, newspaper, or TV. Apart from whatever other meanings subsequent development has attached, such an object relations style, freighted as it is with libidinal and aggressive drive derivatives, often reflects the early crystallization of mother-infant drive definition. Consider also the person whose mother contributed to the infantile dyad a sense of withdrawal in the face of the infant's activated libidinal or aggressive need states. Need we be surprised that for this person as an adult (we assume no reparation has occurred in the course of development) the silence of withdrawal of his partner at times of great emotional need or conflict is felt as an experience of emotional isolation and abandonment of the first water.

Similarly what do we make of the drive/object relations character style of a person who as an adult must always have his food prepared for him, a person who literally and figuratively cannot feed himself? And yet in the course of everyday life the attention of others is not called to this basic drive/object formation. Indeed until analysis this person is himself unconscious of a style of gratification/frustration in which overall he must remain somewhat deprived, unfilled, and *unfulfilled* in the midst of plentiful food stuffs and bountiful opportunities for love and libidinal gratification. Can this constellation not tell us much of his early shaping experiences of total aggressive engagement in the midst of dawning libidinal dependence on a nurturer with whom he struggled constantly for more nurturance but who was nonetheless always less than averagely available and less than fulfilling in her nurturing?

Are we surprised when the child of a cold, silent, distant mother seeks treatment as an adult because any potentially intimate partner is eventually, if not immediately, subjected to his cold, silent, withdrawn, often unconscious expressions of rage which have caused a severe atrophy in love and work relations? On the other hand, need we be surprised that the well-matched mother-infant couple's experience is internalized by the child and reflected in the adult by regular, harmonious, personal relations, the rejection of the unharmonious, and the self-confident engagement with self and others? These are schematic descriptions. I hope they have not come across as reductionistic. Obviously much that is telling, shaping, and meaning-giving happens in life after infancy. I am trying to develop a better picture of the "grain" of the mind, the bedrock of experience which provides the structure upon which subsequent altering, shaping, or exaggerating of mental functions and individual character occur. Examples of the distortions in this area are often painfully clear during psychosis and with pathological narcissism.

DISCUSSION

Subego-superego provides an engaging symmetry, but I hope more than that. It may support a model for mental reciprocity, exchange, and continuing potential for growth and change. If this model has clinical value, we might be tempted to replace the ontogenetic model of development in this one aspect and substitute one based on the concept of developmental lines arising in earliest infancy. Rather than seeing structural development as the arising of the id-ego from some undifferentiated psychological state to be capped a few years later by the crystallization of the superego out of the ego, we might consider a state of affairs in which there is a simultaneity in the development of these agencies across the differentiating grade of what we term the ego proper. Positing simultaneous development of course does not imply that these agencies would all develop at the same rate. Nor does it imply equal accessibility to environment during any period. In this regard a case can be made (Downey, 1987) for tracing the roots of superego development to the earliest experiences of guilt originating in the farthest reaches of mother-infant experience. This increases the parity in the argument for a superego, ego, subego structure arising simultaneously from earliest experience.

In Winnicott's (1960) terms, what I am attempting to conceptualize structurally would probably be subsumed in his self psychology under the concept of "true self," that is, a self healthily omnipotent yet largely unconscious. I would emphasize that this is a partial sense of self which requires the contributions of ego and superego for the total sense of self to develop. A subego structure might go awry, depending on whether it receives a final positive or negative balance defined by the mother-infant experience in developing autonomy. This area would also functionally approximate Winnicott's "third area" (1953)—that intermediate space where powerful creative and communicative forces of a primary process nature press for expression and a presence in the external world relatively independent of "higher level" ego functions. The beloving or harshly critical superego represents a sum of the child's interpretation of parental control, criticism, or neglect. So too perhaps the extent to which the child is loved for what he is rather than for what he should be socially (and there is a necessary mix here), and the extent to which he is *reasonably* stimulated and supported in developing his drive potentials produce a subego structure that can best serve to balance the self/other interests of the individual. This eases the toil of the ego. This would be a preverbal imagistic structure which would remain committed throughout life to communicating the basic truths of the heart through the earliest means of conceptualization, visual metaphor. We are familiar with this mode in dreams, art, sports, and love-making. We can sometimes even experience it by staring into the distance or closing our eyes. Then we may be confronted with a lively, ongoing, primary process imagery filtering our current experience of self and others through the visual medium of the subego. This is a constant, visual free association that we may open ourselves up to or we may be blind to, just as certain aspects of subego function may be addressed silently or indirectly in the clinical setting. Rhythm and regularity of sessions, visual milieu, tone of voice, sense of the analyst's presence and attentiveness, and reliance on questions rather than interpretations to facilitate the process may all address the infantile subego colic in ourselves in a manner not possible with words alone.

SUMMARY

This paper began with definitions and it will end with one; albeit a tentative one.

Subego: The postulated realm of the mind derived from the infant-mother experience culminating in the development or maldevelopment of a partial sense of self as sensate, effective, and autonomous. A structure for driving and interpreting experience through largely unconscious visual imagery, a structure in a state of constant communication and overlap with the ego and superego.

Reviewing what I have written leads to this afterword. Perhaps the present conceptualization of the id gives physiology and animal behavior a bad name. Perhaps we would advance structural theory more if we reserved the term "id" for the distorted state of wish fulfillment resulting from compromised parental malnurturing of the "good enough infant." Intrapsychic activities must *to some degree* be inimical. A better conceptual balance needs to be struck between their harmonious and antagonistic functioning.

This condensed preliminary communication was intended to suggest some ways in which, in the spirit of Loewald, experience can give meaning to theory and theory can become a beacon for hardy clinicians seeking new avenues of exploration.

BIBLIOGRAPHY

BRAZELTON, T. B. & ALS, H. (1979). Four early stages in the development of mother-infant interaction. *Psychoanal. Study Child*, 34:349–369.

DOWNEY, T. W. (1987). Notes on play and guilt in child analysis. *Psychoanal. Study Child*, 42:105–125.

FREUD, A. (1936). The ego and the mechanisms of defense. *W.*, 2.

——— (1965). Normality and pathology in childhood. *W.*, 6.

FREUD, S. (1923). The ego and the id. *S.E.*, 19:3–66.

LOEWALD, H. W. (1970). Psychoanalytic theory and the psychoanalytic process. In *Papers on Psychoanalysis*. New Haven: Yale Univ. Press, 1980, pp. 277–301.

——— (1978a). Instinct theory, object relations, and psychic structure formation. *Ibid.*, pp. 207–218.

——— (1978b). *Psychoanalysis and the History of the Individual*. New Haven: Yale Univ. Press.

STERN, D. N. (1985). *The Interpersonal World of the Human Infant*. New York: Basic Books.

WINNICOTT, D. W. (1953). Transitional objects and transitional phenomena. In *Collected Papers*. New York: Basic Books, 1958, pp. 229–242.

——— (1960). Ego distortion in terms of true and false self. In *The Maturational Processes and the Facilitating Environment*. New York: Int. Univ. Press, 1965, pp. 140–152.

Psychoanalytic Neutrality toward Religious Experience

NATHANIEL LAOR, M.D., Ph.D.

CAN A RELIGIOUS PERSON CONSISTENTLY EMBRACE BOTH SCIENCE AND psychoanalysis? Can a scientist consistently embrace both religion and psychoanalysis? Can a psychoanalyst consistently embrace both religion and science? Can each maintain his own identity vis-à-vis the other, without at the same time losing his integrity? This question is of particular importance for practicing psychoanalysts because it applies to psychoanalytic theory, treatment, and technique. In this domain the following questions arise: The theoretical question, how do psychoanalysts understand the analysand's religious discourse and effort? The therapeutic question, given the psychoanalytic formulation, is any modification of the analysand's religious experience and beliefs called for, and, if so, how do psychoanalysts understand what should be aimed at? The technical question, how would psychoanalysts maintain their neutrality vis-à-vis the religious analysand given their own religious makeup and their self-selected psychoanalytic theory of religion and religious experience?

In our Western liberal society that maintains the separation between church and state, most discussions of religious creed are private. The institutional separation between church and state underscores the indifference of the political organ to the parochial one. But the insistence on privacy of religious matters tells us more: it reflects the notion that these matters are precious to one's self; their critical discussion is a sensitive and risky endeavor. Yet the court of reason is public, and to refrain from openly discussing religious matters may unnecessarily deprive us of the opportunity to clarify and refine our sentiments and beliefs.

Yale department of psychiatry, and Child Study Center. Paper read to the Kanzer Seminar, Yale University, November 1985, and to the Denver Psychoanalytic Society, Colorado, December 1987. I am grateful to all those who discussed this paper, particularly to Joseph Agassi, and also Albert J. Solnit, Vann Spruiell, and Lottie Newman.

What is the conflict between psychoanalysis and religion about? One way of understanding this conflict is to see it as part of the difficulty to reconcile religious experience and human rationality. This problem arises when a person can no longer believe in the literal word of the scriptures. The most prevalent alternative is the assumption of some sort of functional-pragmatic attitude toward parochial religion and ignoring altogether its claim on reality. This maneuver conserves the religious sentiment but prevents its further refinement in the light of reason as it safeguards it against tests of reality. For the pragmatists care less about the truth of an assertion concerning reality than about its usefulness.

Freud (1927) viewed (Western theistic) religion as based on fantasy. His psychology may thus constitute an antireligious philosophy where both meet, the radical empiricist scientists who strongly object to the belief in the "spiritual" and the psychoanalysts who strictly follow Freud. The psychoanalysts, however, are not only scientists of the mind; they are also healers. As healers some of them (e.g., Adler, 1933; Loewald, 1953) have observed that some individuals' functioning may be enhanced by religion. These psychoanalysts are often supportive of religion. Here, the pragmatic psychoanalysts and the pragmatic religionists may meet.

The pragmatic approach to science and established religion avoids the clash between them, but it exacts a very high price—both cognitive and moral. When there is a clash between religion and science, it could be avoided by maintaining that the statements made within one of the fields are devoid of any empirical reference and that they could be endorsed as merely useful propositions (Agassi, 1975). Such an intellectual maneuver may cost science its informative content and religion its objects; both lose their moral force. In reality, however, the claim that theoretical statements are useful is empirical and therefore subject to considerations as to truth and propriety. We are again facing the two horns of the dilemma: religion or science? This dilemma has become acute because religion is associated with faith and science with reason. Who in his right mind would give up on reason? But would a religious person give up God?

The religious psychoanalysts facing this dilemma find themselves in a particularly difficult position. They may be unable fully to endorse or completely to abandon their science or religion. As scientists, they seek the universal, secular, and impersonal. They may try to avoid mixing the religious with the scientific, the private with the cosmic, the patients' intimate world of suffering, and the objective theory of illness.

As scientists of the mind, however, the private world is for them their cosmos that needs to be explored.

A few rationalist scientists and philosophers have claimed that science may offer a solid alternative to parochial religion, an experience which is, at the core, nothing short of a religious experience: it opens the door to the comprehension of the secret of the universe (Russell, 1903; Einstein, 1954; Freud, 1927, p. 54). When the secret considered is that of illness, science may claim to displace religion not only as a system of belief but also as a technology of healing.

Freud himself despaired of the hope that psychoanalysis would ever help cure humanity of all its ills. He realistically appreciated the limits on the technological promise of psychoanalysis. The *locus classicus* is *Civilization and Its Discontents* (1930). Freud underscored, however, that if any progress is to be made in the mental capacity of humans, it is science and psychoanalysis and not religion that would bring it about. Religion, as analyzed by Freud, is for the most part regressive. This view brings psychoanalysis into an open conflict with all established Western religion: psychoanalysis and religion seem to be two kinds of explanatory systems and technologies that compete with each other. How should one decide rationally between them?

It has been argued that psychoanalysis as science ought to stay neutral to religious doctrine, and as medicine it ought to stay neutral to religious practice (Guntrip, 1956). But it is precisely religious belief and practice that Freud deemed regressive. As physicians of the mind, the psychoanalysts find it their business to diagnose and cure illness. Admittedly, as philosophers-metaphysicians, psychoanalysts may at times wish to dwell on problems raised by established religious belief and practice and explore the religious dimension as such—but then duty demands that the theories of psychopathology be left behind and not be indiscriminately applied to religion and metaphysics. This requirement may not have posed difficulties for the radical empiricist physicians of the mind, because, according to them, the theory and practice of psychoanalytic therapy are a science, not a metaphysics. Will this separation between science and metaphysics prevent the conflicts between religion, science, and psychoanalysis?

Consider the scientific study of religion in its attempt to prevent conflicts. Theology is the field within which religious thinkers offer theories concerning their religious doctrine and practice in the attempt to justify them rationally. It represents the philosophical attempt to endorse both reason and faith in God. As a science, theology originates in intense self-doubt. Theology thus may harbor the seeds of its own destruction and, for that matter, the destruction of established religion itself. In many ways, the logic of the traditional relationship between theology and science (or rational philosophy) repeats itself in the conflict between religion and psychoanalysis. When the psychological science of religious experience is offered as the modern complement to theology, it intensifies the stress put on the religious student of religion. For a science that claims to uncover the psychological roots of all religious experience may threaten parochial dogma. This may be the reason why religious thinkers often proposed a demarcation between the psychological science of fantasy and the dogmatic metaphysics whose concern is with divine reality.

This will not do. Psychoanalysis, like science, is couched in a metaphysics (Popper, 1963; Agassi, 1975; Wisdom, 1970) and (Western theistic) religion contains empirical claims (e.g., concerning revelation) that are crucial to its foundation. Ignoring these facts may impoverish the cognitive and moral standing of both fields, and reflect nothing but a modern version of the old pragmatist attempt to reconcile science and religion. The implications of such a philosophy are far-reaching. For example, psychoanalysts who are oblivious to Freud's metapsychology may fail to observe that it encourages the reduction of religious phenomena to regressive fantasy; thereby it cannot account for that which turns human thought, feeling, or images religious, as distinct from that which turns them pathological. Similarly, religionists who are oblivious to their empirical claims and to the scientific challenge to them, or those who insist that dogmatic empirical claims can be taken only metaphorically risk that their central doctrines, too, will be taken only metaphorically and thereby be upheld by reference to parochial authority.

In the past, the defensive posture of religious scientists has been regarded as a sign of weakness that could legitimize the declaration of triumph of metaphysicians, devoted to promoting science and combating religion. Yet for some of these metaphysicians science is a new kind of religion: the search for the secret of the universe. Apply the scientist's critique of religion to science itself and both science and religion are either in or out of trouble. Apply the view of science as religion to psychoanalysis, and the psychoanalysts' neutrality toward religious experience is jeopardized. It seems we have reached an impasse. Where has the discussion gone wrong?

The discussion I propose has unfortunately begun with the wrong problem. The problem for rational religious persons to face is not how to reconcile the service of two authorities—faith and reason, science and psychoanalysis, psychoanalysis and the church—but how to reason and act as autonomously as possible, while refining their religious experience. From the psychoanalytic perspective, refining one's religious experience may mean refining one's position vis-à-vis internalized religious objects. This view implies a developmental perspective on religious life (Rizzuto, 1979) and poses a problem for the concerned psychoanalyst: How can individual religious experience be the source of improvement in both autonomy and rationality, and how can individual autonomy and rationality be the source of refinement of religious experience? How can a psychoanalyst maintain neutrality toward religious experience without losing the capacity to help refine it?

The discussion takes us back to my point of origin: to Freud's (1927) interest in human development and its pathology, and to his doubt whether religion can ever be compatible with human maturity, mental health, and personal autonomy. If such a religion were possible, then, according to Freud, there could not be raised a rational objection against the essence of religion, or a plea, like Freud's, to do away with it altogether:

> ... nothing can withstand reason and experience. . . . Even purified religious ideas cannot escape this fate, so long as they try to preserve anything of the consolation of religion. No doubt if they confine themselves to a belief in a higher spiritual being, whose qualities are indefinable and whose purposes cannot be discerned, they will be proof against the challenge of science; but then they will also lose their hold on human interest [p. 54].

This view of religion situates Freud within the tradition of those theologians who, ever since Philo, have aspired to refine the view of God by demythologizing it. Freud believed that performing this operation would radically impoverish religion. But, on his own account, Freud was not personally moved by religious experience to begin with. Can both psychoanalysis and religion independently survive and possibly be enriched by the psychoanalyst's interest?

PSYCHOANALYSIS AND RELIGIOUS EXPERIENCE

Why should a person be free of both religious doctrine and religious experience? The answer to this question lies in the answer to a different though related one: How could a person reason and act as autonomously as possible?

Psychoanalysis underscores the value of autonomy and rationality for the person. It thus threatens all forms of heteronomy and irrationalism embedded in Western parochialism, particularly when it claims to refine the religious experience of the individual. Freud (1927) endorsed Feuerbach's view (1841) of parochial doctrine as projection. Likewise he (1912–13) endorsed James Frazer's view of men having emerged from the realm of magic, developed through that of religion, and reached their intellectual heights through scientific thinking. If we follow Feuerbach on the road to autonomy, the religious object, the transcendent Deity, ought to be fully internalized. This can be done with or without leaving intact the religious overtones attached to the original object. But such a *full* internalization is impossible for a serious believer. In His resurrection solely within a person's psychological sphere, there can be no solace for the religious individual: God as a mere image is no better than as a mere fantasy or as a mere idol. Consequently, religion is viewed as an arbitrary and parochial hindrance, designed to impose heteronomy, or, put in other words, to offer solace through dependence; the very search for autonomy obviously includes the search for a method of dispensing with religion altogether.

This is one alternative view (a) that competes with the following views of religion as (b) conducive to human autonomy; (c) beneficial, conducive to maturation and adaptation of the individual, within a given social context; adaptation may be partly heteronomous, but preferably conducive to increased autonomy; (d) an inescapable evil, part-and-parcel of the human heteronomous condition; and (e) quite indifferent, in essence, to the problem of autonomy; or as conducive to it in some cases, detrimental in others, and indifferent in the rest.

In what follows I shall present the views of some of the most eminent psychoanalytic thinkers, the first generation of the trailblazers and the second generation of the followers in the various psychoanalytic schools. All of them made enormous contributions to psychoanalysis in general and to our understanding of the psychology of the religious experience in particular. My focus has to do with the psychoanalytic view of this experience. We shall see, however, that the psychoanalytic formulations of religious experience and the attitude of the analyst toward it are interdependent. None of the eminent thinkers opted for alternative (e) (which incidentally reflects Freud's insight at the end of *The Future of an Illusion*). The eminent scholars reviewed here maintained and propagated the classical struggle between religion and science, with psychoanalysis as the latter-day representative of science or of religion or of both. Hence, in their hands, there might be a danger that psychoanalysis may become either a theology—theistic or atheistic—or an antitheology. In either view, psychoanalysis defeats its own quest for a neutral position toward human experience which is also compatible with human autonomy.

Following Ludwig Feuerbach, Freud (1912–13, 1927, 1939) viewed all religious experience as illusory and as regressive. He equated it, at times, with that of a neurosis, at other times with that of a psychosis (1930, p. 81). Freud repeatedly refused to see parochial religion in any way other than as a major hindrance to personal growth. At best, he saw it as an infantile solace. Freud wished for the mature adult to dispense with both religious experience and parochial doctrine.

It is precisely because Freud could not see the problem of autonomy as possibly indifferent to religion that he could not be neutral toward it and allow it to occupy a central role in human life. However, I wish to look at religion from a psychoanalytic perspective and at psychoanalysis from a religious perspective. We thus can ask: Can psychoanalysis itself avoid the fate it sees for religion? Can it free itself from theology or, shall we say, psychoanalytic theology? Can it put up with religious experience? Can it put up with parochial doctrine? Or can it at least remain neutral to religion at large and still contribute to human autonomy?

In Adler's view (1933), all human experience is organized around self-deception and fiction. Fiction is normal, he said, insofar as it is practical and socially acceptable. Adler saw theological concepts, human autonomy, and responsibility as mere functional fictions. Established religion—in contrast to the religion of the innovative individual—is thereby granted a respectable and comfortable niche in this psychology. In fact, both occupy a similar pragmatic status, thereby losing their informative content and moral force. This result is the direct outcome of Adler's total disregard of the theological tension and problems as well as of the problems concerning human autonomy. The logic of such a disregard as well as the logic of its failure are common to all of pragmatism. And Adler's pragmatism is all-encompassing: it embraces and undermines science and religion.

Ironically, in the conflict between psychoanalysis and religion, Freud's conservative rationalist outlook led him to hostility toward established religion, whereas Adler's socialism led him through his pragmatist philosophy to the opposite. It was Adler's pragmatism which led him to clash with Freud's radical empiricism.

Sensitive to the empirical claims of both science and religion, Freud expressed the utmost respect for realism—both scientific and re-

ligious—when he reacted to Adler's psychology which followed closely
Hans Vaihinger's philosophy (1911) (see Laor, 1984), and which recommended the view of all theoretical constructs, human autonomy,
and responsibility as well as of God as mere functional fictions: "A man
whose thinking is not influenced by the artifices of philosophy will
never be able to accept it; in such a man's view, the admission that
something is absurd or contrary to reason leaves no more to be said"
(Freud, 1927, p. 29).

The religious psychoanalysts who explore the religious experience
could endorse neither Freud's positivist realism nor Adler's pragmatism. Therefore, they traditionally opted for idealism or fiction-
alism (Laor, 1989), i.e., the view that the human mind cannot transcend its own bounds and reveal any truth about reality—either
empirical or transcendental.

Jung at times occupied Freud's position on religion, at others
Adler's. He was the first and most important psychoanalyst to blur the
boundaries between religion and psychoanalysis, if not to fuse them
with each other. Inconsistencies do not seem to have bothered Jung.
Since later writers on the conflict between religion and psychoanalysis
recapitulate Jung's claim, his claims cannot be ignored.

Jung (1937) viewed religious experience as absolute and its truth as
indisputable and quite compelling (pp. 7–9, 104–105). He found the
nature of religious reality to be rooted in the universal unconscious (p.
50). Indeed, he saw religious experience as delving into the universal
unconscious which is the "shadow" of the human psyche (p. 76f.).
Delving into one's own, and thus into the universal, unconscious is
potentially revitalizing. It is also risky since culture, including established religion, proscribes it. It is barred from immediate experience as
"bad," by science and established religion (p. 43ff.). The shadow, according to Jung, is real, though its proscription makes it an illusion. Yet
the proscription is also real. So, for Jung, the shadow is real illusion: it is
the locus of the God-man currently "descended from its throne" (p.
84).

No one denies that dreams are both real and illusory. They really
occur and their content is actual, but their reference is not. Jung confused sense and reference (p. 104f.). Moreover, there is no doubt that
every experience, even the most illusory one, has a reference of being
experienced. The unreality of the object as if perceived in the experience must be distinguished from the experience which is real, can be
reported and even perceived. Jung demanded that the problem be
silenced. He invited religious experience as the only road to authenticity (p. 43ff.) and precluded any analysis of it. By fusing religious

symbol and psychoanalytic reference, Jung turned psychoanalysis into a new religion.

Jung thus invited his followers to enter into the religious dimension, but at the same time forced them to dwell there. A Jungian analyst or analysand cannot remain secular. Neither can he comfortably stay with traditional established religion—he must join Jung's. But Jung, in his insensitivity to absurdity, simultaneously espoused a realist and a pragmatist view of religion. He refused to see that the fact of an illusion is only as real as the disillusionment from it. Unreal, however, is Jung's respect of the religious person; Jung ends up in condescendence toward him, seeing the common person as inauthentic, heteronomous, and feeble. Jung's real quest is for a human genius as a redeemer (p. 49f.). If we apply Jung's view of religion to his own established dogma, it collapses, or else it stands on his self-appointment as redeemer. What remains, then, is Jung's religious enthrallment while being in the grip of his fascination with the human genius. (His fascination with the Nazi dictatorship is a case in point here.)

FOLLOWERS

What characterizes most of the psychoanalytic discussion on the matter is lack of theoretical self-awareness. Various thinkers, e.g., Fromm (1950), Erikson (1958), Lacan (1973), and Kohut (1971, 1981), have claimed innovation while repeating the logic of the situation when they apply their own innovations in psychoanalysis to the problem of religion. I shall refrain from presenting them and limit myself to the views of Loewald and Winnicott (as applied by Meissner). Each one of these thinkers approaches religion from a different perspective and represents a different school of thought.

Loewald (1953, p. 15) views religion with utmost respect as an integral part of the human condition: "Psychoanalytic treatment, as an educative and re-educative process, implies and appeals consistently to the ego's potentiality for growth. . . . This, in its highest form of awareness, is the freedom for faith and love." Is there a faith psychoanalysis aims at? Loewald views religious experience akin to the early childhood experience of love and warns against disrupting it. He recommends instead refinement. I cannot agree more with Loewald's position. Loewald's view on what refinement might be is, however, thoroughly Feuerbachian: "The mature individual," says Loewald, "being able to reach back into his deep origins and roots of being, finds in himself the oneness from where he stems, and understands this in his freedom as his bond of love with God. The concept of God itself seems to change from that of a blindly omnipotent power to that of the transformation and incarnation of such power in individual freedom and love" (p. 13f.). Loewald no longer advocates faith in doctrine or a transcendent God, but affirms freedom and love. By setting up this ideal for psychoanalytic treatment, Loewald may have transformed religious beliefs into psychoanalytic target symptom-complexes with no surplus value.

It may be possible, however, to regard Loewald's view concerning the process of internalization of God into the human psyche as religious. Loewald (1988, p. 260) deems "the advent of Christianity, initiating the greater intensification of internalization in Western civilization," as significant: "the death of God as incarnated in Christ moves into the center of religious experience. Christ is not only the ultimate love object, which the believer loses as an external object and regains by identification with Him as an ego ideal, He is, in His passion and sacrificial death, the exemplification of complete internalization and sublimation of all earthly relationships and needs." That is to say, the symbol of Jesus as fully destroyed, as dead, comes to represent, according to Loewald, the highest standard for psychic structure formation: the full internalization of Jesus amounts to the total annihilation of the oedipal parental object in the process of superego formation. The price for such perfect achievement is high: asceticism ("The sublimation of all earthly relationships and needs") or the guilt of falling short of it.

Is religious faith an illusion? No, Loewald (1988, p. 70) would say: religion is not necessarily deceptive about reality; religious symbols reveal reality—the reality in question being psychic reality, that of the instincts. Here Loewald (p. 21) identifies the mental and the spiritual and sees their reality as thoroughly sexual. Psychoanalytic reference is thus fused with the religious one. It is due to psychoanalysis, however, that religious symbols can be recognized as such and thus "sublimation turns around upon itself, and as it were against itself—to unmask itself" (p. 43). Psychoanalytic symbolic experience now fully unites with religious experience to render a most refined brand of (psychoanalytic) mysticism. Hence, psychoanalytic-religious experience consists of both "mourning of lost original oneness and a celebration of oneness regained" (p. 81).

Loewald (1978, p. 77), I think, seems to have followed the theologian Bonhoeffer (1951). Both advocate that religious concern and commitment to be expressed in human responsiveness and responsibility. Bonhoeffer, even in his most secular moments, responded to Christ and felt responsible before Him, whereas Loewald advocates that we respond to the id—our own instinct, the stuff spiritual reality is made of. By "respond" Bonhoeffer means "imitate"; not so Loewald. He underscores the duty to respond to the id in a responsible manner. Loewald does not say what makes a particular human response to the id religious. He implies that it is the magical spell of the primal object, eternally lost but symbolically found on a higher level (1988, p. 80f.). But then any system of symbols may convey such a spell—ethical, aesthetic, religious, or psychoanalytic. The transcendent, the theistic religious object, is thereby destroyed if only to be resurrected as pure sexual instinct.

This logic may take us all the way back to Jung: it may allow psychoanalysis and parochial doctrine either mutually to reinforce or to oppose each other. Within such a framework, psychoanalysts may find it difficult to maintain their neutrality.

The problem concerning the theoretical insufficiency in our dealing with religion may not be a minor one. It may reflect some other, deep-seated problems that are rooted in the philosophical framework of psychoanalytic theory. For example, following Heidegger, Loewald (1978, 1980) repeatedly stresses the historical nature of the individual and the value of personal authenticity. Heidegger's moral philosophy is relativist (and thereby could tolerate any moral regression provided it is culturally acceptable); Loewald's is not. Within a relativist framework, Heidegger could justify a regression to becoming an authentic Nazi by reference to the authentic historicity of individuals within their given historical culture. Loewald (1980, pp. xiii–xix), however, washes his hands clean of his teacher. Loewald's proposal (1978, p. 77), that we respond to the id in a responsible manner, may have been his implicit response to Heidegger. But Loewald's (p. 74) fusion of spirituality and instinctuality may invite difficulties in that he introduces both sexuality and aggression into the domain of the spiritual. Unlike Jung, Loewald almost entirely refrains from addressing the problem of instinctual dualism.[1] This, I think, is due to Loewald's more specific theoretical preoccupation with the unity of the psychic apparatus.

Loewald's project takes its origin in the view of the original instinctual unity of the psychic apparatus—hence his need to explain psychic deinstinctualization. This he does by referring to internalization and sublimation, which, when applied to religion, seem not to go beyond the basic unity of sexuality and spirituality. But the view of "science, art, philosophy, religious thought and ritual" on a par, as "sublimations par excellence" (Loewald, 1988, p. 80), may amount to

1. Exceptions are, e.g., Loewald's comments in 1988 (pp. 21, 80).

blurring the difference not only between sexuality and spirituality but also between fantasy and reality. This consequence is not obligatory within Loewald's psychoanalytic framework, but it does reflect the susceptibility due to a rigorous insistence (p. 20f.) on viewing the ego (contra Hartmann, 1955) as fully imbued with the sexual instinct.

In summary, Loewald's psychoanalytic theory is respectful of established religion yet reduces it to be fully absorbed in psychoanalytic reality. Can religion go beyond psychoanalysis? Is there a reality, a space, which belongs with religion and which psychoanalysis can formulate yet remain neutral to? Is there a surplus value to religious reality which need not be viewed as instinctual in nature, can be mentally represented, and need not be mourned?

Next I shall discuss the religious psychoanalysts who endorse parochial doctrine and view religious experience as central to psychoanalytic theory and theology. These scholars view Freud's appreciation of art and depreciation of religion as reflective of his personal weakness and look for the rational limit of psychoanalysis.

Meissner (1984) and others, e.g., Rizzuto (1979) and Pruysner (1974, 1985), endorse Winnicott's theory of the transitional object (1965, 1966, 1971) as the root of cultural phenomena. They use this theory to account psychoanalytically for the religious experience and to resolve the historical conflict between psychoanalysis and religion. In Meissner's hands (see Laor, 1986), God becomes a transitional object for the religious believers; once they mature, so do their images of God.

Similarly, Meissner and others like Rizzuto and Pruysner have made clinical contributions in their study of "the epigenetic and developmental formation . . . and use of the God representation during the course of human life" (Rizzuto, 1979, p. 182). The clinical contribution, however, cannot serve as grounds for religious belief, nor for psychoanalytic neutrality toward it, not even by restating the old Jungian point of view that "Reality and illusion are not contradictory terms" (Rizzuto, 1979, p. 209). It demands a theological complement. Indeed, the religious psychoanalyst who struggles seriously with the problem at hand cannot avoid reasoning about psychoanalytic theory and religious theology or philosophy.

As theologian, Meissner (who in this position has been joined by Leavy, 1988, 1989) argues for the higher epistemological status and the autonomy of parochial doctrine. He says, however, that the religious experience of the great leaders of established religion has a privileged status. It follows that the psychology of the great and their empirical experience prescribe and mirror parochial doctrine. Is this claim about the religious leaders dogmatic or empirical? Meissner does not say, but we know that the claim of traditional theologians and parochial historians is that it is both. How else could they view these great leaders as heretics or reformers? All we have to do is take the empirical aspect as separate from the dogmatic and all these leaders become empirically heretics and dogmatically reformers. A way out, of course, is to declare my religious leader great and yours small; mine capable of a genuine mystic union, yours not; my doctrine sacred, yours a system of illusions. Here, however, another problem of demarcation arises: which one of the claimants for leadership is genuine and whose claim should be endorsed and why? Who is a genuine reformer, a malingerer, or a mere paranoiac? Meissner does not deal with the problem and vacillates between parochialism and universalism, empiricism and pragmatism.

The problem of demarcation will not go away: it is central to both Freudian psychoanalysis and established theology and more. Since Freud, we remember, deemed any religion—even that of the parochially established great leaders—as an instance of either neurosis or psychosis, the problem is barred from Freudian psychoanalysis. The problem of demarcation does come up within, and is indeed central to, any religion: it calls into question the very foundation of parochial doctrine. For parochial doctrine not only mirrors the experience of the great but also conditions the experience of common persons.

We are back with the attempts psychoanalysts have made to resolve the conflict between psychoanalysis and religion, yet these attempts have consistently misplaced or, at best, ignored the problem. Either parochial doctrine is viewed as a transitional phenomenon and loses its privileged status, or religious experience of the common person is granted a respectable realistic status.

Winnicott's theory of culture says nothing at all about the specific aspect of the religious dimension. It is merely interested in establishing autonomy for cultural "fields"—not in solving genuine cultural problems. Furthermore, even when taken within Winnicott's own conceptual framework, the image of God does not fulfill Winnicott's definition of the transitional object inasmuch as its meaning for the believer is never lost. No doubt, some atheists may feel God has been for them a transitional object. Yet turning the Deity into one "transitional object" is a disservice to both religion and psychoanalysis.

Meissner observes that Winnicott's views can implicate psychoanalysis as "transitional" too (so does Rizzuto, 1979, p. 209). This may be dangerous, he feels, since such an implication voids the field of its universal and realistic content. Rather than change it, Meissner proposes the conservative pragmatist peace treaty between psychoanalysis and established religion: each field would accept the autonomy of the other. Yet Meissner indicates that religious doctrine occupies a higher epistemological and moral status than psychoanalysis.

I have come to the end of my commentary on the views of two generations of psychoanalytic thinkers concerning religious experience. We have seen that the analyst's neutral position (A. Freud, 1936) is affected by formulating this experience from various perspectives: the perspective of the superego (Freud), the id (Jung), the pragmatic ego (Adler), the libidinized ego (Loewald), and the transitional object (Winnicott and Meissner). In the next section I shall explore the implications of this commentary and attempt to determine the conditions for a more conflict-free (Hartmann, 1955) psychoanalytic neutrality toward religious experience.

PSYCHOANALYTIC NEUTRALITY TOWARD RELIGIOUS EXPERIENCE

Einstein was both sensitive as a scientist and as a religious individual. For him, "science without religion is lame, religion without science is blind" (1954, p. 46). He wished to resolve the conflict between science and religion. Einstein refused to turn either science or religion into a hollow pragmatic convention. He knew all too well that such a maneuver would deprive science of its informative content and religion of its finest qualities. Einstein therefore relinquished parochial doctrine and held on to Spinoza's principle for religious experience: *Amor intellectualis Dei.*[2] This brief expression tells volumes about Spinoza's value system, of his love of research for its own sake. The cognitive and emotional commitment of the scientist to the scientific inquiry is expressed in an unceasing pursuit of knowledge which is also the aim of the enlightened, universalistic, natural religion. The love of God secures for Einstein, as well as for Spinoza, the humanistic ethical counterpart of the commitment.

What might the intellectual love of God mean? For Spinoza, the pantheist, it meant the intellectual love of the universe, namely, the love which is the attraction expressed as the search for the secret of (i.e., the Essence of) the universe. No wonder that his system of thought has been traditionally indicted by established religion as systematized atheism. His dictum, however, was not: it is borrowed from religious sources—philosophical as well as cabalistic. Within the estab-

---

2. This dictum goes back to Philo and was introduced into the modern scientific community by Robert Boyle (1659).

lished framework, it invites a host of images which can be viewed as idolatrous to their root. The traditional parochial defense is that such images—not the very dictum itself—can only be taken as metaphors.

Freud could not let metaphors pass by without examining their roots and then interpreting them in the light of his theory. To resist the interpretation and insist that metaphors are solely and unambiguously abstract are dual errors. It would render the normal speakers linguistically concrete and leave them psychologically restricted. According to traditional psychoanalysis, the love of God—whether the love of a personal God, the concrete universe, its fleeting reality, or any manifestation thereof—is, at best, nothing but the love of the missing mother or the prohibiting father, or else instinctual and nonspecific.

This, then, is the significance of Freud's criticism of religion. According to Freud, one cannot worship the divine but as one's fantasy. Religiously speaking, any religious experience that puts forward any claim concerning the supernatural reality is, in essence, a mere case of idolatry. Here the aims of the psychoanalytic critique of religion and of negative theology coalesce.[3] Both, in the name of reason, demand a refinement of the religious belief and experience. (I leave the discussion of the theological roots of the conflict between psychoanalysis and religion to a later occasion.)

Incidentally, Freud's endorsement of science as his own rational religion (1927, p. 54) is not irrelevant to my discussion. Peter Gay (1987) attempts to explain Freud's references to "our God *Logos*" (p. 54). He views Freud as an atheist, as the last philosophe who created in the tradition of the Deists. The Enlightenment Deist tradition itself, however, obliges us to take literally Freud's expressions about science as a rational religion.

The most rational scholars of our age (e.g., Einstein, Russell, and Freud), who have repeatedly expressed their commitment to the idea of and the progress in rationality, and even contributed to it, have also expressed their religious feelings. The most noble expression of this combination has been Spinoza's. From our modern, more critical perspective we have seen that, though Spinoza's natural religion refers to science as its foundation, it may not be cognitively or religiously on a much higher status than traditional established religion. For, in Spinoza's hands, God's attributes are, at least in part, natural; as we see them today, they are human-made—i.e., given by science. Freud's critique of established religion—even of its social order—may apply

---

3. Philo laid the foundation of Western negative theology which concerns the ineffability of God (Wolfson, 1947).

here too. Can one maintain one's autonomy as well as one's rationality and religion?

I shall be looking for those conditions that could satisfy us as an answer to this question and thereby also constitute the minimum (universal) requirement for a religious experience that would conflict neither with reason nor with psychoanalytic neutrality nor with a developmental view of the religious experience. These conditions and requirements I shall view as constitutive of the religious register.

Psychoanalysis may demand a refinement of our religious experience. Such refinement may prove crucial for our capacity to empathize with the religious analysand. Religious love, fear, and even awe are feelings which seem to have become, in the light of psychoanalysis, affectively laden; even as religious constructs they have become overly charged. What, then, remains of religious experience? It is commonly believed that Freud's view was that once libidinal ties to parental figures are given up, all religious experience is turned into naught. A closer reading of his texts may lead to a different conclusion:

> The last figure in the series that began with the parents is the dark power of Destiny which only the fewest of us are able to look upon as impersonal. There is little to be said against . . . Multatuli when he replaces . . . the Destiny of the Greeks by the divine pair . . . Reason and Necessity; but all who transfer the guidance of the world to Providence, to God, or to God and Nature, arouse a suspicion that they still look upon these ultimate and remotest powers as a parental couple, in a mythological sense, and believe themselves linked to them by libidinal ties [1924, p. 168].

Thus perceived, the religious experience may be viewed as rooted in neurotic libidinal anxiety. The fear of God and the realistic fear of death can be derived from "the same parental view of fate" which is so "very hard to free oneself from" (*ibid.*). This is so because death is "an abstract concept with a negative content for which no unconscious correlative can be found" and thus, for its representation, "the ego relinquishes its narcissistic libidinal cathexis in a very large measure . . . it gives up itself, just as it gives up some *external* object in other cases in which it feels anxiety" (1923, p. 58). Freud concludes that this dynamics occurs between the ego and the superego. The alternative, it is implied, is the effective internalization through mourning and the facing of death as an instance of Reason and Necessity.

What kind of conflict-free personal experience is entailed by this Freudian position vis-à-vis Reason and Necessity, vis-à-vis a Deity that, like death, can be for humans a mere abstract concept with negative content? Is this experience religious? Can it go beyond Reason and

Necessity? Here is where Freud (1927, p. 54) declared his total indifference on the matter.

If we follow Freud's critique, it is possible that the experience of wondering could remain as the common, potentially conflict-free core of the religious feeling in conjunction with the autonomy to wonder about its very psychological structure. Wondering—wonderment as such—may at times come together with yearning for, curiosity about, and even fear and awe of that which is beyond any empirical limit. Insofar as wondering is rooted in desire, it is desire turned on itself, eternally frustrated. The traditional outcome of such a logic was asceticism (see, for example, Schopenhauer, 1819). The concept of wondering, I believe, can replace any kind of asceticism with the recognition of the irrelevance of any human desire for that which can never be what a human thinks or imagines it to be.

It may well be that the minimum requirement for the religious register at large could be defined by the position of wondering vis à vis a *concept* of God who ought not to be what we think or imagine a Deity to be. This requirement, however, puts a limit on the extent of mourning for the Deity as prescribed by Freud (following Feuerbach) which is, of necessity, an integral part of refining one's religious experience. Although such a concept of the Deity has neither unconscious nor empirical correlatives, although such a concept is abstract with a mere negative content, it is constitutive of a whole register of universal human experience. Hence, it may well be that the tenuousness of the realist value (reference) of the concept of God is that which gives rise to and partly constitutes the religious experience for individuals. Traditional religious experience, mysticism, dogmatism, and religious crisis can be viewed as phenomena, objects for investigation, within the register thus defined.

In other words, the actual owning up to one's capacity for religious experience assumes the very subtle position one can maintain vis-à-vis one's own empirical religious position. The religious register is logically prior to the empirical religious experience and thus constitutes its meta-level. Viewed from the meta-level perspective, psychoanalysts could neutrally regard each kind of parochial religion as both an expression and an alleviation of the tenuousness of the religious meta-position. From this perspective, one's effort to refine one's creed and religious experience can be neutrally explored as a struggle on the matter of reality—physical as well as mental—as it both limits and is limited by the anguish of mourning.

It may well be that such an experience and such a concept of the Divine, by being indifferent to parochialism, science, and ethics, could allow the promotion of human autonomy. Consequently, it may well be that religion, in a sense, ought to lie beyond reason for reason to develop freely to its fullest extent. This, ironically, still leaves religion within the limits of reason. The question concerning the limits of religion, science, and rationality therefore remains context-dependent and level-dependent and thereby multiply open.

Such a view of the religious register, by being general enough yet nonetheless religious at its core, would be enlightened by and complement psychoanalytic theory, practice, and experience. It may enhance the empathic understanding of and the respectful communication with the religious individuals.

Psychoanalysis may demand a refinement of the scientific position as well. It may call upon psychoanalysts as scientists to maintain their neutrality vis-à-vis theory (Laor, 1989) and to suspend religious love and remain both concerned and critically contained vis-à-vis opinions and sentiments. Yesterday's paradigms and communal commitments of scientists, à la Polanyi (1958) and Kuhn (1970), are tomorrow's dogmas and herd affiliations. If this view is correct, then some of the most advanced and liberal views of science—and by implication, also of psychoanalysis as science—need to be superseded (Agassi, 1981; Laor, 1985a). The religious experience of the researcher is not science.

Psychoanalysis may demand a refinement of its own classical position. The most advanced and humanistic psychoanalytic view of religion as solely illusory needs to be superseded. Once censored (or even allowed in) as mere illusion, religion, being thus suppressed, could indiscriminately color psychoanalytic theory and practice and thereby turn both into mere dogmatic symbols and rituals. A more mature, less dismissive view of religion would be more consistent with psychoanalysis as clinical science (Laor, 1985b, 1988; Laor and Agassi, 1986, 1988). The mere requirement, which I consider minimal, for respect for the religious convictions and experience (of the more or less sophisticated analysand) already amounts to a modification of Freud's views of religion as well as of psychoanalysis as science. For the view of the religious register I propose—a view which I consider minimal—allows regarding the religious belief and practice of any individual not merely as reflective of one's regression but also as one's continuous effort to stand vis-à-vis that which is beyond any possible human reach.

A precondition for such an obviously desirable state of affairs is that psychoanalysis develop as a science neutral to, yet not oblivious of, religion, where the neutrality spells respect for both the religious and the irreligious, so that it can sensitively help them both to refine their sentiments and opinions.

BIBLIOGRAPHY

ADLER, A. (1933). Religion and individual psychology. In *Superiority and Social Interest*. New York: Norton, 1964, pp. 271–308.

AGASSI, J. (1975). *Science in Flux*. Dordrecht, The Netherlands: Reidel.

—— (1981). *Science and Society*. Dordrecht, The Netherlands: Reidel.

BONHOEFFER, D. (1951). *Letters and Papers from Prison*. New York: Macmillan, 1953.

BOYLE, R. (1659). *The Works of the Honorable Robert Boyle*. London: W. Jonson et al., 1772.

EINSTEIN, A. (1954). *Ideas and Opinions*. New York: Crown.

ERIKSON, E. H. (1958). *Young Man Luther*. New York: Norton.

FEUERBACH, L. A. (1841). *The Essence of Christianity*. London: Chapman, 1854.

FREUD, A. (1936). The ego and the mechanisms of defense. *W.*, 2.

FREUD, S. (1910). From the history of an infantile neurosis. *S.E.*, 17:3–122.

—— (1912–13). Totem and taboo. *S.E.*, 13:1–161.

—— (1923). The ego and the id. *S.E.*, 19:3–66.

—— (1924). The economic problem of masochism. *S.E.*, 19:157–170.

—— (1927). The future of an illusion. *S.E.*, 21:5–56.

—— (1930). Civilization and its discontents. *S.E.*, 21:59–145.

—— (1939). Moses and monotheism. *S.E.*, 23:7–137.

FROMM, E. (1950). *Psychoanalysis and Religion*. New Haven: Yale Univ. Press.

GAY, P. (1987). *A Godless Jew*. New Haven: Yale Univ. Press.

GUNTRIP, H. (1956). *Psychotherapy and Religion*. New York: Harper & Brothers.

HARTMANN, H. (1955). Notes on the theory of sublimation. *Psychoanal. Study Child*, 10:9–29.

JUNG, C. G. (1937). Psychology and religion In *The Collected Works of C. G. Jung*, 2:3–105. Princeton Univ. Press, 1969.

KOHUT, H. (1971). *The Analysis of the Self*. New York: Int. Univ. Press.

—— (1981). Religion, ethics and values. In *Self Psychology and the Humanities*, ed. C. B. Strozier. New York: Norton, 1985, pp. 261–262.

KUHN, T. S. (1970). *The Structure of Scientific Revolutions*. Chicago Univ. Press.

LACAN, J. (1973). *The Four Fundamental Concepts of Psychoanalysis*. New York: Norton, 1981.

LAOR, N. (1984). Common sense, ethics and psychiatry. *Psychiatry*, 47:135–150.

—— (1985a). Prometheus the imposter. *British Med. J.*, 290:681–684.

—— (1985b). Psychoanalysis as science. *J. Amer. Psychoanal. Assn.*, 33:149–166.

—— (1986). Review of *Psychoanalysis and Religious Experience*, W. W. Meissner. *Psychoanal. Q.*, 55:672–678.

—— (1988). Psychoanalysis without shame. *Israel J. Psychiat. & Rel. Sci.*, 24:257–264.

—— (1989). The prision-house of fiction: review of *Freud*, ed. P. E. Stepansky (in press).

—— & AGASSI, J. (1986). Lacan contra Freud. *Psychoanal. Contemp. Thought*, 9:465–492.

————— ————— (1988). The grand protestor. *Philos. Soc. Sci.*, 18:73–100.

LEAVY, S. A. (1988). *In the Image of God.* New Haven: Yale Univ. Press.

————— (1989). Reality in religion and psychoanalysis. In *Psychiatry and the Humanities*, ed. J. Smith. New Haven: Yale Univ. Press (in press).

LOEWALD, H. W. (1953). Psychoanalysis and modern views on human existence and religious experience. *J. Past. Care*, 7:1–15.

————— (1978). *Psychoanalysis and the History of the Individual.* New Haven: Yale Univ. Press.

————— (1980). *Papers on Psychoanalysis.* New Haven: Yale Univ. Press.

————— (1988). *Sublimation.* New Haven: Yale Univ. Press.

MEISSNER, W. W. (1984). *Psychoanalysis and Religious Experience.* New Haven: Yale Univ. Press.

POLANYI, M. (1958). *Personal Knowledge.* London: Routledge & Kegan Paul, 1962.

POPPER, K. R. (1963). *Conjectures and Refutations.* New York: Harper & Row.

PRUYSNER, P. R. (1974). *The Play of the Imagination.* New York: Int. Univ. Press.

————— (1985). Forms and functions of the imagination in religion. *Bull. Menninger Clin.*, 49:353–370.

RIZZUTO, A-M. (1979). *The Birth of the Living God.* Chicago Univ. Press.

RUSSELL, B. (1903). A free man's worship. In *Why I Am Not a Christian.* New York: Simon & Schuster, 1957, pp. 40–47.

SCHOPENHAUER, A. (1819). *The World as Will and Representation.* New York: Dover, 1969.

SPINOZA, B. (1670). A theologico-political treatise. In *Works of Spinoza*, vol. 1. New York: Dover.

VAIHINGER, H. (1911). *The Philosophy of 'As If.'* New York: Harcourt, Brace, 1924.

WINNICOTT, D. W. (1965). *The Maturational Processes and the Facilitating Environment.* New York: Int. Univ. Press.

————— (1966). The location of cultural experience. *Int. J. Psychoanal.*, 48:368–72.

————— (1971). *Playing and Reality.* Harmondsworth: Penguin, 1974.

WISDOM, J. O. (1970). Freud and Melanie Klein. In *Psychoanalysis and Philosophy*, ed. C. Hanly & M. Lazanowitz. New York: Int. Univ. Press, pp. 327–362.

WOLFSON, H. A. (1947). *Philo.* Cambridge: Harvard Univ. Press.

Time and World in the Thought of Hans W. Loewald

STANLEY A. LEAVY, M.D.

IF WE ENTER ANY FIELD OF THOUGHT, A POINT OF VIEW IS NECESSARY AND inevitable. Total innocence, meaning mere observation without applying references already present in the observer's mind, if it existed, would be totally unproductive. This has nothing to do with an idealistic denial of the independent reality of the external world. It does mean that for the psychoanalyst everything, even the most objective brute fact of experience, needs to find a place in the intricate network of meaning that is unique for every individual. I understand that I have thereby stated a point of view and have thereby revealed an aspect of my own position toward the analysis of experience, affecting all that I bring to bear on the words I hear and the actions I witness in the consulting room. It would be incorrect, however, to name the sum of all constituents of a point of view a "philosophy"; philosophy is a rational discipline, not just an attitude toward life or psychology. There may be hidden philosophies in many points of view, affecting the process of discrimination of observed facts through the structures of thought that they uphold. These philosophies may actually be concealed by more common, even trivial attitudes: for example, to say that we regard everything we hear from our patients as true in some fashion, or that everything said is a distortion of something unsaid, are both bits of analytic folk wisdom which may be based on more fundamental and rational positions genuinely philosophical in nature.

All this applies equally to psychoanalytic theory and practice. It has always seemed to me to have been a serious loss for psychology in general and psychoanalysis in particular that it was cut off from its philosophical underpinnings. In William James, on the contrary, we see the value of the constant critical engagement of a philosophical mind with psychology. Even the limited uses to which logic may be put serve as beneficial pruning actions on the efflorescences of psychology; of greater pertinence to us might be the philosophical demonstration of the limitations of the natural scientific method in understanding human experience. It is curious, in that regard, that in recent years analysts, not ordinarily eager to enlist the aid of philosophers in correcting their theory, have congregated in large numbers to listen to certain philosophers, whose understanding of psychoanalysis is unimpressive, but who enjoy berating psychoanalysis for not succeeding as the natural science *they* demand it to be.

Hans Loewald is a rare exception among us because he is a philosophically trained and philosophically conscious psychoanalyst, who has made a profound and yet also subtle impact on our theory. It is profound in that he demands of us that we reexamine our presuppositions, subtle in that he is the least revolutionary or neologistic of innovators, and has always remained in continuity with Freud's teachings as Freud pronounced them. I would remark here that I am not myself sure whether this subtlety, which suggests a greater conservatism than the substance of Loewald's thought conveys, has been useful or not. However that may be, we must take him for what he is and be grateful.

The figure of modern philosophy to whom Loewald points is Martin Heidegger, whom neither Loewald nor anyone else can admire without ambivalence on account of Heidegger's appalling period of defection to the criminal state. Heidegger scratched out the name of his Jewish teacher Husserl from the dedication of his *Sein und Zeit* in the edition published under the Nazi regime. It is to Loewald's credit that on the contrary, he has always acknowledged his indebtedness to Heidegger, only after Freud, as his teacher. I have taken as my task in this essay to examine Loewald's writings for some evidences of this philosophical influence. It is a task that would be more appropriately undertaken by an analyst more expert in philosophy than I am, especially in Heidegger's work, or for a philosopher who has learned to undertake the practical work of psychoanalyzing. I can only hope that this effort may inspire someone more qualified to go further than I can.

On the face of it, Loewald's writing is not strikingly innovative with respect to terminology or even to basic psychoanalytic theory. Topographical and structural theories, libido theory, castration complex and oedipus complex are operative everywhere in the papers he has given us. If he protests here and there against certain excesses of ego psychology,[1] he is far from opposition to its general application. Traditional formulations of libido theory and psychic structure abound in

---

1. See, for example, references to the work of Hartmann (1939, 1964) in Loewald (1980, p. 81). Unless indicated, all page references refer to this book.

certain papers, such as the following statement, which would be comfortably met with in any classic writing on psychoanalytic theory: "The relinquishment of Oedipal objects and their 'restitution' in the ego, as a precipitate or differentiating grade constituting the superego, is a process of desexualization of libidinal cathexis, so that object cathexis becomes transformed into neutralized, narcissistic cathexis" (p. 331). In advance of more detailed discussion it is worth noting here that such seemingly unmodified classical theory appears more prominently in Loewald's discussions of the oedipus complex such as the one from which my quotation was drawn, than in those analyzing the deeper preoedipal epoch into which he has made his most original investigations. One could, although to no particular purpose, pile on the examples of Loewald's conservatism, especially of language, but all of his readers are probably sufficiently familiar with it. I may be permitted, however, to refer to his very characteristic demurrer against the attempt of George Klein and others to present metapsychology as nonpsychoanalytic or nonpsychological, in which he says: "I wish to make it clear that I do not share that position. At the same time I do think that what goes under the name of metapsychology both needs and deserves renewed thought, elaboration, and reinterpretations" (p. 148).

It is against the background of this evident determination of Loewald's to maintain continuity with what has become the language of psychoanalysis that any inquiry into the very important modifications he has made should begin. We are not dealing here with an innovator like Kohut whose new emphases apparently require a whole shift of focus on the transference, for example, and a modified vocabulary to suit it. A yet more strained contrast with Lacan would make this position even plainer, but is hardly needed for the point I wish to make.

There is only one extended reference to Heidegger's philosophy in Loewald's writings, beyond the grateful but critical mention in the preface to the collected papers, although other philosophers come up from time to time: Kant, Kierkegaard, Augustine, among others not often met with in the writings of psychoanalysts. This one is in his short book containing the Freud lectures delivered at Yale in 1978, *Psychoanalysis and the History of the Individual*. Here in lectures addressed to an audience united by a common psychoanalytic and humanistic concern, Loewald moves easily between a fairly technical psychoanalytic language and one of more philosophical inclination than he has shown elsewhere. He describes the development of the individual from a lower to a higher level as "a continuous appropriation of the unconscious levels of functioning, an owning up to them as potentially *me*, ego," and calls this integrating process "in a different framework, an existential task." Here then comes the rare direct reference to his early mentor: "I believe that Heidegger's concepts of *Geworfenheit*—man is thrown into the world, unplanned and unintended by himself—and *Entwerfen*—the taking over and actively developing the potentialities of this fact—have grown in the same soil" (p. 19) (the same soil, that is, as Loewald's description of human development).

In a footnote to this remark, Loewald takes pains to distinguish between Heidegger's philosophical discourse and his own psychological one, particularly noting something that must always be borne in mind in comparing psychoanalytic points of view with those of Heidegger and other phenomenologists: namely, that these philosophers do not make the distinction between conscious and unconscious which is fundamental in any psychoanalytic theory worth the name. Nevertheless, as Loewald summarizes, psychoanalyst and philosopher are at one in the classic dictum: "Become what you are." This becoming, this living out of potentiality (if I may thereby paraphrase Heidegger's specialized language), carries with it the implication that the person being-there, the *Dasein*, possesses his or her own future, as a "project" to be fulfilled, or not fulfilled, since Heidegger is not a determinist.[2]

There is much more than meets the eye in this seemingly commonplace remark. It contains in a nutshell one of the essential guidelines to his psychoanalytic thought, and can serve as an example of the uses to which a philosophic position may be put in our work. While it would be absurd to read even a fragment of Loewald's writings in the light of this single philosophic statement, the concepts quoted by him are drawn from a larger mosaic of Heidegger's thought where they represent a distinct trend. It is not my purpose to take up Heidegger's philosophy at length, and actually the best way to refer to specific aspects of it will be with reference to some of Loewald's ideas as they are put forth in his papers. Very briefly, the phenomenology on which Heidegger's work stands is in contrast to the prevailing scientific view that opposes an observing subject to a world of objects. Such a splitting has undoubtedly been fruitful in producing the understanding of our existence that we find through the natural sciences. It often appears to be implicit also in the psychological sciences including psychoanalysis, with insufficient appreciation of the reality that the observer and the observed are aspects of a unity, rather than a dichotomous pair. "Being-there" is being committed to a world that is neither internal nor external to oneself. In George Steiner's words (1978), this is "radical

2. See Heidegger (1927), especially p. 185f.

immanence, . . . embeddedness," or as Heidegger (1927) calls it, "In-der-Welt-sein," "being-in-the-world" (p. 83).

Heidegger's account of the nature of this "world" is necessarily one of philosophical abstraction, and it is going to be Loewald's fleshing it out with the real life of psychoanalytic experience that will be my main theme. Perhaps it is not so much a definition of "world" that we need as a reminder that it is not to be conceived of as that which exists apart from human concern; to the contrary, "world" is that which *concerns* the person-there. One of the consequences of concern is temporality, another of the concepts which Loewald has dealt with originally. To be concerned about anything or anyone (and it is a personal world that is mainly at stake here) is to be interested in it, him, her, as another being-in-the-world who has experienced a past and anticipates a future (Heidegger, 1927, p. 278).

Let us leave the philosopher for a while and return to the psycho-analyst. I proposed that Loewald has been guided by concepts put forward by Heidegger, mainly in his early and most important book, *Being and Time*, of which I have given only the smallest sample. For another thing, it is the whole impact of this massive work in its immense complexity relating many unfamiliar concepts to one another, that we sense in following Loewald's application of them. It is indeed more than an application, but an extension into a sphere of understanding foreign to their creator, the sphere of human development, and of the unconscious life in which the past survives, and the future is in process of becoming.

What, to continue, do the concepts of thrownness and project have to do with Loewald's point of view? As long ago as 1949, in his paper "Ego and Reality," and continuing in the study "The Problem of Defense and the Neurotic Interpretation of Reality" (1951), Loewald convincingly distinguished the meaning of "reality" accepted in psycho-analysis until then from another more fundamental one. *It is not by opposition of the ego to the external world that we acquire our basic knowledge of reality*, that is, the reality acquired through the fear of castration by the father. The underlying reality is that of primary narcissism, when child and mother are in a yet undisturbed unity. Our theory has been influenced by a powerful cultural attitude, "the hostile, submissive-rebellious manipulation of the environment" (p. 29).[3] This obsessional picture of the world has been taken as the normal. It is a picture of an alienated ego, its structures formed defensively. If, on the other hand,

---

3. It is of interest that this inherent disturbance of our culture was a paramount concern of Heidegger's too. See, for example, (1949–53).

we stay with the given fact of human experience, our "thrownness" is better conceived as one into a world that is prior to defense. Not only the infant lives in this unitary world; the parents also, especially the mother, have the wherewithal, the persisting capacity, to "regress" to the infantile level sufficiently to be one with the child. Interaction with the environment at this stage is not defensive. The growth of defensive structures is of course inevitable; the primary unity itself can become a threat for the emerging individual, and the environment personified in the father assumes at once its protective and its threatening role. But, and this is Loewald's insistent point, what is primary may be built upon and may be distorted, but it is not superseded.

Reality, the "real world," is, then, to begin with a subject-object unity. Both subject and object partake of one another. The "instincts" are motivations, psychic in nature, although powered by neural energies, and these motivations come to be *"organized as such through interactions within a psychic field consisting originally of the mother-child (psychic) unit"* (p. 128).

The making of the world of the child goes on continuously. As Loewald put it in his "Perspectives on Memory" with regard to internalization: "I conceive of it, broadly speaking, as the process by which interactions within the original mother-child psychic matrix, and later between the growing individual and his environment, become transmuted into internal interactions constituting the individual psyche . . . and developing an internal world" (p. 167). Here too the language is familiar enough, but the emphasis has the difference special to its author. The inner-outer world of the matrix is paradigmatic, and it is one that is philosophically organized in association with Heidegger's concepts of the finding of the individual being within a world that it makes its own. The thrownness of the infant is into a world of interactions. I shall examine a bit later Loewald's acute inquiry into the temporality of these processes. Internalization, which is the making of a world, "is conceived as the basic way of functioning of the psyche, not as one of its functions" (p. 71).

There runs throughout these statements, and the careful theoretical reasoning from which they emerge, a view of psyche as action or, in Heidegger's word, as "project." Loewald here also expresses his indebtedness to Nietzsche's concept of internalization as an active process. In all these instances the point at issue, which we have seen earlier too, is that reality does not stand primarily in opposition to the ego; it is this environment, this *Umwelt*, out of which the inner world is organized and enriched. Internalization is not a defense. Not quite to our purpose here, but of equal moment, is the further generalization of

Loewald's that internalization is also in fact the opposite of repression, and that it operates contrary to the Nirvana principle, moving toward more life, rather than toward a state of rest. Experience makes for structure, and structure itself organizes; it is not primarily engaged in tension reduction (see Schur, 1966; Loewald, 1980, p. 58ff., p. 177).

More than a by-product of Loewald's concern with the organizing work of the mother-child unity (and this is a concept that unifies *his* work too) is the significance he attaches to its repetition in the psychoanalytic situation. Actually one might well suppose that it was his reflections on the psychoanalytic situation that encouraged him to look for its prototype in the original unity. To begin with, the whole analytic enterprise depends on the ability of the analyst to join his or her patient when the latter relaxes the grip of the secondary process and makes the primary process accessible. The "global" interaction of mother and child is revived in the analysis (p. 180; p. 237ff.). While the analysis of adults is necessarily conducted in language that is an attainment of the secondary process, intersubjectivity (not a term used by Loewald) comes about through "the creation of an identity of experience in two systems of different levels of ego organization" (p. 239), which precisely parallels the mother-child matrix.

From the beginning of his published work, Loewald has pointed out the contrast between the preoedipal and the oedipal reality, or "world." In the early "Ego and Reality," he offered a "dialectical" reading of the two: (1) the positive, narcissistic relation with the mother, the aspect which underlies the discussion of the basic matrix, but at the same time presents the danger of being lost in the womb; and (2) the positive identifying relation with the father, out of which on the other hand the castration threat arises. Advance to a grasp of reality as an existence outside the matrix does not, however, begin with the oedipal "objectivity," but is greatly enhanced by it. It begins in the earlier recognition shared by mother and infant of the otherness of each, which in turn is associated with the care for the child by the mother as one "being-there" not identical with herself. Secondary process of thought has the same origins in the presentation of a differentiated world. Loewald also said: "the more alive people are, . . . the broader their range of ego-reality," that is, the greater their capacity for holding to both worlds (p. 20). I need only repeat here that it is in this analysis that Loewald brings Heidegger's conceptualizations to life by installing them in a developmental psychological reference. Care is another such concept that Heidegger dealt with extensively in *Being and Time,* from which we may extract the following: "Because Being-in-the-world is essentially care, Being-alongside the ready-to-hand (sc. "objects" in the most general sense) could be taken . . . as *concern,* and Being with the Dasein-with of Others as we encounter it within-the-world could be taken as *solicitude*" (p. 237). That appears to say, in more comfortable psychoanalytic language, that there is a continuity between maternal solicitude and the recognition of the external world, to which Loewald adds the development of the secondary process.

The question of time has obviously attracted Hans Loewald's attention for many years. Time in the most banal sense of duration has been of psychoanalytic interest mainly in its relation to development and its phases, although there have also been studies of changes in the sense of time under varying psychological and pathological conditions. Loewald's interest is of another sort. It is not linear, objective time with which he has been concerned, the time that is apparent from change and mobility. It is psychic time, in which past and future are at work in the present, the past by reminiscence, the future by anticipation. In "Superego and Time," Loewald proposed that psychic structures are temporal in nature. The superego he saw as a future mode of the ego preeminently: "only insofar as we are in advance of ourselves—conceive of ourselves as potentially more, stronger, better, or as less, weaker, worse than we are at present—can we be said to have a superego" (p. 46). Moreover, "the superego . . . would represent the past as seen from a future" (p. 49). In an earlier paper, in which his focus was on internalization, this was expressed still more explicitly and in greater detail. He also shows how this aspect of temporality is acquired through "parental expectations, fears, and hopes, the guidance and examples of authorities," etc., all of which, as permanently present in the child's psyche, are so to speak an embedded future (see especially p. 273).

From another study, we learn that the past, although we think of it as fixed if we conceive of it only objectively, as a psychic function living within the individual world, is subject to influence by the present, as the psychoanalytic rewriting of history amply demonstrates (p. 360). In the same paper, Loewald understands that the "regression" of the transference "conjoins the patient's experiential past . . . with his experiential present," while concurrently, by differentiating the past from the present, the analyst's interpretations influence the future (p. 367). Any modification of the experience of the sequences of time are therefore changes in the lived world of the analysand (p. 144).

Loewald's awareness of the philosophical background of his picture of temporality in the psychoanalytic construction of psychic life is significantly alluded to in a footnote (p. 146), in which he refers the reader to the famous chapter 20 on time in Book XI of the *Confessions* of St. Augustine. That fourth-century study of time does indeed take in its essence the phenomenological approach that Loewald also urges: thus, "there are three times, a present time of things past, a present time of things present, a present time of things to come. . . . The presence of things past is memory, the presence of things present is perception, the presence of things to come is expectation." As I read Heidegger, according to William Richardson (1974, p. 85ff.), whose commentary on Heidegger I follow at this point, the author of *Being and Time* extends Augustine's analysis of time in this way:

1. The kind of world that Heidegger intends, and that Loewald writes about, and that I am discussing here, is a world of human comprehension. No doubt that it exists in itself, in objective space and time, but whatever being we attribute to it, whatever we can know about, derives from human experience, past or present. We may justly say that its being is constituted by our being-there, or someone's being-there. But to be-there is to be interested, concerned, caring. Care (to use the most personal word) always anticipates and retrospects. It is temporal by nature. It is also concerned with others' being-there; that is, others are made manifest, even to themselves, by being recognized and addressed.

2. Being-there (*Dasein*) is processive, it has direction, it is becoming. That is its future. But it becomes what it is itself in its being thrown into the world. It has only its own history. So while we conceive of it as advancing into an unknown future, we also know that this future is a coming to be of a self that has already been, a historical being. Future and past are reciprocal: being-there means coming to be what has been in its original thrownness. Richardson (1974) writes: "Existence consists in the coming (future) of Being to a self that already is (past), rendering manifest the Being of beings with which it is concerned (present)" (p. 87). And, as Heidegger put it: "Temporality reveals itself as the meaning of authentic care" (p. 374). The past in this sense is existential: it exists now as having been; the other sense of past is of that which once was but is no more, in the objective world.

I have already given examples of Loewald's psychoanalytic understanding of time. They are formulated within the terms of psychoanalytic theory, and with close attention to the observable phenomena of our experience. But I think that it is equally clear that they have been structured philosophically in a different way from the more familiar positivistic theory. In his paper on memory, he goes further into the temporal aspect of mind, with the proposal, "through psychoanalysis man may become a truly historical being . . . the higher forms of memorial activity make us create a history of ourselves as a race and as individuals" (p. 171). That is, the appropriation of the unconscious past—itself not a topic of interest to Heidegger—continues the process of individuation that originates in the mother-child matrix and makes one's hitherto abandoned history part of oneself. Time as memory is constitutive of the inner world, the "being-there" that projects itself into the future, and that will in turn from its new horizon look back on a more ample history of itself. How far all this is from the model of a psychic system that finds its goal in a state of rest!

Let me conclude these remarks on philosophy and psychoanalysis with a warning. They ought not suggest that Loewald has superimposed a philosophical system on psychoanalytic theory, or conversely stretched the theory to fit a philosophical structure. We have earlier had in the "existential psychoanalysis" of Binswanger, Boss, and others examples of the way in which a primary adherence to Heideggerian thought alienated those thinkers from their Freudian origins; in their cases the concept of the unconscious itself has been largely eroded away, whatever other valuable insights they may have offered. Loewald's philosophical background has rather served as a methodological corrective to the unexamined positivism of psychoanalysis. He stands squarely in the Freudian tradition, but as one who has advanced it by critical reinterpretation from within. Of Loewald it may be said, in Goethe's phrase, that which he has inherited he has made his own.

BIBLIOGRAPHY

HARTMANN, H. (1939). *Ego Psychology and the Problem of Adaptation.* New York: Int. Univ. Press, 1958.

——— (1964). *Essays on Ego Psychology.* New York: Int. Univ. Press.

HEIDEGGER, M. (1927). *Being and Time,* tr. J. Macquarrie & E. Robinson. New York: Harper & Row, 1962.

——— (1949–53). The question concerning technology. In *Basic Writings,* tr. D. Krell. New York: Harper & Row, 1977, pp. 283–318.

LOEWALD, H. W. (1978), *Psychoanalysis and the History of the Individual.* New Haven: Yale Univ. Press.

——— (1980). *Papers on Psychoanalysis.* New Haven: Yale Univ. Press.

RICHARDSON, W. J. (1974). *Heidegger: Through Phenomenology to Thought.* The Hague: Martinus Nijhoff.

SCHUR, M. (1966). *The Regulatory Principles of Mental Functioning.* New York: Int. Univ. Press.

STEINER, G. (1978). *Martin Heidegger.* New York: Viking Press.

On Blaming

An Entry to the Question of Values

VANN SPRUIELL, M.D.

> . . . psychoanalytic findings and theory . . . are promi-
> nently concerned with man as a moral being . . . it is
> the scope of psychoanalysis to consider human nature
> in the fullness of the individual's concrete existence.
>
> LOEWALD (1978, p 5f)

HUMANS HAVE PREFERENCES, SOMETIMES OVERWHELMING ONES. THEY
have sets of realistic, aesthetic and moral values which may be volatile
or relatively stable, depending upon changing inner states and outer
circumstances. Values are everywhere in mental life—and psychoanalysts tread gingerly about them.

Any intellectual discipline makes fundamental assumptions to which
it holds. Simultaneously, it makes every effort to put aside personal
values while making empirical observations. This is particularly urgent
for psychoanalysts because of the nature of their work, which, to paraphrase Fenichel, tries to deal with irrational content without *becoming*
irrational. Among all professionals, psychoanalysts are probably the
most self-reflective and watchful in their efforts to identify and correct
the distorting influences of prejudices and private beliefs. At the same
time, psychoanalysts cannot forget that values, especially moral values,
are a large part of the very stuff of their own and their patients' lives. If
values are a major part of the "fullness of the individual's concrete
existence," then the investigation of the analyst's and analysand's values cannot be ignored. To ignore them would be less "scientific," not
more. To evade the subject would amount to a travesty of science.

President of the New Orleans Psychoanalytic Institute; clinical professor of psychiatry,
Tulane Medical School; and clinical professor of psychiatry, Louisiana State University
School of Medicine.

Heinz Hartmann, whose theories in some respects were very differ-ent from those of Loewald, summarized several of the most important of these issues in *Psychoanalysis and Moral Values* (1960). Unfortunately, that little book tends to be remembered merely as a cautionary homily (Spruiell, 1989). But it is much more. Hartmann discussed tendencies in people to "agglutinate" their values, combining values which vary in rationality. Values can seem to become "contagious." The good can be seen simultaneously and contradictorily as the ideal and as the average or mean. And not only psychoanalytic theory, but analytic techniques themselves are sometimes misapplied as prescriptions of behavior in the nontherapeutic world—with consequences which are sometimes ludicrous and occasionally tragic.

Hartmann criticizes "health morality" and, like Freud, does not be-lieve that psychoanalysis can provide, by itself, a valid *Weltanschauung* (the term I prefer to this variously defined German word is *folk philoso-phy*). He made it clear, however, that psychoanalysis may have a role in understanding how values are created, applied, how means, ends, and consequences are assessed, and that potential psychoanalytic contribu-tions might enrich a rational ethical philosophy. And in this he is joined by Loewald.

Values have existence as immaterial entities. As such they are fit subjects for scientific investigation insofar as they can be investigated. Even if there is no way currently available to do that, we do not wear blinders and declare all nonscientific knowledge to be invalid. Quite often, we have to acknowledge antinomies: for example, we cannot do without a concept of personal intentionality on conscious and uncon-scious levels, just as we cannot do without some version of scientific determinism.

A host of related interests will demand our attention in the future: the psychological nature of valuations, validations, their retention or replacement, stability, the depth and strength with which they are held, how they can be compartmentalized within appropriate situa-tions, how contradictions and conflicts among them can be governed. And we may have to endure unanswerable questions about the gener-alizability of value contents for a long time—or forever. Are they strict-ly relative in nature? Are they strictly utilitarian? Is it possible that there are social structures in many or all cultures which are to some extent products of universal moral interests? Might there be some ways the values of all human beings, insofar as they are developed, resemble each other?

I am specifically concerned here with the moral spectrum, and leave to the side all the others of a realistic, self-centered, aesthetic, or social nature. This essay, in honor of Hans Loewald, reopens old questions and speculates about some possible answers. My interests are my own. While they have been enormously stimulated and influenced by Loewald's work, they do not necessarily reflect his own formulations and solutions.

An examination of blaming, an almost ubiquitous and apparently simple human phenomenon, is one way to approach the subject. Blaming is an operation which is expectable in early stages of life, and is "normal" also in adults who live in traditional societies which have fixed rules defining free will and evil. Among adults who have had an opportunity to mature in posttraditional, relatively free societies, however, blaming is not necessarily "normal" at all, except in some emergency situations. In such societies, at least a few adults replace *blaming systems* with *responsibility systems*.

I also use blame and blaming to illustrate questions of individual group values and their organization and disorganization. My intention is to demonstrate that psychoanalysis can play an essential part—but only a part—in the future construction of a nondeistic theory of values, a theory which would have general validity rather than mere social serviceability.

To Blame: Some Possible Meanings

Blaming: a commonplace human quality; usually found obnoxious by its targets; it is the designation of the source of evil. The evil agent may be enemy, human or otherwise, even one's own self. The blamer assumes his victim is malevolent and chooses the bad. Blaming is a judgment of *deliberate* evil. It imputes power to the blamed—not to speak of power to the blamer as soothsayer: thus good authority to the blamer (who hopes others will join the blame-group); thus evil authority to the accused.

Blame is an onus. If communicated to the human target, it is apt to stir him up in one way or another. If the blamed one accepts the charge, he may feel guilt, or at least pretend so. If he rejects the stigma, he feels falsely accused, outraged, hurt, treated unfairly. He may try to mollify his accuser. He may openly or furtively counterattack—by ejecting the blame, returning it to its sender, smearing it on someone else. One common tactic to dodge blame is to say, "It wasn't me, it was somebody or something else. And whoever says it was me is a liar. He or she is evil, not me."

Or the blame might be accepted. The blamed person may try to expiate his wrongness; feel bad; accept punishment as his rightful due; support the righteousness of his accuser.

An observer thinks about "blame" differently if he is external to the field of observation than if he is within it. The observer not only thinks differently but feels differently if he is in one way or another involved as an active participant. Because of the nature of our discipline, most psychoanalysts tend to think "internally" about a psychological event like blaming. They think of the simultaneous operation and compromises of the four great springs of human motivation, discussed with variations of emphases by Waelder (1930), who includes the repetition compulsion as a separate source of motivation, and Brenner (1982): (1) the manifold influences of the id; (2) the ego ideal and superego at all levels of development and regression; (3) ego operations and phenomena having to do with conceptions of one's own self and of other people and relations with them; with control and modulations systems; and with the final pathways to action, etc; (4) apprehensions of the external worlds in which the person lives which exert influences on him. External perceptions are tucked into remembered contexts—the representations of subjects and objects in action, who, if not strangers, share conventions and beliefs about external realities.

Proscriptive rules in psychological systems set boundaries. They are usually more numerous and explicit, at least in relatively free societies, than the other category of rules, *prescriptive rules*. The latter define what must be done in various circumstances. In regard to particular actions, prescriptive rules abrogate freedom; in contrast, proscriptive rules define the limits of freedom. Prescriptive rules predominate in the hive and the herd; proscriptive rules predominate in groups of higher mammals, particularly humans, who have many options.

This classification of rules is for convenience. Of course, prescriptive and proscriptive rules cannot always be delineated. Many are arbitrary pairs; there are many regularities of behavior which can be identified either way; one statement for what must be done; an obverse statement for what cannot be.

Blame refers to particular acts of judgment in a field within a coherent human system. If blame is consensually agreed by a group to be appropriate and just, then it is one element of what is assumed "by everybody" to be external reality. Such "external" versions of reality have variable influences on "inner" constructions of reality. The variables have to do with the relative strength of the external impingements on the one hand, and the developmental maturity and autonomy of the individual's intrapsychic operations on the other.

Even God can be and gets blamed. The stars. Uncanny influences.

Governments. But individual people are seen no less magically as evil-doers. Parents and children, spouses and siblings, authorities, peers and siblings, especially psychoanalysts—all get blamed. Patterns of blaming may become deeply rooted as a consequence of group influence (for example, if practically everybody else in a given culture indulges in blaming), and as a consequence of the structuring of character traits (which arise out of early identifications).

On the other hand, some people have character traits which make them appear incapable of blaming. If the incapacity to blame is actual, a fixed defensive stance rather than a transiently defensive denial, a very serious illness, is probable. The statement may become clearer in what follows. In any event, society often rewards both blame-seekers and blamers, regardless of whether they are individually pathological or not.

But among reasonably well-educated people in our culture, calculated blame is "known" to be irrational. To blame is to lose a more accurate view of a differentiated world and of the interactions of forces in causal networks within it. To blame is to retain or revert to childish modes, by definition, immaturely narcissistic modes—especially in relation to the aggressive aspects of babyish narcissism. There is a reversion to a psychic state of seeming oneness between self and other, like the actual or seeming lack of differentiation within the mother-infant unity or field. I believe that such regressions, if they do not become fixed, are at times adaptive (E. Kris, 1950).

To blame is not the same as the discovery of defects or inefficiencies within a causal network, or the discovery of faults or breaks in a system. To blame is magically to short-circuit the recognition of multiple determinants or actual defects in the system itself. To blame is a leap to "discover" simple causes which are thought to be acts of intentional evil. In the sense that psychoanalysis sees events as psychologically determined, the search for single sources of evil is absurd. But in the sense that psychoanalysis retains concepts of freedom of choice, then, of course, one can imagine choices by individuals which at least most people would regard as evil. Perhaps this apparent antinomy can be resolved if traditional concepts of morality itself can be rethought. Perhaps blaming systems can be replaced by responsibility systems.

At least in our culture, the acts of chronic blamers and blame-seekers are primarily motivated by defensive reactions aimed to suppress and contain imperative id and superego motivations. The result is a violation of inner integrity—and attempts to control behavior by mastery and repression rather than as a result of the buffering, interacting elements of a free mind.

As pathological or immature as blame can appear when viewed rationally, it is evident that some consistent systems of blaming can be, and often are, stabilizing in given cultures. Such systems silently define coherent patterns which determine where evil (the simple "cause") is, whom or what to blame, and what might be done about it. These patterns of blame are largely unconscious conventions which infiltrate societies. They may not be reasonable in themselves, but they help hold groups together.

But when these social systems of blaming break down—as is the case in contemporary Western societies—and are not replaced by any other consistent ordering devices, social authority breaks down too. Not only is society put at risk, but so is the individual. An environment gone amok no longer can support a person's shared folk philosophy (Spruiell, 1988), his largely unconscious notions of practical reliability about what he calls external reality or commonsense morality. The individual loses bare safety of orientation.

THE VIRGIN SPRING—SIN AND EXPIATION

Most people think of narcissistic traits in terms of sin. Ingmar Bergman's movie, *The Virgin Spring,* based on an old Swedish legend, is relevant to blame. A nubile and flirtatious adolescent girl, who simultaneously seems uncannily beautiful and pure, is allowed to take offerings to a shrine a day's walk through the medieval forest. Her stern father, patriarch of the medieval farm, worships the girl and his judgment is clouded by her charm. The mother, also a slave, flutters before her pure and clean angel-product. In the little world encased within the dour stockade, only a servant girl, pregnant, is not consumed by the positive idealization of the child. Like a dying sailor she drinks the urine of her own envy; in her bitter spite she too is a slave.

The virgin, dressed in splendor, rides alone through the forest. She is unaware that the servant, frightened by terrible wishes of her own, trails behind. Just before the latter catches up, the young pilgrim comes across three youths, filthy, hungry, and homeless. The oldest is a mute whose tongue had been cut out; the youngest is a pubescent boy. Ugly, unattached except to each other, these goatherds are like subhuman creatures to her, alien to anything she has ever known. She is fascinated, romantically charmed by them, and stops to share her food. Her patronizing Christian ministrations are first accepted, then interrupted by a sudden recognition of danger, evil. She is trapped, held by the young men, brutally raped, finally by the tongueless man. The boy, transfixed, watches. The servant, hiding in the bushes above, watching also, is perversely thrilled. Suddenly, in the thrall of the rape, ecstasy transfigures the child-woman's face. Afterwards, stunned, she weeps—then stares, unbelieving and believing, as one of the young men begins to club her to death.

The boy's fixed stare is broken. Left for a time by his brothers, he tries ineffectually to cover the girl's body. Then he tries to eat a bite of her bread. He vomits. The serving girl's posture of thrill turns to shudders.

Later, the wanderers find shelter in the family farm. There is no sign that they know or bother to wonder if it might be the girl's home. They are taken in and fed. But during the night the young man who can speak offers to sell the mother an elaborately sewn shift. To his blandishments she is silent; she sees that the shift had been the virgin's. Later she finds the rest of the bloody belongings and lets the father-husband know. He prepares himself. His measured, vengeant butchery of the grown brothers, followed by the lifting of the whole body of the young boy and smashing it like a club against the wall is almost unbearable to watch. When the father is finished, a passing expression of prideful pleasure crosses his face.

The family and servants make a processional to the awful site of the daughter's death. The blame clearly falls upon each—including the angel-child-woman. Blame and remorse are accepted by each of the living. As they pray, a virgin spring wells up from the spot where she had rested. The father vows to build a shrine there. Undone authority is restored; God's place is fixed.

The audience can see that if there is blame, there is a nexus of blame. If there is blame, each is to blame. Anyone of them, including the virgin, could have prevented the crime if only there had not been the selfish concerns, sinful in the legend, narcissistic to us: the idealized enthrallment and barely hidden possessiveness of the parents—in the father so clearly and intolerably erotic; in the mother, beneath surface doting, so hateful; corrosive envy and spite in the servant girl; the perverse lust for both sexes coupled with murderousness in the two goatherds, with their blindness for people, sight for things; the boy at puberty, in a roar of impulses and fears, shaking with unbearable wishes which have to be vomited; to be them all: the innocent, the rapist, the murderer, the avenger of hunger—and he who is raped and killed; the virgin girl herself, who embodied the special, stupid vanity of the omnipotent and totally indulged beginner in genitality.

But at least the characters in the legend had the certainties of faith, the knowledge of sin and how to find it, the belief in expiation and forgiveness. At least their system of blaming was consistent, coherent, and believable. It is not so simple for us.

NORMAL AND PATHOLOGICAL ASSESSMENT: INDIVIDUALS AND GROUPS

Blame can be as insignificant as a passing sniff, as palpable as a black oven awaiting its spark. Blamers are all of us sometimes. And blamers are the inquisitors, the great and mad leaders of history. Blamers are people harassed by emergency circumstance. They may be hostile and guilty obsessionals. They may be injustice collectors or other kinds of angry narcissists. In particular, blamers are among the unhappy souls with congenital defects or bodily deformities. They are the oppressed and easily identifiable minority groups. Blamers may have any diagnosis.

But in our society, the most common forms of obviously distorted blaming are found among sadomasochistic, paranoid, and depressed people, people whose childish catastrophic fantasies were stimulated, at least, by external reality, and seem to continue to be confirmed by it. They live lives in terms of being able to blame themselves or others. Or worse still, they surrender to temporary or permanent helplessness, irrationally incapable of blaming. These are people, the strong and the weak, obsessed by questions of who has the power, and what is its quality—from the overwhelmingly catastrophic and magical to ordinary blackmail operations within a family. They believe they are internally possessed by mindless systems of monstrous goodness or by other systems between or among themselves and other people which are implacable.

The subject of blaming is too broad, blaming too widespread, to be identified with specific diagnostic categories or characterological types. But it is useful to explore ways of thinking about the various phenomena herded together under the term. Then we wind a path from the rational, to the infantile, and thus to the narcissistic. At all levels we can see that the act of blaming is the servant of many masters, many motivations which may conflict and must somehow be compromised and interdigitated.

We need the bridge uniting intrapsychic psychology (made up of the influences and integrations and compromises of these four sources of motivations), and a compatible interactional psychology (Spruiell, 1983). The usual approach is to postulate two psychologies, one intrapsychic, seen heuristically as a closed system; the other a compatible group or interactional psychology, made up of multiple closed systems which communicate, negotiate, battle, and cooperate across space. In this view, the individual and his group are like figure to ground, or ground to figure. The aim of development is thought to be to distinguish self from object.

But there can be another approach: that individuals are only apparently as separate as their bodies seem to be, that psychological worlds are made up of fields of forces in which only more or less differentiated centers of organization exist. It is only the external observer who sees them as individual people, separated by empty space, communicating across it by signals. I do not know how to do without both views—intrapsychic-interpersonal psychology, and the unitary psychology toward which Freud leaned in his later years. In this essay, I take this second heuristic point of view, from the "inside," so to speak, and take into account the oscillations between partial separations and partial returns to original oneness postulated by Hans Loewald (1971). This view has to do with simultaneous life within the mind and lives among minds. The fields encompassing individual centers of activity remain.

In truth, we cannot delineate precisely what we mean by "individual" or by "group," anymore than we can be precise about "intentionality" or "freedom." We know in general what we mean, and in fact cannot function as analysts without drawing upon these meanings, simultaneously evocative within us, vaguely understood among us. We can, however, recognize that extreme versions of "individualism" and "socialization" express philosophical assumptions which are in radical conflict with each other in regard to responsibility, intentionality, and the nature of good and evil.

THE PSYCHOANALYTIC CONTRIBUTION TO MORAL VALUES

Of the philosophers who attempted to construct nondeistic ethical systems, Aristotle and Kant made the most notable efforts. Each began by basing his system on the realities, as he understood them, of the strengths and limitations of actual human beings. A conception of mind is the most important part of that nature.

It would be as absurd to demand that a human have magical mental powers in order to be moral as it would be absurd to demand that he have wings in order that he could fly. Unless we draw upon the chancy gods of our magical unconscious wishes, we must, as Aristotle and Kant knew, draw upon what *is* present in mortal bodies and minds. All aspects of mind have to be taken into account, but for morality the most relevant discoveries of psychoanalysis have to do with the existence of the dynamic unconscious, the relationship of internalization processes to the acquisition of layers of more and more highly organized psychic structures, the increasing complexity of drive-object relations, and the acquisition of more and more complex systems. All of these understandings are essential. No scientific discipline has studied individual human beings as deeply as psychoanalysis. What it has to offer has to do with insights into the nature of man—but not a complete view of the values he should have.

It is true that values can be smuggled into analytic situations. Examples are the "healthy morality" which Hartmann (1960) warned about, the conception of "normality" as an ideal, and all sorts of subtle and gross infiltrations of prejudices, opinions, and even specific political dogmas. But the most serious contaminations of psychoanalysis with values which are in fact antianalytic have to do with evasions of the painful truths of life, particularly as they refer to the realities of the dynamic unconscious, the continued effects of infantile sexuality, and the extent and persistence of aggressive destruction. All these distortions and more can subvert analytic work. That is why analysts pay such assiduous attention to them.

Among the manifestations of countertransference phenomena, psychoanalysts can also become blamers—and can even accept irrational blame of themselves. Analysts in the past particularly blamed individual parents, and it is a common observation that analysts tend to blame each other for all sorts of things. To blame is not to analyze. To analyze is to peer into seeming chaos and find connections and order—and constraints to freedom of thought and affect. From the aspect of mind, to analyze is to look at and finally begin to comprehend the network of associations which underlie any particular act, whether physical, verbal, fantasy, or dream. What a thrill it is to be able to do that! To analyze is to try to see the interrelationships, and even the "nodal points" in the associations (Freud, 1900; Loewald, 1971), the unexpected intersections of lines of thought from differing modalities: past, present, future; the worlds of transference, past intimacies, and contemporary external life; experiences of being from immediate to the abstract; "outside life"; blessings and curses of desire; ranges from rational to nonrational to irrational.

Ultimately, to analyze is to seek (and to whatever extent possible, find) one's own person as a whole, thus embrace the responsibility for the whole person, what Freud meant by *Gesamt-Ich*. And it means the ferreting out of what might be called pseudo-responsibility—the distortion implied when a person purloins responsibilities which rightfully belong to others. True responsibility for all psychic acts must come to be seen to reside more and more "within" the person, despite the inevitable helplessness, imperfections, faults, and deficits which also live in that place within the field. It means to find whatever there is of conscious and unconscious freedom of choice, and expand it as much as possible. If it was the fate of psychoanalysis to demonstrate to man that his ego was not master in its own house, it nevertheless is central to the psychoanalytic endeavor that it expand whatever freedom there is: to make into ego where id was. Psychoanalysis could not endure if it imagined analysands were slaves or robots.

It is one of the tragedies of being human that what is demanded of a mature person is the absolute maximum of responsibility for himself (even for those matters within his purview in the face of which he feels helpless), while recognizing that his actual rather than pretended freedom is more constrained than had ever had been assumed in past times. It is only in the area of that small portion of actual freedom—that portion which practicality rather than philosophical proof forces us to assume—that one can rationally speak of moral choice in the old, traditional way. Psychoanalysis has little or nothing to say about good and evil in this sense because it is not able to determine the relative extent of this freedom. It cannot measure it, even in comparison to the other multiple determinants of psychic acts. All it can say is that there *is* choice, and freedom is to be cherished.

It is, of course, a temptation to think of morality in terms of one part of the structural point of view of mind, the superego, which traffics in ideas and feelings of good and evil. But it is obvious that any moral system must take into account all the other structures of mind, all the other motivations deriving from id, ego, and internal maps of the external world. All is process—and even the superego is in a state of constant flux and change. To illustrate, individual superego maturation—in relation to all the other psychic elements—results in the gradual buffering (but not loss!) of rigid, dogmatic generalizations, which apply at first to mother and child, then to family, eventually to the outside social world. In the middle of adolescence healthy superego maturation implies a structural revolution: the harsh superego of latency is partly replaced by a more adult form of the ego ideal. Naturally, if this is to occur, it also depends upon object relations becoming more clearly organized in terms of intimacy—just as these alterations of object relations depend upon the alterations of drives and their modulations. Superego maturation potentially even moves away from the supposedly pragmatic necessities of the (mostly silent) rules defining conventional social relationships. Individual ego and superego maturation may reach a point at which the individual can make choices among prevailing social rules, or allow healthy hypocrisy in relation to them, or, if necessary, allow outright defiance.

Thus, the maturing individual acquires more choices. Put another way, there is less dependence upon automatic, infantile, simple, and categorical rules—particularly those rules which are socially prescriptive (how a person is supposed to do things just so) rather socially proscriptive (the boundary-setting limits of permissible behavior). Yet if maturity is genuine, not the pseudomaturity of hyperrationality, the factors leading to unconscious and conscious choice remain accessible to and interdigitated with all the preceding layers of one's psychic being, and all the layers of a person's sense of separateness and oneness.

Psychoanalysis, even though it cannot exist without humane values, rationality, and a belief in freedom, cannot provide the content of a moral system. But it can encourage human endeavors which are apt to facilitate humane and constructive moral development. And, in the other direction, psychoanalysis certainly can play a part in informing others of practices of child rearing which are harmful. It can play a part in documenting those social conditions which are apt to contribute to eventual acts of cruelty and destructiveness.

In particular, psychoanalysis demonstrates the limitations of "will power" as it pertains to inner life. At the same time, it demonstrates— as everyone who experienced a successful therapeutic analysis knows— that inner change is indeed possible and at least partially understandable. It did not take analysts long to understand that they could not "make" their patients "grow up," nor could they correct or extirpate pathological elements. They learned that infantile wishes never disappear. They are not simply "given up." Instead, if all goes well, they remain conscious and accessible, but are overlain and buffered and even infiltrated by *other* fantasies, including the restoration to the wholeness of life of previously suppressed and repressed impulses and fantasies along with the acquisition of more elaborate and complex and mature new versions.

The resulting integration of the "lowest" and the "highest" can save the individual from the aridity of empty intellectualizations to the one side and the sumps of adult infantilism on the other hand. Instead of "helping" analysands in traditional styles of "help," analysts can provide an amazing situation, like no other, in which it is safe for the analysand to discover himself and accept his own responsibilities and thus integrity—without blame, and eventually, for the most part, without shame.

In the past, it was supposed that the results of successful ordinary development (and the results of successful analyses) would result in reaching the stage of "genitality," which succeeded the dissolution of the oedipus complex and should allow the individual to both love sexually and work successfully as an adult. Genitality is hardly mentioned in the contemporary literature, partly because few, if any psychoanalysts now believe the oedipus complex is ever "dissolved," and partly because there are such enormous differences between postoedipal children, early and late adolescents, and adults of various ages, chronological and psychological. Another reason for the lack of popularity of the term is that "genitality" can be confused with phallic narcissism, mixed up with questions of gender, and misinterpreted reductionistically. Nevertheless, there is a metaphorical advantage to the use of "genitality," just as there was a metaphorical advantage to insist that the Freudian conception of sexuality should include experiences which many would have preferred to call "sensual."

Genitality is not merely established, it evolves. An adult stage of genitality evolving ultimately toward death is the fate of lucky men and women. The same state of evolving maturity is alluded to by some (but not all) cults of phallicism, found in cultures about the world, and referring to the celebration of male and female sexuality, fertility, generativity—and usually in a disguised way, to death. The evolution of genitality (or Eros and death) implies the evolution of responsibility. The rules governing responsibility are highlighted by the very celebrations and fiestas which allow them to be broken in circumscribed ways. The Dionysian symbol Phallos is a representation of these collective agreements, but needs to be sharply distinguished from the more "penis-oriented" immaturity known as phallicism (in the everyday sense) and phallic narcissism.

In the celebration of maturity is the loss, temporarily, of aloneness of parts of the mind from the whole and the loss of separateness from other people. One might say it is the grief of maturity to recognize our essential aloneness and incapacity to fully integrate our parts. Our health lies in the ability to oscillate between these states—to some extent according to our own volition. Our illnesses lie in the fixations in one place or another. The capacity to reach temporary experiences of wholeness—and to separate again—is an important way to distinguish what might be thought of as genuinely normal maturation from pseudomaturations in which the earlier stages of development seem to be lost from experience and no longer are interdigitated with all the other levels in undisguised ways.

> To own up to our own history, to be responsible for our unconscious . . . means to bring unconscious forms of experiencing into the context and onto the level of the more mature, more lucid life of the adult

mind. Our drives, our basic needs, in such transformation, are not relinquished, nor are traumatic and distorting childhood experiences made conscious in order to be deplored and undone—even if that were possible. They are part of the stuff our lives are made of. What is possible is to engage in the task of actively reorganizing, reworking, creatively transforming those early experiences [Loewald, 1978, p. 21].

The successful living by a whole person, waxing and waning, implies that a reliable inner sense of authority has been established within— and allowed to wane in the father in favor of its waxing in the sons. If humane and reliable superego functions are internalized and subsequently modified in the direction of rationality, more autonomy and freedom can exist for the individual; there is less dependence on controls from the environment. There is more to be had from life.

I am sure that psychoanalysts will differ in regard to this or that aspect of general maturation, but not about its fundamental nature. For me, it is a perspective which is central not only to psychoanalytic theory but to human morality. Whatever facilitates growth toward states in which more and more choices are available for the individual—and from which the individual is capable of selecting—by definition furthers the possibility that constructive as opposed to destructive choices will be made in the course of ordinary life.

The question of sublimation is another matter. Dale Boesky (1986) has written a valuable and incisive survey of the many contradictory usages of the term *sublimation*. His "Questions about Sublimation" should demonstrate to any reader just how complex "sublimation" is— and yet how persistent the need for its use. Sublimation has been used as simply another "defense mechanism" and as something "higher" and "more normal" than a defense mechanism. It has been used in terms of one form of Freud's concepts of drives and in terms of other analysts' concepts of drives, e.g., those of Loewald, which Boesky believes are incompatible with Freud's meanings. Sublimation has been used as practically synonymous with the "neutralization" of sexual and aggressive drives and as somehow a different process. And it has been used by some as the extreme expression of individuation and by others as a creative—not a neurotic—return to the original wholeness characterized by the mother-infant unity. Boesky particularly criticizes Loewald's use of sublimation in this sense because he believes such a use does not adequately distinguish it from normal development.

The criticisms of Loewald's use of sublimation are debatable and important, because they relate to central theoretical conceptions of the nature of reality—in particular, nonmaterial reality. But I cannot do justice to the debate here. My concern is limited to blaming and responsibility systems as they refer to the question of values.

Occasionally we observe dramatic changes within an analysis which do not seem to represent the undoing of a chronic regression, or the achievement of some new level of normal organization. It is probable that there are more such happenings than we recognize. I am referring to changes which we are inclined to label as sublimations, and they represent fascinating processes. There are regular elements in these processes, although they do not necessarily take place in the order I shall list: an older sexual-aggressive organization, including more or less fixed motivational elements and systems of resolution, becomes disrupted; a period of disorganization supervenes; there are evidences of transitory regressions, which besides having obvious defensive uses may contain extraordinarily rich, evocative images or fantasies which are more like primary than secondary process mentation; the individual appears to be much more self-preoccupied; erotic and aggressive fantasies may temporarily seem much more "narcissistic"—in fact, contain more perverse qualities which seem to have little to do with other people as actual persons at all; at these times, everything in life seems to be put aside, in particular many of the ordinary, restraining, proscriptive and prescriptive rules governing behavior; there may be much more anxiety and restlessness; and then, quite often, there is a sudden resolution—a "surprise," a "Eureka," or an "all the pieces fit together" experience. There is almost always a feeling of pleasure; sometimes there is a feeling of awe; there is almost always at least a feeling of wholeness.

While the new acquisition is intensely felt, it seems to have nothing directly to do with sexual or aggressive elements—although it can be utilized indirectly for purposes of derivatives. And while the sublimatory experience can certainly be drawn into defensive operations, as anything human can be, defensive uses do not appear to be primary. But it is not "neutral" either.

These states quite often oscillate with more mundane neurotic (or perverse, or psychotic) ways of being. Finally, we know that during the extremes of sublimatory triumphs, the individual—whether good or evil—is apt to be involved in passionate states which transcend his own sense of egoistic preoccupations; he is apt to feel at one with a larger collective, or even that he *is* that larger body.

This process is certainly like that in creative acts, and it is easy to see how the regressions, disorganizations, and access to infantile levels of drive derivatives provide opportunities to observe the "nodal points" described by Freud when patterns of association from different levels intersect. I think many major creative acts are sublimations, but sublimations are not necessarily artistic or scientific acts. And the process is certainly like that which precedes major new insights in analysis—and major new insights often are sublimations. Probably the process occurs in a variety of special situations in ordinary life.

We can be certain of no one-to-one correlation between evil sublimatory states and what we regard as "good" and "constructive acts." Fiendish destructions can come out of complex states which cannot be distinguished qualitatively in terms of their elements from those that result in the greatest gifts to mankind. We know too little about the distinctions. We believe, however, that maturational developments broadly distributed among the functions of the psyche—cognitive, affective, drive-related, object-related—are more apt to lead to constructive and compassionate actions than monstrously dehumanized actions, which are apt to be related to perverse or psychotic fixations.

Sublimation seems to Loewald (1981) to take part in a a form of nonmaterial inner reality, "psychic reality" itself. But while Freud was considering psychic reality, he remained devoted to scientific materialism. It was difficult or impossible then (and now) to demonstrate, as opposed to postulate, close causal connections between psychic reality and the brain. Much of the difficulty with the concept of sublimation has to do with just this question: if material reality is seen as the only authentic reality, sublimation must be seen only in terms of illusions which are inherently false.

The concept of sublimation, in Loewald's words (1988), is "at once privileged and suspect": privileged in the nearly universal view of man as uniquely valuable; suspect in terms of the scientific need to analyze man's development impartially as a resultant of more primary (and allegedly more "real") components. Sublimation in this sense is not a "mystical" or "oceanic" experience, not a state of mental life with distinct boundaries, not one to be conjured up by specific exercises or "mantras." It may or may not seem to be limited by specific periods of time. It may or may not be associated with the creation of any external product. Yet, it is a recognizable state of mind, and with it goes a unique, unmistakable experience of meaning and integration—one which has been described many times by many observers in many cultures. Yet it is one which cannot be described in words very well. It is better known through some experiences in solitude, in intimate relations, and in communion with art.

I agree with Loewald (1981, 1988) that there are qualitative differences between genuine sublimations ("passion transformed") and what might be called pseudosublimations (primarily the results of unconscious defensive reactions to intense infantile wishes, which often happen to be rewarded by the world).

It is morally valid to favor and encourage states of life which make true individuation and sublimation more possible, more likely. To provide only one example of what I mean: individuation-deindividuation processes and sublimation are more possible in societies in which there is freedom of thought and expression and less likely in authoritarian societies.

It should be noted that the concept of sublimation used here is the very antithesis to regressive processes of desublimation—like blaming.

In summary, the fundamental theories of psychoanalysis, having to do with the most important aspects of man's nature, must play a contextual part in any rational moral theory. The understandings of human individuation and deindividuation, together with a particular view of sublimation, should play an important part in future general theories of morality.

A JOURNEY INTO GROUP PSYCHOLOGY

It is dangerous for psychoanalysts to venture away from their own stockades in the wilderness, which seem cheerless to outsiders, but rich with warmth and sadness for those inside. We know things about the clinical practice of analysis and we have an admirable and useful theory of intrapsychic life. But few of us are more than amateurs in other fields: philosophy, folk philosophy, anthropology, sociology, mythology, physics, or the neural sciences. The danger of excursions into these woods is that they will become flights; they might make too much of what is apt to be a small fund of knowledge. But some risks are worth taking.

Patterns of blaming and the rules governing blaming which involve specific values, standards, and ideals are usually acquired through identifications with parents and other authorities, although individuals can also internalize their own creative constructions. These patterns of blaming have to do with ego functions (being "realistic") and superego prohibitory and idealistic functions. There is another element in the acquisition of values which is often ignored except in reference to adolescence: the enormous needs children have to be like their peers, to be accepted by them, to be at one with them, their brothers and sisters. From babyhood there is an eagerness to know how to do things, how big kids act, what is the right way and what is the wrong way, what is fair. The dialectic between conformity and freedom continues through all but the earliest developmental levels.

Most if not all moral restraints, or their lack, and dull or shining ideals (no matter how well internalized) depend upon regular reinforcements from the outside world's versions of social reality—and prescriptions and proscriptions of behavior embedded within these versions. Traditions, conventions, standards, principles, values—all can be usefully examined by the utilization of formal rule theory (Spruiell, 1983). Rule theory can supplement the insights of Freud (1921) into group psychology, for example, the embodiment of shared values by a leader.

Shared values provide the binding which holds small and large groups together (Spruiell, 1988). But compliance may be only superficial. There may be inner freedoms held tenaciously. Deeply held private values, which have been truly internalized and are at least somewhat independent of the external contemporary group, may persist as banked fires, with potential to flame forth as agents of change.

In our own past, most of the masses—Protestants, Catholics, Jews, and the irreligious—were overtly in general agreement about good and evil. This was because there was a public consensus claimed about the material and moral world—a *folk philosophy,* expressed consciously in religion and patriotism. It varied slightly in content from place to place, and of course there were different levels of sophistication from class to class. The folk philosophy was supported by authority (probably cynically by most individual leaders). A socially useful hypocrisy prevailed. Those followers and leaders who did not seem to accept "self-evident" rights and wrongs were apt to be branded outlaws and fit subjects for torture. The masses could be suppressed; old leaders could be overthrown by new ones with more plausible pretenses. Not so many official laws were needed to define evil because covert and overt common rules defined it without an appeal process. This is no longer true.

For all the dangers posed by the disorganization of social rule systems, such as the state of blaming, there are certain advantages. Our present world allows for an unprecedented amount of freedom in "inner reality," available to an unprecedented number of people. On a mass scale, too, it may be that sublimation can exist.

A RETURN TO DIRECT PSYCHOANALYTIC OBSERVATIONS

For all the worries (and promises) about our condition, and for all the arguments that blaming is an absurd, unreasonable, and inappropriate activity when applied to the world at large, the psychoanalyst needs to touch base with clinical experience. From that position it is evident that, for practical psychological purposes, blamings will always be with us as subjective phenomena, invoked in emergencies and in our most immediate relationships. If an adolescent pokes a gun in my ribs on Conti Street in New Orleans, I certainly will blame him. I will not care in the least about his motives, or his unfortunate past. At that moment I will not even care about him as a human being. Only if he were neutralized, no immediate threat, could I afford to be more objective, conceivably even compassionate. Nevertheless, my regression to blaming, provided it was temporary, would have been immediately adaptive.

A child cannot be expected to have any objective understanding of the disparate realistic or neurotic reasons behind his mistreatments, especially on the part of his parents. Only when the adult is able to overlay his childish self with more mature patterns of being—and thus to some extent transcend childhood, and to some extent recontact his childhood on a higher level—will he be able to forgive his past, no longer blame his past as a way of escaping present responsibility.

These are all transformations of narcissism, from the viewpoint of the drives and from the viewpoint of object relations. Blaming, especially, has to do with aggressive actions, thus the omnipotent strand of narcissism. In the best of worlds, as development proceeds, the earliest omnipotence gives way to more and more elaborate alterations. The process moves from magic omnipotence, through the delegated omnipotence to authorities, to the boundlessness of adolescent fantasies, to true adult potency. Still, the certainties of at least temporary regressions are always there, in everybody. And some kinds of regression—perhaps to distinguish them from flights of terror we should call them inward historical pilgrimages—are necessary for a life to be whole and in process.

The origins of blame are in the sense of reproach the infant feels toward his mother for whatever unpleasure he experiences. He can do this when the mother becomes at least partially distinguished from himself. Blame and blaming come into their own with the anal struggles between the ages of 1½ and 3—the period described by Mahler et al. (1975) in terms of the rapprochement subphase of separation-individuation. Thus the development of a capacity to blame is crucial. It is one signal of the development of relations with others—and it is missing from those horribly mistreated individuals described by Shengold (1979) as victims of "soul murder" in childhood. These people as children were quite unable to imagine blame, much less blame their cruel parents.

It is during the period just preceding and including the climax of the oedipal passions that blame and blaming mechanisms come to be internally codified. Taboos and ideals become specified and stratified in importance. There are strong pressures against behaving "babyishly" beyond one's time. On the other hand, major blame can become associated with trivial indiscretions because of links to incestuous and murderous taboos.

Blaming as a fantasy is one thing, blaming as an act is another. The former may become replaced by other fantasies, or the targets of blame might be shifted, or the fantasy become frozen as a character trait—perhaps a pattern of grudges. Pathological blaming is a chronic maneuver in the inner world involving disavowal, denial, isolation, and projection. But acts in the interactional "outside" world related to these fantasies cause harm to other human beings. Childish acts of blame are hostile and often sadistic, indulged in by children and adults who are terrified of the consequences of forbidden wishes and of real or fantastic punishments, sadistically eager to divert these consequences to others. They are acts particularly seen among siblings in competition for the love of authoritarian parents, and in competition to avoid censure by the same authorities.

Typically, the blamer tries to recruit others to identify a victim. A successful group of blamers can become a group of persecutors, even a fundamental part of the actual external world of the targeted person or group. To whatever tendencies already exist to neurotically accept blame, there may be additional needs to avoid acknowledgment of perceptions of evil in the external world; the result may be a dangerous paralysis of aggressive impulses, a self-destructive response well-known to concentration camp victims and to some of the prisoners of war—for example, in the hideous prisons of both sides during the American Civil War.

PHILOSOPHICAL AND FOLK PHILOSOPHICAL CONSIDERATIONS

Bernard Williams (1985) has written a brilliant book about the current state of nondeistic philosophical considerations of ethics. It summarizes the profound but partially failed efforts of Aristotle and Kant, along with contemporary philosophical efforts, documenting their limits. The title, *Ethics*, is perhaps not as important as the subtitle, *Limits of Philosophy*. Williams too characterizes blame, the location of deliberately evil actions, as a central type of negative ethical reaction in response to the conduct of others. He too believes blame springs "from a deeply rooted misconception of life." But philosophy, he admits modestly, can play only a part in correcting those misconceptions.

Systems of blaming are supported by the rules of the dominant folk philosophies of a society. They are affected little, if at all, by the careful thoughts of philosophers and theologians, much less by the essays of psychoanalysts. Williams admires the moral systems of Aristotle and Kant, but cannot totally accept their metapsychological assumptions. He does not mention Whitehead (1929), who developed the only twentieth-century extensive morality embedded in a new metaphysics, with its emphasis on process and spiraling increases in organization of systems.

Nevertheless, is there hope for a more rational folk philosophy? An ethical mechanism to replace blaming? I believe there are many grounds for such hopes, but I am aware of the distinction between "my" moral beliefs and what might be "ours." In any event, it would be a terrible misconception to rely only on man's "highest" levels of rationality, and utilize them to deny what psychoanalysts know more about than anyone else; what seems to be the "lowest" in man may also be the language of the heart. It is only when the language of the intellect is married to the language of the heart that authentic reason—the God-child, Logos—comes into being.

SUMMARY

In this paper I have considered acts of blaming as an approach to a psychoanalytic contribution to a theory of moral values—a search for a way of thinking about the mental processes mediating values and valuations. Many modern philosophers do not believe their own discipline will be able to develop complete, valid, acceptable, and workable nondeistic ethical understandings alone. Psychoanalysts cannot either, but psychoanalysis can contribute necessary components in its unique understandings of mental operations.

The study of blaming as a part of a larger system of values can also be an avenue to the study of intrapsychic-interactional theoretical propositions. The stability or lack of stability of the "worlds" in which we live has influences on all of us, especially those who are most vulnerable to "external" influences.

Empirically, in addition to responses to immediate threats from the outside world, an internal world of blaming always remains. The self may be blamed for its failure to live up to its own standards and rules. Often this internal blaming and acceptance of the blame—thus guilt—operate unrealistically. Nevertheless, some such operations continue in even the most mature people, but in mature people it is possible to transform blaming systems into responsibility systems. Along with other transformations that accompany sublimations, the wholeness of personality can be restored in part.

One of the faces of a responsibility system is turned toward inner, passionate, often contradictory animal needs which remain in us all. Unless "owned," channeled, restrained, some wishes would be externally disastrous if converted directly into behavior and personally disastrous if totally repressed instead of channeled. Not only this, their disguised expressions can again become externally harmful to oneself and others when projected outward in the form of blame.

The other face is turned toward the ways the individuals' motives join (or rejoin) the affairs of the collective "other"—some of which have to do with the most transcendent qualities in man.

BIBLIOGRAPHY

Boesky, D. (1986). Questions about sublimation. In *Psychoanalysis*, ed. A. Richards & M. S. Willick. Hillsdale, N.J.: Analytic Press, pp. 153–176.

Brenner, C. (1982). *The Mind in Conflict*. New York: Int. Univ. Press.

Freud, S. (1900). The interpretation of dreams, *S.E.*, 4 & 5.

——— (1921). Group psychology and the analysis of the ego. *S.E.*, 18:69–143.

Hartmann, H. (1960). *Psychoanalysis and Moral Values*. New York: Int. Univ. Press.

Kris, A. (1982). *Free Association*. New Haven: Yale Univ. Press.

Kris, E. (1950). On preconscious mental processes. In *Psychoanalytic Explorations in Art*. New York: Int. Univ. Press, 1952, pp. 303–318.

Loewald, H. W. (1971). On motivation and instinct theory. *Psychoanal. Study Child*, 26:91–128.

——— (1978). *Psychoanalysis and the History of the Individual*. New Haven: Yale Univ. Press.

——— (1979). The waning of the oedipus complex. *J. Amer. Psychoanal. Assn.*, 27:751–775.

——— (1980). *Papers on Psychoanalysis*. New Haven: Yale Univ. Press.

——— (1981). Sublimation. Freud lecture, New York Psychoanalytic Society. Reported by D. Berger in *Psychoanal. Q.*, 52:319–321.

——— (1988). *Sublimation*. New Haven: Yale Univ. Press.

Mahler, M.S., Pine, F., & Bergman, A. (1975). *The Psychological Birth of the Human Infant*. New York: Basic Books.

Shengold, L. (1979). Child abuse and deprivation. *J. Amer. Psychoanal. Assn.*, 27:533–559.

Spruiell, V. (1983). The rules and frames of the psychoanalytic situation. *Psychoanal. Q.*, 52:1–33.

——— (1988). Crowd psychology and ideology. *Int. J. Psychoanal.*, 69:171–178.

——— (1989). Neglected classics: Hartmann's *Psychoanalysis and Moral Values*. *Psychoanal. Q.* (in press).

WAELDER, R. (1930). The principle of multiple function. In *Psychoanalysis: Observation, Theory, Application*. New York: Int. Univ. Press, 1976, pp. 68–83.

WHITEHEAD, A. N. (1929). *Process and Reality*. New York: Free Press, 1978.

WILLIAMS, B. (1985). *Ethics and the Limits of Philosophy*. Cambridge: Harvard Univ. Press.

IN HONOR OF
SAMUEL RITVO

Daughters and Mothers

Oedipal Aspects of the Witch-Mother

E. KIRSTEN DAHL, Ph.D.

CURRENT LITERATURE CONCERNING THE VICISSITUDES OF FEMALE DEVEL-
opment emphasizes the centrality of the girl's long dependence on the
mother. Usually what is commented on is the tenacity of the daughter's
attachment and the difficulty she seems to have in relinquishing it.
Because of the apparent hostility and sadism which seem to characterize this tenacity, the prominence of envy rather than jealousy, the
girl's insistence on dyadic as opposed to triadic issues, and the girl's
attachment to her mother are often understood as primarily preoedipal. From this point of view, the girl's difficulties lie in the arena of
separation-individuation, and the fantasies are seen as having to do
with the archaic omnipotent mother. For example, Bernstein and
Warner (1984) state, "The shadow of the preoedipal mother falls constantly upon the girl's representational world during the oedipal period" (p. 54).

I think that the fantasy of the fascinating and terrifying "witch-
mother" that is so frequently associated with the daughter's tenacious,
hostile attachment to her mother is better understood as an oedipal
fantasy configuration. This paper presents clinical material from the
analyses of several adult women, an adolescent girl, and a prepubertal
girl, illustrating a configuration of fantasies about the mother that
include: a secret excited longing for the mother and her body which
the daughter experiences as putting her at risk to be taken over by the
mother for the mother's pleasure; the projection onto the mother of
the envious, hostile, jealous, and possessive aspects of the daughter's
love; the experience of the mother as malignantly destructive of the
daughter's efforts to obtain genital pleasure from other sources; and

Harris assistant professor of child psychoanalysis, Yale University Child Study Center,
New Haven, Connecticut.

the oscillation between the wish to be the mother's erotic partner and the fear that the mother would destroy the daughter if she knew the daughter had an alternative erotic object in the tie to the man. After the clinical material I discuss what seem to be the common elements in these fantasies: the view of the mother as envious and hostile; the emphasis on bodily experience; and the use of silence and secrets within the transference. Finally I argue that these fantasies are the result of a reworking of earlier fantasies now in an oedipal context in an effort to postpone an acceptance of oedipal reality: that is, the acceptance of generational as well as genital differences.

I have made no effort to present the scope of the individual analyses or the dynamics of each patient. Rather, I have selected the material because it most clearly presents the particular fantasies I want to understand.

CLINICAL MATERIAL

Although the decision to undertake an analysis was motivated by discomfort with quite differing symptom pictures and character structures, over the years several of my adult female patients have expressed a common pattern as their analyses unfolded. These women described a deeply unsatisfying relationship with their actual mother (somewhat better in the present than in the past) in which the daughter experienced her mother as withholding or withdrawn and as hostile and destructive to those interests of the daughter which did not coincide with the mother's interests. At the same time, the daughter perceived her mother as "fascinating," "vivid," "charming," and powerfully effective in her own life. The now adult daughter found herself, to her continual unpleasant surprise, still seeking her mother's love and approval and feeling once again disappointed by her failure to capture her mother's attention.

Although more pressing current difficulties in adult life were the conscious spur to seek an analysis, each of these women was adamant in her wish for a woman analyst, feeling that "only a woman" could understand the inner world of another woman. As the transference developed over time, each of these women experienced her analyst as hostile and destructive of the patient's interests and yet all-consuming and demanding as if the patient/daughter could be neither comfortably close to nor happily independent from her female analyst. The ready availability of what seemed to be a prepared transference functioned as a resistance to the analysis but also contained the wish for a cure via the relationship to the analyst; both the prepared transference and the wish for a "transference cure" served to defend against oedipal wishes.

1. Twenty-five-year-old Maggie, toward the close of the second year of her analysis, felt herself uncomfortably preoccupied with her analyst; much to her own irritation, she often found herself wishing her analyst would tell her how to manage difficult situations; or she was "childishly" curious about her analyst's life outside the sessions. Associations to a series of dreams suggested a secret, excited longing for the mother and her body which Maggie experienced as leaving her helpless and messy, overwhelmed by excitement, at risk of being either taken over by the mother for the mother's pleasure or left to stew in her own mess. Maggie could imagine no "middle ground"—only one of them could "win" or succeed in getting the upper hand over the other.

The central theme in an hour following the reporting of the dreams was Maggie's experience of her mother as envious and destructive of Maggie's pleasure with her boyfriend. Maggie felt her pleasurable activities with her boyfriend were better kept secret from her mother or her mother would find some subtle way of spoiling things. Maggie's associations suggested an oscillation between her wish for the exciting, forbidden, body-to-body attachment to the mother and her anxiety that she would have to relinquish the erotic tie to the man in order to satisfy her mother. The hour was replete with images having to do with being cheated either by her mother or by the analyst, of being cut short, and of lacking something. These images were used to represent both the mother's destructive power and Maggie's fear that she could not be an adequate partner for her mother or the analyst. Maggie reported an episode in which she experienced her mother's actions as directed at spoiling Maggie's pleasure with her boyfriend. Maggie had responded by turning to activity independent from her mother, but she had also arranged things so that she was unavailable to her boyfriend as well. She felt as though she had won something and lost something: she had the satisfaction of being autonomous from her mother, but she had lost out on any fun with her boyfriend. She then reported having had the thought in the preceding hour that the analyst had cheated her; Maggie thought the analyst had gotten bored listening to her describe her pleasure with her boyfriend and had cut the hour short. Her thoughts turned to plans she and her boyfriend had made for the coming weekend, and then she fell quite silent. I wondered if her silence was a way of protecting her secret pleasure; she worried if I knew about *how much* pleasure she experienced being alone with her boyfriend, I would be envious and try to spoil it. Maggie reported having had the fantasy in the preceding hour that I brought fresh flowers to the office because I knew she would like them. She once again fell silent. I commented that it seemed as if that thought had made her anxious—her wish that I give her flowers, followed by her silence, suggested that she felt afraid I would extract something in return. Maggie responded by saying that the fantasy about the flowers had been the last thought of the preceding hour; "I had the thought you'd done it just for me, just because you knew I'd like it. But I didn't want to tell you. I was silent. And then as I was leaving, I had the thought you'd cheated me on the time. You cut me short!"

2. Brenda was referred at age 15 for analysis because of her suicidal thoughts and subsequent withdrawal from social life. At the time of referral Brenda said she thought her problem was that her chronic rage at her mother was out of proportion to the situation: "I mean it's one thing to get angry at your mother for nagging you, but when my mother asks me to vacuum, I feel like I'm going to kill her. That doesn't make any sense, so I just try to supress my feelings and then somehow I get depressed." Brenda was aware of being anxiously preoccupied with her mother; she felt that her parents were so involved with one another, they had taken little notice of her until her depression had become less severe.

In this material Brenda presents herself as fighting off a mother who jealously holds onto her. She simultaneously gives over her body to her mother's care and tries to be the sole mistress of her own body through battles with her mother around its care. As with Maggie, the man is only hinted at, a secret attachment that must be protected from the mother's powerfully destructive jealousy.

Early in her second year of analysis, Brenda began an hour by announcing that her parents had left the previous night on vacation. She reported angrily that her mother had insisted on knowing where Brenda was going to be "every minute—even if I am not there, she wants to know." After a brief pause, Brenda said that her mother had decided to stop Brenda's art lessons for the summer because she felt Brenda needed a vacation. Brenda thought this did not make sense as she would paint anyway; *she* did not feel she needed a break from what she loved most—her painting. Then Brenda thought of her two girlfriends and how irritated she felt with them right now. She wondered if "It's all in my mind—that it's really my problem. Because I just feel *too* angry with them. Just the way I do with my mother." She thought about the previous night. She had wanted to go out, but not with her sister and her sister's boyfriend because she would just feel like "a third wheel." But her two girlfriends just could not make up their minds; they were very "dithery." Brenda got all ready to go and at the last minute the two decided not to go out. But how could she feel so angry with them when a lot of the time she felt like she was just pretending with them anyway? She thought her girlfriends did not notice her irritation and that in the past Brenda would not have noticed it either. She wondered if she had changed and added that her mother said Brenda never changed. "Like, everyone else grows up, but not me. My mother doesn't *want* me to grow up." Brenda thought maybe she had changed, but she could not be sure. I commented that it sounded as though it was hard for her to notice ways in which she might be different from her mother. Brenda agreed. After a silence she added that she was letting her hair grow. Her mother did not like it, but she had won this battle. Now her hair was in "the awkward stage"; she thought it probably did not look very good, but Brenda was not going to cut it just to give in to her mother. I said that it was hard for Brenda to know whether her hair looked pretty when it felt so connected to her mother. Brenda agreed and added forcefully, "Wearing my hair like this is what my mother *doesn't* want. I can't see what *I* want. I just get lost in the battle with her." She then went on to talk about her battles with her mother over clothing. Her mother liked her to dress in "little girl" clothes, while Brenda liked "darker colors." Her sister used to dress like a tomboy, but now she was very feminine and their mother loved everything the sister did. "My mother thinks what I like is masculine— there's no middle ground—it's either *very* feminine or *very* masculine!"

Brenda was nearly mute over the next three sessions. In the fourth hour, she mentioned a big blow-up with her sister, focusing on how emotionally disturbed she thought her sister was. Her sister really had not been able to separate from their mother. Brenda felt lucky she had gotten into analysis; she felt she had a real chance to become independent from her mother. Brenda then looked sad and said she felt very guilty that she could "get away" and her sister could not. Now, Brenda thought, maybe there would not be any need for her to have a a big dramatic break from her parents; maybe she could just "fade away" while her parents were so preoccupied with her sister.

In the next hour Brenda reported having gotten into a fight with her mother in the car. Her mother would not let her have any privacy or any secrets. She recalled with some feeling how her mother had discovered her diary several months ago and this had ruined it for Brenda. Brenda had thrown the diary away. I commented that the mother's finding the diary had also involved the mother's and my discovery of Brenda's secret cutting of herself, an activity that had felt like an exciting, secret possession of her own body. Brenda yawned and said her mind seemed to be drifting; she fell silent.

In a session a month later, Brenda came in very upset. She had had a terrible battle with her mother over her friends. Her mother simply did not trust her. "It's just the way it was with the diary—she never understands what *I* need—she thinks what I need is crazy! But this time I'm not going to back down—even if she's right!" Brenda reported that "for once" her father had stuck up for her; *he* was able to understand. Brenda felt that her mother demanded, "Me or your friends." "My mother doesn't understand the importance of privacy. She can't understand I can't be her good little girl anymore. She makes me feel crazy. She wants me to be just the same as her—there's no room for me to be anything else." Brenda became teary as she recalled her father's defense of her. He used to defend her when she was little, but then he had stopped. "Somehow I feel I can survive the break from my mother knowing this one time he was there for me. He is the most important person in my life and my mother knows this. And that's what makes it so dangerous—not just for me but for him too. But I'm going to hold firm this time."

3. Lucy, age 12, was referred for analysis following a collapse in school in which she felt overwhelmed by suicidal thoughts of cutting herself; she found herself unable to return to school and preoccupied with obsessive thoughts concerning all the "bad" things she had ever done and a compulsion to confess to her parents. Lucy's parents had separated when she was 5 and divorced when she was 7. The parents had agreed that Lucy and her brother would remain with their father; mother visited the children on weekends. At the time of referral, Lucy felt she must speak to her mother several times a day and had frequent, anxious thoughts that her mother might die in a car accident. Lucy had not yet reached menarche, but she had been told by her pediatrician that she soon would; she felt quite terrified about menstruation. After several months of conducting her analysis by sitting and talking with me, Lucy brought a board game from home, introducing it by saying it was a game she had often played with her mother and it would make her feel more comfortable to play a game while we talked. She said she did not like leaving her hours feeling upset and she thought the board game would help her confine her feelings to the sessions. She was quite resistant to any further exploration of the meaning of the game.

The latent image in these two sessions involved a fantasy configuration concerning the erotic tie to the powerful, witch-mother. Lucy seemed to employ the longing for the mother as a protection against feeling helpless in the face of sexual excitement with the man. However, the fantasy of being an adequate partner for the mother awakened Lucy's fear that she would succumb to a homosexual object choice. The theme of keeping balanced between exciting but dangerous alternatives was central.

In the ninth month of her analysis, Lucy came to a session wearing an uncharacteristically frilly blouse, reminiscent of the frilly party dresses of preschool girls. She drew my attention to the blouse, commenting that she did not usually wear it, but her best friend, Kelly, "loved it" and talked her into wearing it. (I remembered that it was Kelly's comment that Lucy should spend more time with her mother rather than with Kelly that had been the manifest cause of Lucy's breakdown in school.) Lucy then got out the game and as she was setting it up, I reminded her of several changes in her appointment times for the next week necessitated by her father's work schedule. Lucy responded in a characteristic way, blandly listening as if she were used to the endless jumbling of schedules in her family's life. She then laughed as she told me she felt really tired, having been out late roller skating the night before; "and my feet are really killing me!" (She had told me in the preceding hour that she and Kelly were going skating in anticipation of Lucy's thirteenth birthday the following week. I also remembered that she had decided not to visit her mother this weekend, so that Lucy could spend more time with Kelly.) "Boy, was it fun! But you know I'm starting to get those upset feelings about Kelly again. It's funny—now that I *can* see her [Kelly had been grounded for a month], I get these thoughts that I don't want to—I *know* that's not how I really feel, so I just try to put those thoughts out of my mind." I wondered what she thought about feeling worried that she might be getting too close to Kelly. Lucy said it reminded her about her bad, sexual thoughts about her Dad, about his penis. She added that she never had upsetting feelings like this about her mother because "I don't see her that much." (This last was a striking denial because the preceding months had been occupied by Lucy's increasing awareness of how painful the repeated separations from her mother had been.) She said she sort of was guessing, but she wondered "if it's sort of like I get worried they will leave me; so I get the thought I'll leave them first, so I don't get hurt." I commented that it *was* very painful for her to be left by someone she loved, that it reminded her of what she felt with her mother. Lucy became teary and said, "Yes, that's what I *do* think because I *do* want to be friends with Kelly, but it scares me and I wonder if somehow that's what happened with Mary." (Mary, now in her 20s, had been Lucy's babysitter when Lucy was younger. Lucy referred to Mary as her "second mother" and during the analysis alternately longed for Mary and felt furious that Mary, although devoted to Lucy, was so involved with her boyfriend. The situation with Mary was a remarkable parallel to Lucy's situation with her mother, although Lucy had been able to express her feelings about Mary much more directly than about her mother.) Lucy continued, "But with Mary it's all sort of foggy and mixed up in my mind, but maybe with Mary it's something like that too." Lucy then returned to playing the board game for a while, keeping careful score and expressing pleasure every time she beat me in a round. As she won one round, she grinned broadly and exclaimed, "There! That evens things up!" I commented, "You like it that sometimes I win and sometimes you win—the game evens things up between us." She grinned again and added, "Yeah, it makes for a closer game between us." I said, "It keeps us close, but not too close; you like to maintain a very even balance between winning and losing." Lucy smiled, relaxed slightly, and said, "Yeah, I like it that way; that's why I like to play this game with you. Today Kelly and I are going shopping and we're gonna spend everything we've got! I *love* having my own money—then *I* get to decide how I'm going to spend it." She recalled a time when she and Kelly had gone into an expensive woman's clothing store and been chased out by "an ugly old woman."

Another session a month and a half later, Lucy began in good spirits, not commenting on the fact that I had unexpectedly canceled the preceding hour. "Last Friday night was kind of upsetting, but it was sort of okay and fun too. I went to the Mall with Karen, Annie, Joe, and Jack. We met this girl who had a paper cup full of vodka, and she passed it around. I didn't drink any, though. Neither did Joe; he's the son of the police chief so he has to behave. But everybody else did. I felt kind of scared, but it was sort of funny too." Lucy described the new girl as "hanging all over Joe"; Lucy and Joe had devised ways of preventing this. Lucy said she thought the girl was pretty "silly." She wondered if Karen and Annie might have been tipsy too.

The next day Lucy had talked with her Dad; she felt worried about what she should have done about the drinking. He told her that as long as *she* did not drink, she should not worry about it. Lucy wondered what Kelly would have done if *she* had been there. It was very upsetting that Kelly was away; Lucy said she felt kind of let down. I commented that perhaps she felt let down by me—she had expected to see me the next day and had not. "Yeah, I really did. It was a surprise, you know. I'm always surprised that I feel upset when I don't see you— I don't expect to, but then I did—I do feel upset. And my Dad was away too, and I felt sad about that and wanted someone to talk to about Friday night—about what I should have done." I wondered if she had felt left behind in an exciting and scary situation. Lucy giggled and went on to say that Mary had stayed with her while her father was away. Mary had decided not to go to work, which Lucy thought was really nice. "She's kind of mad at Mike, her boyfriend, right now because she made him promise not to drink, but she found out that he did. If he can't keep a little promise like that, how can he keep a bigger one? So we decided if he called, we wouldn't talk to him." I said, "Sounds like it was very comforting when you felt left behind by Kelly, Mom, and me to have Mary all to yourself—no Mike—as a way of making up for the disappointment with the rest of us women." Lucy laughed very broadly and said she and Mary had gone to see *Sleeping Beauty* together; "we were the only people who weren't parents or little kids, so it was sort of weird. But it was really fun." She sighed and blushed as she said, "It was so wonderful when we came home—we were dancing all over with Mary's cats. We felt so good and we weren't going to speak to Mike if he called. Just us! But then that night I had this sort of weird dream. *I dreamed I was a man and there was a big party. Everyone was in costume and dancing around, and I was dancing with this woman. It was very romantic and then I began kissing her. That really scared me, so I woke up.* But I don't think it means I'm a lesbian. I think I had the dream because of the movie and dancing around with Mary." I said, "That's an old worry of yours—that your passionate feelings for women mean you are a lesbian—what do you make of that?" Lucy responded immediately, "Oh it makes me think of my great aunt—my mother's mother's sister. Did I tell you she's a lesbian? We saw her last Christmas. She's really very nice. Actually I like her a lot. She taught me how to play this game. Actually, she was the one who gave this game to me!" For a moment I felt as if the meaning of the game were crystal clear to me and I said, "That helps us understand a little bit more about why this game is so good for keeping us close, but not too close." Lucy laughed delightedly, nodding her head.

DISCUSSION

Several fantasies concerning the mother were reflected both in Maggie's dream thoughts and in her experience of the transference. Most prominent was a configuration that involved a secret, excited longing for the mother and her body. Maggie experienced this configuration as leaving her helpless, awash in her own excitement, a dirty mess, at risk of either being taken over by the mother for the mother's pleasure or of being rejected, left to flounder in her own mess. Both mother and daughter were seen as seeking to possess each other through domination. In the hour reported Maggie's experience of the mother as envious and destructive of Maggie's pleasure with the man was clearer.

The pleasure with the man could only be insured if it was kept secret from the mother and therefore protected from her malignant power. Independence and autonomy appear as nonpleasurable attempts to ward off both the longing for the forbidden, body-to-body, exciting attachment to the mother and the mother's envy. Images of bodily damage were prominent, and the damage seemed to be associated with having a female body. There was the strong suggestion that the mother would damage the daughter's body by taking something away or cutting her.

Brenda experienced herself as fighting off a mother who jealously held onto her even as the mother also possessed the father. She simultaneously involved her mother with her body and attempted to be sole mistress of her own body through the battles around her hair and in her secret cutting of her body. Brenda seemed to experience her body as in danger of becoming her mother's little possession; she expressed confusion as to whether her body was her own to do with as she pleased or whether it had to please her mother. At moments she seemed to experience her body primarily as a negative or reversed image of her mother's body. Paradoxically the battling with her mother represented both an attempt to fend off what she perceived as her mother's claims and an avenue for bodily closeness. She expressed disappointment and rage that she could only be either unsuccessfully masculine or a little girl for her mother; in her rage at her failure to please her mother one can detect her longing to be her mother's adequate partner. The father appeared in the manifest content as protection from the mother; however, the latent meaning seemed to be Brenda's anticipation of how dangerous the mother would become if she appreciated Brenda's attachment to her father; Brenda believed her mother would tolerate no rivals for Brenda's love.

For Lucy her attachment to Kelly appeared as a displacement from her erotic longing for her father. But the penis also represented a connection to the mother; if Lucy had a penis, like her father, her mother's boyfriend, and Mary's boyfriend, maybe then she could keep the mother for herself. The fantasy of being an adequate partner for her mother unleashed Lucy's fear that she would be taken over by the mother or that she would succumb to a homosexual object choice. She searched for a way to keep the relationship to the mother balanced between winning and losing, between pleasure and destruction, between heterosexuality and homosexuality. At the same time Lucy seemed to employ the longing for the mother as a protection against feeling helpless in the face of sexual excitement with the man. It was Lucy who employed the Sleeping Beauty imagery, emphasizing Beauty's dancing with the animals which in the Disney movie (to which she referred) was depicted as a prelude to her erotic encounter with the Prince. Lucy, as Sleeping Beauty, denied the encounter with the Prince, insisting that all she wanted was the witch-mother. Finally, Lucy, as did Maggie and Brenda, depicted the mother as envious and potentially destructive of Lucy's experiences of bodily pleasure.

The fantasies of Maggie, Brenda, and Lucy all reflect rapid oscillations between representations of the body, experiences of pleasure, and images of the mother. The latent fantasy configuration seems to be of a jealously possessive, envious, and malignantly destructive witch-mother whom the daughter cannot let go and who will not let go of the daughter. This fascinating and terrifying witch-mother is seen by the daughter as the regulator of the daughter's body and her pleasure. How can we understand the sources that power this fantasy?

The biologically based upsurge in the drives that usher in the early pubertal period reawakens in the child all the earlier sources of libidinal and aggressive modes of gratification. These earlier modes have a strong pregenital stamp and carry with them as well the valence of the infantile tie to the mother which derives its intensity and strength from her bodily care. The special significance of the preoedipal phase as it is reevoked in early adolescence is that during this infantile period, via the experience of the mother's bodily care, the girl's relationship to her own body became established (M. E. Laufer, 1986). For the girl this is especially problematic and experienced as dangerous, because these experiences of bodily pleasure at the hands of the mother now take on a homosexual charge. For some especially vulnerable girls, as both Deutsch (1944) and Blos (1962) describe, the danger of this regressive tie to the mother of infancy is warded off by a pathologically precocious turn to compulsive or delinquent heterosexuality. For most girls, however, this attempt at a solution through flight to reality is inhibited by superego disapproval. The failure of the turn to reality intensifies the girl's conflict over the nature of her attachment to her internalized mother and her relationship to her own body. As the girl turns toward the father, she wavers between the mother and the father, wanting to have them both. The bisexual valence of this situation can be seen in the girl's continual intrapsychic oscillation between her mother and her father and their substitutes. Nowhere is this bisexual "hovering" more clearly expressed than in the best friend who, in fantasy, is simultaneously girlfriend and boyfriend. This is vividly presented by Lucy when she associates her upset feelings about her girlfriend to her disturbing erotic thoughts about her father. In actuality, the best friend may serve as a link to the first heterosexual encounters as well, her presence helping the girl to maintain an acceptable balance between impulse and inhibition and providing a safe haven when action becomes too exciting. Finally, the best friend is simultaneously agent of the mother, a substitute for the mother, and a companion on the way to relinquishing the tie to the mother.

The biological changes experienced by the girl during the early puberty period forcefully turn her attention back to her body. As Ritvo (1984) points out, "The inescapable need to integrate the representation of the sexually mature body" into the rest of the psychic structure generates intense and painful conflict. It is in this context that the girl turns back to the bodily ego for representation and expression of psychic conflict (p. 468). Both Maggie and Brenda demonstrate how the genital aspects of bodily experience are denied and instead experienced in infantile, particularly anal, terms.

The associative pathway between representations of the mother and representations of the body occur because with the physical changes of puberty, the girl begins to possess a body which is identified with the mother's body (Laufer and Laufer, 1984). This situation threatens to intensify the closeness to the mother and to stimulate fantasies of merging and oneness as well as fears of being overwhelmed (Ritvo, 1988). At the same time, relinquishing this infantile tie to the mother may be experienced by the daughter either as necessitating a renunciation of future bodily pleasure or as a dangerous and destructive surpassing of the mother (Ritvo, 1988). The "solution" that daughters like Maggie, Brenda, and Lucy seem to try on via fantasy is one of *postponement* (M. E. Laufer, 1986) in which the preoedipal attachment to the mother is recast in an oedipal configuration, but a configuration that denies both differences between the sexes and between generations (Chasseguet-Smirgel, 1986). In this fantasy, the daughter's earlier experience of bodily pleasure through maternal care, her envy of the mother's capacity to provide gratification through her active ministrations, and the daughter's wish to provide such satisfactions to the mother spur her to take her mother as erotic object. In an effort to keep from awareness her inadequacy as mother's partner she projects onto the mother the envious, hostile, jealous, and possessive aspects of her love, creating the image of the witch-mother who fascinates and imprisons the daughter. It is now the *mother* who is experienced as malignantly destructive of the *daughter's* efforts to obtain pleasure from the man, as if the mother believed the daughter to be an adequate erotic partner and the man to be the mother's rival. This fantasy is rooted in the denial of the generational difference as well as in the denial of the knowledge that the daughter's body is not adequate to the task of providing full genital satisfaction to the mother (Chasseguet-Smirgel, 1986). The fact that the girl possesses this knowledge but denies it is revealed in the frequent references to being lesser, lacking, and/or damaged. This stance on the daughter's part allows her to postpone the grief she anticipates if she were to acknowledge the anatomical and generational differences and to accept that she cannot keep her mother's love to herself.

This fantasy configuration can be understood as preoedipal only if the specific role of silence and secret keeping is ignored. For all three patients actively keeping silent during a session was revealed as having the meaning in the transference of preventing the mother from learning of the daughter's secret: her alternate possibility of bodily gratification through the erotic tie to the man. The content of this secret is in the manifest content of Maggie's hour and expressed via displacement to the best friend by Brenda and Lucy. It is the fear that the mother will discover this secret, erotic attachment and destroy it as well as the attempt to deny knowledge of the mother's erotic attachment to the father that give the fantasies about the internalized mother their malignant, witchlike valence, and stamp them as oedipal rather than preoedipal. In addition, the creation of the internalized witch-mother and the anal-sadistic attachment to her function as a kind of preoedipal camouflage in the service of masking the daughter's secret, her erotic longing for the father. As she presents herself to her mother as a disgusting mess, unable to regulate her body and its sensations, the daughter's apparent preoedipal attachment conceals and protects the tie to the man from the jealous destructiveness of the internalized mother. It is in this context that Lucy employs the Sleeping Beauty story, in her fantasy insisting that all Beauty wishes for is the endless postponement offered by the witch's magic spell, thereby concealing Beauty's secret—that she has already danced with the Prince.

BIBLIOGRAPHY

BERNSTEIN, A. E. & WARNER, G. M. (1984). *Women Treating Women.* New York: Int. Univ. Press.

BLOS, P. (1962). *On Adolescence.* New York: Free Press.

CHASSEGUET-SMIRGEL, J. (1986). *Sexuality and Mind.* New York: New York Univ. Press.

DEUTSCH, H. (1944). *The Psychology of Women,* vol. 1. New York: Grune & Stratton.

LAUFER, M. (1982). The formation and shaping of the oedipus complex. *Int. J. Psychoanal.,* 63:217–227.

——— & LAUFER, M. E. (1984). *Adolescence and Developmental Breakdown.* New Haven: Yale Univ. Press.

LAUFER, M. E. (1982). Female masturbation in adolescence and the development of the relationship to the body. *Int. J. Psychoanal.*, 63:295–301.

——— (1986). The female oedipus complex and the relationship to the body. *Psychoanal. Study Child,* 41: 259–276.

RITVO, S. (1976). Adolescent to woman. *J. Amer. Psychoanal. Assn. Suppl.,* 24(5):127–138.

——— (1984). The image and uses of the body in psychic conflict. *Psychoanal. Study Child,* 39:449–469.

——— (1988). Observations on the mother-daughter relationship in adolescent development as seen in eating disorders (in press).

Adolescent Sexuality

A Body/Mind Continuum

MOSES LAUFER, Ph.D.

IN THE TREATMENT OF SEVERELY DISTURBED ADOLESCENTS I HAVE BEEN struck time and again by a simple but critical observation, and it is one which I believe to be central to the theme of adolescent sexuality and the body/mind continuum. That observation is: in whichever way the seriously disturbed adolescent tries to alter his body or its image, it is never right for him or her. There is a constant and urgent need to seek answers which can never quite be found, except if the person distorts his body and its sexual role or, as Freud (1924) described it, disavows the experience of the external world and how he sees himself in relation to it. When I refer to the distortion of the body and its sexual role, and use the description of "disavowal," I am obviously referring to the perversions and the psychoses, both of which are signs of severe mental disorder and both of which become organized and irreversibly established (irreversible without treatment) during the period of adolescence. It is with this that I want to begin the examination and the understanding of that process or processes which affect the body/mind continuum in adolescence or which damage or destroy the relationship to one's body.

I want first to describe my way of thinking about adolescence and psychopathology during adolescence, so that the clinical material and the meaning I have put to this material will be seen within a specific framework. Physical sexual maturity, that is, the beginning of the period of adolescence, means not only a fundamental change in the person's relationship to his body, but it means that from puberty onward psychopathology *requires* the availability of the sexually mature body for its expression, that is, for the living out in a predictable and a compelling way of those fantasies which are at the core of the pa-

Director, Centre for Research into Adolescent Breakdown/Brent Consultation Centre, London.

I wish to acknowledge the help of my wife, Eglé, in the preparation of this paper.

thology. But, this use of the sexually mature body for the expression of the pathology—and I will make this more explicit when I describe two adolescents who have been treated and studied at our Adolescent Centre in London—while ensuring gratification, *also destroys genitality*. It might be more correct to state that one essential function of pathology in adolescence—or more specifically, of the development to perversion, or of the break with reality and with one's sexual body as in psychosis—is this destruction of genitality, that is, the destruction of a continuum. It is also the ingredient which is always present in the transference and which faces the adolescent and the analyst with seemingly insurmountable problems during the treatment of these seriously disturbed people.

The development of one's sexuality during the period of adolescence has an integrating function, independent of whether that integration which takes place is normal or has a pathological direction. The presence of a physically mature body at the time of puberty means, in physical terms, the ability to impregnate or the ability to grow a child in one's body. But this process of becoming a sexual male or sexual female, and then enabling oneself to experience the reality of fatherhood or motherhood, depends on the ability to alter the image of one's body during adolescence to include the functioning genitals—which in turn depends on the ability to gratify the oedipal incestuous wishes in ways which are removed psychically from the oedipal parents, that is, from the incestuous objects (Loewald, 1979). Without this, sexuality during adolescence becomes, instead, a psychically painful, frightening, and anxiety-ridden area of experience which participates or results in the psychic destruction of the person as a functioning male or functioning female (Ritvo, 1984).

The variations of psychopathology which we observe in the treatment of adolescents have a very limited repertoire (perversion, the in-between state of uncertainty between perverse or psychotic, and psychosis). The unconscious choice of pathology and what it expresses in adolescence can be understood if, in terms of the theme of body/mind continuum, we think not only of body and mind, but "Which body?" and "Whose body?"—questions which are being examined in our study of Mental Breakdown in Adolescence.

The Study

Some years ago, we undertook a pilot study, through psychoanalytic treatment, of a number of adolescents who had attempted suicide.[1] We

---

1. At the Centre for Research into Adolescent Breakdown.

wanted then to make sense of a well-known but not well-understood observation, which is that attempted suicide or actual suicide becomes a more definite risk as well as a social problem from the time of puberty, that is, from the time the person reaches physical sexual maturity. We hoped that this study would lead us toward a greater understanding of the developmental function of adolescence, and of the specific part played by the sexually mature body in pathology. In the course of this pilot study, we also began to realize that, as part of our contact with many adolescents who came to our walk-in service for help,[2] we were meeting many, very vulnerable, young people who had reached or seemed to be on the way to severe and established pathology, but who had not attempted suicide and where there was little risk of suicide. This left us with the awareness, but not with the understanding, of the fact that the attack on the physically mature body, as exists in suicide or attempted suicide, was only one of the ways of expressing the hatred or rejection or disappointment or shame of that body which these adolescents felt to be the reservoir of their bewildering and often frightening thoughts and feelings.

We then undertook a second study, through psychoanalytic treatment, which would include other adolescents showing signs of the likelihood of the presence of serious psychopathology. Three "types" of adolescents distinguished by the way in which they used the sexually mature body to express the pathology would be treated: (1) those who had attempted suicide; (2) those whose relationships were of a perverse nature, as in homosexuality and fetishism; and (3) those whose behavior showed signs of severe disturbance in functioning (psychotic functioning)—that is, whose fantasies distorted the adolescent's relationship to the outside world; or whose relationships to people are characterized by extreme suspiciousness, accusation, blaming, and violence; or whose fantasies are expressed mainly via the body itself, as in anorexia, bulimia, obesity, and drug-taking. The adolescents accepted for this study were to be between the ages of 15 and 19 at the start of treatment, ages which represented our view about the characteristics of the beginning and the end of adolescence.[3]

We had observed that it is very unusual for adolescents below the age

2. The Brent Consultation Centre.

3. A maximum of 15 adolescents would be in psychoanalytic treatment at any one time as part of this study. This number was decided by the financial resources of the Research Centre and by our awareness that we needed to keep this study to a size which would permit us to address the extremely difficult and predictable problems of treatment in regular weekly clinical discussions. Such a decision also acknowledged, from the outset, the anxieties evoked in the analysts undertaking the treatment of such vulnerable adolescents.

of about 15 to seek help of their own accord. The decision to seek help for himself might represent the adolescent's beginning ability to experience anxiety about himself, without having to rely on others to experience it for him; it might also represent the adolescent's feeling that he could now be responsible for his own body and his emotions. We have assumed that adolescence as a developmental period ends at about the age of 21; this seems to be the time when responses to anxiety become much more predictable, representing a more fixed internal structure and an established relationship to oneself as a sexually mature person. We decided therefore to limit the upper age to 19, assuming that this would enable us to intervene some time before the psychopathology had become fixed.

CASE 1

Mark was 19 when he had a severe mental breakdown. He was seen by his doctor, who referred him to the local psychiatric hospital, where he was diagnosed as being paranoid schizophrenic and admission was recommended. From past experience the family knew that physical treatment did not produce a lasting change, and they looked for a place where he could have therapy or analysis. During this time they heard of the Centre.

When Mark came to the Centre, he was barely able to cope. He was afraid to leave the house, he could not sleep alone, he spent hours washing his "dirty" hands, especially after having defecated. He rarely attended college classes. His sexual life consisted of compulsive masturbation. When he came to the Centre, he was frightened to be left alone with the interviewer; he heard voices that accused him of spreading scurrilous stories about his family, and he was frightened to give in to the voices that told him to jump out of the window or kill himself. He felt sure that he was being followed by agents of the American and Russian governments, and in one interview at the Centre he was unable to leave the building because he felt certain that they were waiting for him.

Soon after the analysis began,[4] Mark began to refer to his anxieties about contamination, experiencing analytic intervention as harmful substances that were being pushed into his mind and driving him crazy. An internal world barely existed for him at this time; everything was being done to him by outside agents. But he talked of his compulsive masturbation, which he felt he had to do to rid himself of tension; otherwise there was the risk of raping a girl or be raped

4. The analyst was K. Mehra, Ph.D.

himself. By looking at naked pictures during masturbation, he tried to sort out his confused ideas about the male and female anatomy; he believed that each sex had both male and female organs. Masturbation proved that he was normal, not only sexually but in his mind as well. His attempts to control his perverse thoughts, however, were not successful; he was assailed by sexual thoughts about men, women, children, and animals. In a desperate attempt to prove his normality, he made friends with a young woman, hoping that sexual intercourse would free him of his perverse ideas, but then he could not have intercourse because of a fear that he might penetrate her anus. This idea also referred to his thoughts about being penetrated by the analyst and, in order to control them, he would masturbate before his session.

After 18 months of treatment, his mental state worsened; he was convinced that men had anal intercourse with one another. He had to turn around in sessions to look at the analyst to be assured that the analyst was not masturbating and that the analyst's penis was not in Mark's anus. It was at this time that Mark had to be admitted to a mental hospital, where he stayed for two months, and where the analyst visited to maintain contact and to ensure the future of the analysis.

It was only in the third year of treatment that Mark could risk showing irritation with the analyst, and that he could begin to think of how he used his body to express emotion. Instead of saying he was angry with the analyst, he thought of ejaculating on him or strangling him; when he was angry with a woman, he imagined her "cunt," and it was only then that he could begin to allow any connection between his thoughts and how he felt.

But it was following the analysis of the erotization of his thought processes that there was a change in Mark's mental state. The early "disputes" which perpetually occupied his thinking could begin to be examined in relation to who was responsible for making him do things—his own mind, or the analyst who had the power to cure him or to make him ill again. But it was only when the psychotic thinking became concentrated more within the transference that Mark could begin to risk seeing any connection between what he thought and what he did either to himself or to others. For example, when the analyst used the word "afraid," Mark became very upset and wanted the analyst to take back what he had said. Or when the analyst referred to Mark's depressed mood, he reacted with panic, afraid that he might be pulled back into the withdrawn and comatose state he had experienced in the past.

It was through these kinds of experiences in the transference that he could begin to feel confident to speak the thoughts that went through his mind. Automobile accidents, attractive women, detached sexual organs could begin to be put into words without the feeling that his body would, without him knowing, do something for which he would then be blamed.

With this also came the danger that he might take risks while driving a car, or that he might involve himself in petty cheating and get himself into trouble and be punished. His ability to begin to speak his thoughts and not to have to believe that he would be sent away, imprisoned, or killed also meant that his grandiosity needed to be understood, but this was only partly successful. He could understand interpretations, but he could not quite use the knowledge to change his behavior. The danger continued that spoken words took on a concrete quality, endowed with the power of the images attached to these words. Talking of his homosexual wishes and his anal masturbation became, for Mark, the recognition that he was homosexual, that men were after him because of what he did, and that his anal masturbation was what he wanted and needed because it kept his life from being bleak.

But what also needs to be added is that Mark has never tried to kill himself but has instead used his sexually mature body and what he feels it does to him as the explanation of what he has to do and think: it is as if he can continue to feel that his body has a way of functioning and has needs, and his mind is entered by this body. It is as if his body is both the persecutor and his ally.[5]

CASE 2

Susan, aged 18, was included in the research study because she had made two suicide attempts in the past 18 months after having run away from home.[6] She had left home at 16 because she felt unable to remain in control of her reactions in response to her mother's demands on her and her mother's constant blaming and abusing of Susan. Susan had been a very gifted child, and her mother made enormous demands on her to work and study. Susan had enjoyed her academic success but felt dominated and controlled by her fear of her mother.

After puberty, as Susan tried to feel that she could act independently of her mother, her mother's physical attacks on Susan became more violent and Susan tried to get satisfaction out of showing her mother that she was strong enough to withstand anything her mother did or said to her without letting her see that it hurt. The sense of power that Susan could experience when she could show her mother that nothing

5. We have been able to understand this state only marginally.
6. The analyst is M. Eglé Laufer.

mother did or said could "penetrate or get inside" her was a source of secret excitement and guilt for Susan. She felt at times that she had no right to live; that there was nothing wrong with her except that she was bad, lazy, and not making enough of an effort. She would try to mobilize herself into activity but, independently of what the activity was— washing herself, dieting, writing, etc.—she would begin to feel out of control and it would take on a manic quality.

This manic behavior had already been noted by the interviewer who saw Susan originally. She noted that Susan used jargon and intellectualization when talking about herself in a bombastic way that eventually left the interviewer feeling overwhelmed. The manic excitement that Susan could experience in this way served as a defense against her feeling of misery and deadness.

When Susan was seen by the interviewer, she actively portrayed her confused relationship to her body in the way she presented herself. She complained of being fat but in fact wore shapeless clothes that disguised how thin she was. She was potentially an attractive girl, but she had cut her hair in a distorted fashion and changed the color constantly. She wore thin summer clothes in the winter and in summer would come in heavy sweaters, complaining of being hot. She suffered from numerous psychosomatic complaints and allergies, most of which were "inherited" from her mother and which necessitated constant medical interventions and medication. When the psychiatrist prescribed major tranquilizers to try to control her manic behavior, Susan used the medication as another way of being able to confuse herself about her bodily perceptions (being hot, sleepy, hungry). She complained of having no sexual feelings now, even though she had felt excited when she had been together with a boy she was fond of when she was younger. Now, she said, she wouldn't mind what she felt, heterosexual or homosexual; it would be better than nothing. It seemed as if the fantasy was of having destroyed all feeling in her efforts to control her body. She felt as if her body was dead or not her own.

Before she started analysis she had become so withdrawn and unable to function that she had had to be hospitalized. She was diagnosed as manic depressive with the possibility of schizophrenia. As she emerged from her withdrawn state, she became more out of control and at times violent. She cut her arms and said she was interested in seeing what was inside her if she were to cut deeply enough. When the analyst took up her attack on herself, Susan's response was to mock the analyst for showing concern. "What I do is nothing compared to what I think about doing to myself." She then proceeded to tell of horrifying visual images of herself with a cut throat and blood pouring out, or jumping off high buildings, and so on. Susan's constant effort in the analytic session was to show the analyst that there was nothing wrong with her. She was just morally bad or lazy. For her to have to recognize herself as mentally disturbed meant feeling hopeless and as if her mother had now really got inside her and taken over both her body and her mind.

Throughout the time since she had run away from home Susan had continued her studies and each year had failed to complete the year and had to begin again. Her thinking was confused and out of her control despite manic efforts to control it. Her thought processes were dominated by the struggle with her body which she felt she was constantly involved with. Yet, the sense of deadness she experienced when she felt her body as being under her control made her feel compelled to seek excitement from her destructive attacks on her body. These she justified with the comment that, as long as she was attacking herself and not her mother, "why should anyone be bothered." At the same time Susan appeared relieved at the analyst's persistence in using the attacks on her body as evidence of her mentally disturbed state and her need for treatment, rather than allowing Susan to destroy the treatment as well as herself.

In the first weeks of her analysis, Susan came to her sessions talking excitedly while trying not to show how frightened and anxious she felt. Unable to allow herself or the analyst to recognize the extent of her fear and the effort she was having to make to come to the sessions, she broke off her treatment twice through being taken to the hospital following an overdose.

It seemed as if, in starting analysis, she was compelled to live out with her body the fantasy she said she used to have as an adolescent before she ran away from home—of carrying out all her mother's demands on her without any sign of anger, but with the result that she would eventually drop dead from exhaustion at her mother's feet. Her analysis continues.

DISCUSSION

I chose to describe Mark and Susan because they came with very different signs of severe pathology, but with neither of them evoking much hope. Although we were very anxious about undertaking their treatment, we knew that they had everything to gain if we succeeded, that we could learn very much even if we failed, and that neither they nor we had anything to lose, whatever the outcome. The initial picture and prognosis were, to say the least, dim for both Mark and Susan, but we decided to try.

I will explain what I mean by this. The initial assumption of our study was that a developmental breakdown occurred at puberty, and that this breakdown is characterized by the rejection of the sexually mature body. Although itself correct in a rather global sense, this assumption did not take into account some of the clinical observations which point to a much more ominous break in the relationship to the sexually mature body, and which contain characteristics that may be the ingredients of psychotic functioning or later psychosis. Rejection of the sexually mature body, as in attempted suicide, allows for an *active* relationship to that body, even though the body is experienced as an enemy, the disturber of the peace, the reservoir of perverse wishes or fantasies or potential actions. But some of the adolescents in our study, as was the case with Mark and somewhat with Susan, already seemed to have taken another step in the process of rejecting the sexually mature body. It is one which represents the presence of a more defined dis-owning of the body and a separation from it which interferes in the sexually mature body's ability to be used actively for the expression of fantasy. Instead of there being an active conflict taking place between the superego and the regressive/perverse wishes, some of our adolescents feel themselves persecuted or forced to act by an enemy which is separated off from the rest of themselves. They have given up the active battle, but instead experience themselves as the passive victims of fantasies and forces which now have a life of their own. They try to silence their persecutors by allowing something "good" to destroy the image of the physically potent body (as in anorexia, drug-taking, bulimia, alcoholism, obesity); or they live out the fantasy of union with an idealized part of themselves (being male and female at the same time) through various forms of autoerotic activity which maintains the defensive withdrawal from objects (through anal masturbation in males, or through compulsive rocking, hitting one's own body, dis-figuring one's own body through cutting, pulling out one's hair).

These different ways in which some of the adolescents whom we are studying *alienate themselves from their sexually mature bodies,* that is, give up the active battle with the body—as was the case with Mark, but not yet wholly with Susan—have important diagnostic and prognostic im-plications because it is beginning to become clearer to us that these adolescents' relationship to the external world is severely damaged and is prone to be overwhelmed by uncontrollable fantasy. For adolescents like Mark, and perhaps Susan, there is a much greater danger of a fixed break with the internalized oedipal objects, with the result that they feel they have capitulated to the persecutors or to the hated and threatening castrater.

In differentiating "alienation from the sexually mature body" from "rejection of the sexually mature body," and implying that alienation is a move nearer to a psychotic organization, I want to call attention to an interference or break in an essential developmental process where the sexually mature body is of primary importance. For some of our adolescents, physical sexual maturity and the ability for incestuous fantasies to be enacted result in the idealized body (the preoedipal/ nonincestuous body) and the postpubertal, sexually mature body to become split off from one another. Instead of the postpubertal, sexually mature body being available for the expression of the central masturbation fantasy and for the integration of this fantasy into the new sexual body image, as would be the case in normal development, alienation from the sexually mature body means that the fantasies which are expressed via the body are the preoedipal/nonincestuous fantasies via the split-off, nonsexual, idealized body. This then results by the end of adolescence or earlier in the integration of the regressive preoedipal fantasies into the new body image and the simultaneous destruction of the possibility of integrating the functioning genitals as part of the sexual body image—in other words, resulting in established perversion, a combined perverse/psychotic organization (psychotic functioning) or psychosis (Laufer and Laufer, 1984, pp. 36–48; pp. 64–75).

I now assume that if there is to be the likelihood of a continuing and active relationship between the mind and the body, the central masturbation fantasy *must* be able to find expression through the sexually mature body, whether or not it is partially expressed in the relationship to objects or in various forms of displaced or sublimated activities. The need to disown the sexually mature body by some adolescents means disowning the functioning genitals and results, by the end of adolescence, in the integration of a body image without sexually functioning genitals.

Role of Treatment

If the description of the meaning of the presence of severe psychopathology in adolescence is correct, it then also should enable us to define how psychoanalytic treatment, or more specifically how the experience within the transference, may be able to reestablish that continuum of body and mind which is essential for the undoing of psychopathology and which can then also protect the adolescent from future severe disorder. Each adolescent in our study came for help at a time when he either was using his relationships as a vehicle for living out his abnormal sexual fantasies, or he had become aware that he was at risk of expressing these fantasies in ways that could result in his death by suicide. A new kind of internal reasoning began when the treatment, through the use of the transference, addressed itself to those emotions and the constant projections which continued to damage his relationship to himself. Once the adolescent was able to get in touch with his pathological development, he could begin to risk experiencing again the (temporary?) break with reality that took place at the onset of puberty and continued to act as a traumatic warning throughout adolescence. The madness the adolescent felt at puberty had been repressed, but it continued to act as a frightening reminder of the power of the breakdown. Reexperiencing the developmental breakdown in the transference could enable him to understand why he *had to have* the breakdown, and he could then begin to risk reviving his relationship to his body which he had felt compelled to reject or destroy at the time of the breakdown.

An essential characteristic of the pathology of these adolescents is their need to maintain the rupture that had taken place with their pasts, a rupture that was acute at the time of puberty, when it was intended to strengthen the unconscious belief that they could maintain a relationship to their fantasied omnipotent image of themselves. Analytic treatment was threatening or even dangerous because it questioned their need to use this rupture defensively. Puberty and adolescence confronted them unconsciously with the reality of their "failed" sexually mature body and their illusory image of themselves as omnipotent, an image which they could maintain up to the time that they became sexually mature. Before puberty they could maintain the belief that they did not have to be male or female or that they could be omnipotent without being sexual. Physical sexual maturity suddenly shattered this illusion and confronted them with the reality of their body as being inadequate and dangerous at the same time. Their central masturbation fantasy forced them to a sexual answer which sought gratifications that were pregenital and safe but which also removed them from the real world.

If the adolescent's breakdown is to be understood and is to have a chance of becoming integrated as part of his history, the possibility must exist for him to risk allowing continuity between his present and past life. Instead of keeping his past isolated, populated by monsters that must never be confronted, the adolescent can begin to find it possible, as part of his treatment experience, to question what he has done to the memory of his past and to understand the need for his distortions of his experiences and perceptions. This is by no means an academic exercise; the experience and the understanding of the transference enable the adolescent to confront himself with the defensive reasons for the distortions of his relationship to his body in the present and allow him the internal freedom to claim his sexuality as his own rather than as something made up of violence, destructiveness, madness, or thoughts and wishes that perpetuate the attack on his genital sexuality.

But reestablishing a continuity between body and mind in the lives of such severely disturbed adolescents is by no means a certainty, and often results either in partial success or in failure. For example, with Mark the analytic treatment altered his life as regards his ability to study and work. He was able to undertake a course of study, graduated at degree standard, and then was able to find and maintain work. But he was helped less in overcoming his inability to function sexually as a male. In some of our adolescents, as was the case with Mark, their anal masturbation contained the core of their sexuality and enabled them to live out, via their bodies, the belief that they did not have to alter the image of the body because they were complete within themselves. This could be described and dismissed as a resistance to change, but such a description would miss the point. It would be more correct to say that Mark was not able to give up the dependence on the distorted body image, thus still leaving open the possibility of the need to establish perverse sexual relationships. But, at the same time, what has been reestablished through the treatment is the belief that he could establish and maintain an object relationship—a belief which was lost to him before treatment. His life was transformed not only by his new-found ability to study and work, but he could experience the ability to think in a more organized and directed way. It is likely that the danger of severe psychopathology is less than before treatment because he now has some conscious control over his previous helpless feeling of being compelled to behave in certain ways.

Susan's treatment is still going on. She feels that she can now appear normal to others and says she has no need to cut herself or pull out her hair, as if she has lost her need to use this way of showing her internal state to others. But she still does not feel normal. She is aware of her mood swings, and that her active happy times become confused with manic excited states where she loses control over the excitement of using "effort" as a source of gratification. But she is afraid of the depression that she feels she will sink into, which she fantasizes as a state of total inertia where she would feel unable to move or do anything to keep herself alive. The last holiday break, when she felt herself beginning to become depressed and giving up, she resolved her anxiety by the conviction that she had to do the only thing she could still do perfectly, which was to kill herself. She began preparing to do so by tidying up her flat and writing her will. But she was able to become frightened, and told a friend of what she was doing, and said that she needed to be admitted to a hospital.

COMMENT

What can our clinical observations add to the understanding of the body/mind continuum, and specifically to the way in which the developmental function of adolescence is affected when this continuum is disrupted? We have clinical evidence from our adolescents to show that, in each case, a developmental breakdown took place at puberty, and that this developmental breakdown created a serious risk to the adolescent's ability either to maintain a nonpsychotic relation to the external world or to avoid attacking his or her body as a means of removing the reservoir of the perverse or persecuting fantasies.[7] Our clinical experience also suggests, however, that the direction and the severity of the developmental breakdown depend on whether the acute breakdown takes place at the time of puberty or whether the response at puberty is the result of, or reaction to, a pathological oedipal resolution which has led to the establishment of a distorted body image. We think that if the severe disruption took place before puberty, the availability at puberty of physically mature, functioning genitals acts as the organizer toward a perverse or a psychoticlike solution—a solution used defensively to contain the overwhelming anxiety aroused by pubertal development. For these adolescents, the confrontation with the real presence of their mature male or female genitals is experienced as an attack and a potential destruction of the idealized but distorted body image—a prepubertal body image which, in fantasy, contained the perfect but pathological solution.

If this is so, it would help to explain why our therapeutic efforts have been successful in certain areas of their lives, but have been very limited or virtually nil in other areas of their lives, specifically in their sexual lives. We might say that the gratifications obtained from their perverse or psychoticlike solutions are used defensively to ward off the unconscious belief that genital sexuality would mean their own destruction or would unleash a violence which would destroy the sexual

---

7. Some of this is documented in a book (in press) prepared by some of the staff of the Research Centre (see Laufer and Laufer, 1989).

partner or the oedipal parent. This may well be so, and in this sense these young people remain vulnerable to crippling pathology in later life. Stated differently, it may be that the rupture with the past can never really be established emotionally because this would, for them, be to risk being destroyed. The dilemma for them is always there, as expressed by the violence which was common to all of the adolescents, and which was present in their relationships to themselves, to objects, and within the transference. By violence I mean attacks on their own bodies or minds, rather than attacks on people or property, but it is nevertheless a violence which, although it may be gratifying, also expresses the presence of a persecutor who can never quite be silenced.

An associated observation, and perhaps one which is also linked to the reestablishment of a continuum in their developmental lives, is that none of the adolescents in our study killed themselves. This fact has a range of theoretical and clinical explanations, one being that these adolescents experience the Centre's commitment to them as our belief that they are not worthless and that we are not frightened of their hatred of themselves or of the hatred they felt for their fantasied enemies. Our commitment also meant that they no longer had to be alone or feel alone with their pathology.

We are aware that we are only just at the beginning of understanding some of the meanings of the presence of psychopathology in adolescence—or more specifically, of the meaning of the compelling need for some adolescents to destroy their genitality. But we are becoming more convinced that the continued study of the adolescent's relationship to his body, and the reasons why he feels compelled to alter that body and its use, may bring answers to those unknowns which, at present, still limit our ability to stand in the way of crippling pathology.

BIBLIOGRAPHY

FREUD, S. (1924). The loss of reality in neurosis and psychosis. *S.E.*, 19:183–187.

LAUFER, M. (1986). Adolescence and psychosis. *Int. J. Psychoanal.*, 67:367–372.

——— & LAUFER, M. E. (1984). *Adolescence and Developmental Breakdown*. New Haven: Yale Univ. Press.

——— eds. (1989). *Developmental Breakdown and Psychoanalytic Treatment in Adolescence*. New Haven: Yale Univ. Press.

LOEWALD, H. W. (1979). The waning of the oedipus complex. *J. Amer. Psychoanal. Assn.*, 27:751–775.

RITVO, S. (1984). The image and uses of the body in psychic conflict. *Psychoanal. Study Child*, 39:449–469.

APPLIED PSYCHOANALYSIS

Child Analysis and *The Little Prince*

STEVEN LURIA ABLON, M.D.

Moments when the original poet in each of us created
the outside world for us, by finding the familiar in the
unfamiliar, are perhaps forgotten by most people; or
else they are guarded in some secret place of memory
because they are too much like visitations of the gods to
be mixed with everyday thinking.
MILNER, QUOTED BY WINNICOTT (1971b, p. 39)

THE LITTLE PRINCE BY ANTOINE DE SAINT EXUPÉRY (1942) TELLS THE
story of a pilot who, because of an accident with his plane, lands in the
Sahara desert and meets the little prince. This story, which has been
translated into many languages and has been loved by readers young
and old, evokes feelings and concerns that are important to many of us.
I was impressed with how among other powerful themes *The Little
Prince* explores uses of play, imagination, creativity, and integration.
From this perspective *The Little Prince* impressed me as a vehicle for
extending our understanding of play in child analysis. Here, my focus
is primarily on noninterpretive aspects and interventions in analysis.
Bibring (1954) clearly outlines different groups of basic therapeutic
techniques. Technical considerations concerning interpretation and
verbal insight have been discussed at length in the analytic literature. I
would like to use this compelling story to illustrate the way a child uses
the structure of play with the analyst in the analytic setting, that is, to
play with some ideas about play. Although *The Little Prince* has been

I would like to express my appreciation to the Study Group on "The Many Meanings
of Play" sponsored by the Psychoanalytic Research and Development Fund and to the
Ninth International Scientific Colloquium (1987) at the Anna Freud Centre on "Play and
Playing."

helpful to me in thinking about play in child analysis, I would be distressed if such an approach detracted from the importance of St. Exupéry's sensibility and use of language in *The Little Prince*. In addition, although I focus on child analysis, I believe that what is being explored applies equally well to adult analysis and psychoanalytic psychotherapies. Here I agree with Winnicott (1971b): "Whatever I say about children playing really applies to adults as well, only the matter is more difficult to describe when the patient's material appears mainly in terms of verbal communication. I suggest that we must expect to find playing just as evident in the analyses of adults as it is in the case of our work with children. It manifests itself, for instance, in the choice of words, in the inflections of the voice, and indeed in the sense of humour" (p. 46).

In the first chapter of *The Little Prince* St. Exupéry describes how he made "Drawing Number One" (fig. 1) of a boa constrictor digesting an elephant. When he showed this drawing to adults and asked if they were frightened, they answered, "Frighten? Why should any one be frightened by a hat?" St. Exupéry describes how when he drew figure 2, grown-ups discouraged him from making these drawings, suggest-

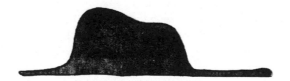

Figure 1.   Drawing Number One

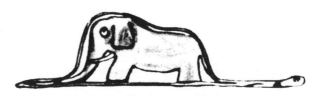

Figure 2.   Drawing Number Two

ing instead that he devote himself to "geography, history, arithmetic and grammar." As a result, St. Exupéry writes, "at the age of six, I gave up what might have been a magnificent career as a painter. I had been disheartened by the failure of my Drawing Number One and my Drawing Number Two. Grown-ups never understand anything by themselves, and it is tiresome for children to be always and forever explaining things to them" (p. 4). Subsequently St. Exupéry adds, "In the course of this life I have had a great many encounters with a great many people who have been concerned with matters of consequence. I have lived a great deal among grown-ups. I have seen them intimately, close at hand. And that hasn't much improved my opinion of them.

"Whenever I met one of them who seemed to me at all clear-sighted, I tried the experiment of showing him my Drawing Number One, which I have always kept. I would try to find out, so, if this was a person of true understanding. But, whoever it was, he, or she, would always say: 'That is a hat.'

"Then I would never talk to that person about boa constrictors, or primeval forests, or stars. I would bring myself down to his level. I would talk to him about bridge, and golf, and politics, and neckties. And the grown-up would be greatly pleased to have met such a sensible man" (p. 5).

The beginning of the story reminded me how difficult it is not to impose our ideas and psychological theories on our child analysands until the children talk to us about "bridge, and golf, and politics." St. Exupéry says, "Boa constrictors swallow their prey whole, without chewing it. After that they are not able to move, and they sleep through six months that they need for digestion" (p. 3). This is perhaps not so different from the time and patience necessary to understand our analysands' play and the importance of not biting in our frustration. Other important themes seem to be the incomprehensibility for the adult of the child's perspective, the child's wish to keep his world to himself, the bitterness of not being understood that one experiences in St. Exupéry's tone and in the metaphor of the snake eating the elephant. This highlights how in the analytic setting the analyst undertakes to try and understand and respect the child's internal world as it is represented in the play. This can be thought of as reflecting the mother's emphatic understanding of the infant, facilitating self-object differentiation and a mutual valuing of the transitional object and the child's play and creativity.

In the second chapter St. Exupéry describes how he has lived alone "without anyone that I could really talk to" (p. 5) until he had an accident with his plane in the Sahara. "Something was broken in my engine. . . . I set myself to attempt the difficult repairs all alone. It was a question of life or death for me." He was "more isolated than a ship-wrecked sailor on a raft in the middle of the ocean" (p. 6). Although usually not explicitly verbalized or conscious, our child analysands often come to us under similar circumstances. St. Exupéry is awakened by the little prince saying, "If you please—draw me a sheep!" Joining in play and creativity are offered as a process on the path of repair. St. Exupéry struggles to draw a sheep that satisfies the little prince. In his attempt to understand the little prince St. Exupéry draws a box with the sheep inside. They are both confident, as Winnicott (1971a) de-scribes, that they are communicating significantly (p. 19). Perhaps this box can also be seen as representing what Winnicott calls the holding environment. The dialogue between St. Exupéry and the little prince about the sheep is reminiscent of how at the beginning of an analysis the analyst sees the analysand's productions as communicative and the child analysand will only gradually and with increasing consciousness share this view. As the dialogue unfolds, the little prince sometimes sounds like an errant analyst, "The little prince, who asked me so many questions, never seemed to hear the ones I asked him. It was from words dropped by chance that, little by little, everything was revealed to me" (p. 10f.). St. Exupéry was fascinated by the planet the little prince came from, perhaps like we puzzle our child analysands as if we came from another planet, especially at the beginning of an analysis.

As St. Exupéry and the little prince get to know each other, St. Exupéry notes, "To forget a friend is sad. Not every one has had a friend" (p. 18). Is this not part of what Winnicott (1958) refers to as "the paradox that the capacity to be alone is based on the experience of being alone in the presence of someone, and that without a sufficiency of this experience the capacity to be alone cannot develop? . . . Now, if I am right in the matter of this paradox, it is interesting to examine the nature of the relationship of the infant to the mother, that which for the purposes of this paper I have called ego-relatedness. It will be seen that I attach a great importance to this relationship, as I consider that it is the stuff out of which friendship is made. It may turn out to be the *matrix of transference*" (p. 418). This aspect of friendship or the physi-cianly attitude is elaborated by Stone (1981); it is an important part of the analytic work and is intertwined with the transference and alliance in a complex way. "The 'love' implicit in empathy, listening and trying to understand, in nonseductive devotion to the task, the sense of full acceptance, respect, and sometimes the homely phenomenon of sheer dependable patience, extending over long periods of time, may take their place as equal or nearly equal in importance to sheer interpretive skill" (p. 114). St. Exupéry reflects the complex interplay of therapeutic alliance and transference. In terms of the alliance, he says, "The proof that the little prince existed is that he was charming, that he laughed, and that he was looking for a sheep. If anybody wants a sheep, that is a proof that he exists" (p. 17). The added aspect of transference can be seen in "I shall certainly try to make my portraits as true to life as possible. But I am not at all sure of success. One drawing goes along all right, and another has no resemblance to its subject. I make some errors, too, in the little prince's height: in one place he is too tall and in another too short. And I feel some doubts about the color of his costume" (p. 19).

As St. Exupéry learns more about the little prince, the subjects that they discuss can be seen as important issues in analysis. First the little prince explains how there are good plants and bad plants coming from good seeds and bad seeds that "sleep deep in the heart of the earth's darkness, until some one among them is seized with the desire to awaken" (p. 21). The little prince explains how the bad seeds give rise to the dangerous, destructive baobab tree. St. Exupéry acknowledges the importance of splitting, anger, and destruction, while emphasizing the urgent and compelling nature of these affects. "Perhaps you will ask me, 'Why are there no other drawings in this book as magnificent and impressive as this drawing of the baobabs?'

"The reply is simple. . . . When I made the drawing of the baobabs I was carried beyond myself by the inspiring force of urgent necessity" (p. 24).

By now the analysis is well under way. St. Exupéry was worried about his breakdown, but with the little prince's help St. Exupéry learns to answer "with the first thing that came into my head" (p. 27) and not to disregard issues such as what use are thorns on flowers because they don't seem to be "Matters of consequence" (p. 28). In this way as an analysis progresses with the help of analyzing defenses, the dialogue moves more toward verbalization and a back and forth between action, fantasy, and language (Santostefano, 1989). This leads to a central theme in *The Little Prince* as well as in analysis. This theme has to do with the centrality of affect, affect as a motivating force (Tompkins, 1962–63, 1981) and play and analysis as ways to communicate, defend against, and transform affect states. This is related to the mother of fusion (Chasseguet-Smirgel, 1984) as well as the oedipal mother. "If some one loves a flower, of which just one single blossom grows in all the millions and millions of stars, it is enough to make him happy just to look at the stars. He can say to himself: 'Somewhere, my flower is there. . .' But if the sheep eats the flower, in one moment all the stars will be darkened . . . And you think that is not important!"

"He could not say anything more. His words were choked by sobbing" (p. 29f.).

> The night had fallen. I had let my tools drop from my hands. Of what moment now was my hammer, my bolt, or thirst, or death? On one star, one planet, my planet, the Earth, there was a little prince to be comforted. I took him in my arms, and rocked him. I said to him:
> "The flower that you love is not in danger. I will draw you a muzzle for your sheep. I will draw you a railing to put around your flower. I will—"
> I did not know what to say to him. I felt awkward and blundering. I did not know how I could reach him, where I could overtake him and go on hand and hand with him once more.
> It is such a secret place, the land of tears [p. 31].

The little prince describes his attempts to understand the flower and his love for her. The flower says, "Of course I love you" (p. 40), but the little prince has decided to go away and leave the planet, a condensed metaphor suggestive of the process of separation and individuation. As the little prince struggles to solve his problems, St. Exupéry's plane needs repairs. Is this not like the workings of displacement, projection, externalization, and the transference in analysis? At the same time the little prince is like different internalized objects that are part of St. Exupéry's efforts at repair and part of the dialogue between inner objects in analysis. In addition, the way in which St. Exupéry and the little prince both grow and repair is not unlike the effects of the dialogue between the analysand and the analyst. Reading *The Little Prince* one wonders where the sexual aspects of the love in this dialogue are. Is it idealized love, romantic love, pregenital love, and why? The little prince leaves his planet "in order to add to his knowledge" (p. 41). First the little prince meets a king whose "rule was not only absolute: it was also universal" (p. 44). For this to be possible, however, the king must only order what is reasonable from other people's point of view. On the other planets the little prince meets a conceited man, a tippler, a businessman, a lamplighter, and a geographer. Does this voyage add to the little prince's knowledge of his different selves, the omnipotent, narcissistic, addicted, obsessive-compulsive, delusional, or absurd and phobic selves? Perhaps the development of a cohesive sense of self takes priority over genital sexuality?

Finally the little prince comes to earth, and when asked why, he replies, "I have been having some trouble with a flower" (p. 70). The little prince comes to a town and sees many roses like his flower. "I thought that I was rich, with a flower that was unique in all the world; and all I had was a common rose. A common rose, and three volcanoes that come up to my knees—and one of them perhaps extinct forever . . . That doesn't make me a very great prince.

"And he lay down in the grass and cried" (p. 78).

As the little prince grieves for his lack of omnipotence and uniqueness, he meets a fox who explains how to tame is "To establish ties" (p. 80). The fox explains, "To me, you are still nothing more than a little boy who is just like a hundred thousand other little boys. And I have no need of you. And you, on your part, have no need of me. To you, I am nothing more than a fox like a hundred thousand other foxes. But if you tame me, then we shall need each other. To me, you will be unique in all the world. To you, I shall be unique in all the world.

"I am beginning to understand," said the little prince. "There is a flower . . . I think that she has tamed me" (p. 80). Again, is this not close to the analytic process, the moving from primary to secondary narcissism (Freud, 1914) and the gradual taming of the instincts (Freud, 1927)? The fox insists that the little prince tame him and explains how it is to be done, "You must be very patient . . . First you will sit down at a little distance from me—like that   in the grass. I shall look at you out of the corner of my eye, and you will say nothing. Words are the source of misunderstandings. But you will sit a little closer to me, every day" (p. 84). This echoes Stern's (1985) observations about the limitations of words in capturing preverbal experience. The fox also outlines the importance of the analytic envelope. "It would have been better to come back at the same hour," said the fox. "If, for example, you come at four o'clock in the afternoon, then at three o'clock I shall begin to be happy. I shall feel happier and happier as the hour advances. At four o'clock, I shall already be worrying and jumping about. I shall show you how happy I am! But if you come at just any time, I shall never know at what hour my heart is to be ready to greet you" (p. 84). Stone (1981) puts it this way, "Most important attitudes are imparted nonverbally—by the timing and duration of silences, by tone of voice and rhetorical nuances in interventions, by facial expression at the beginning and end of hours, by the mood in which realities are dealt with: hours, fees, absences, intercurrent life crises, or other important matters" (p. 109). Saying good-bye the fox emphasizes the central importance of affect and putting in the time. "It is only with the heart that one can see rightly; what is essential is invisible to the eye. . . . It is the time you have wasted for your rose that makes your rose so important" (p. 87).

The little prince and St. Exupéry find a well in the desert, drink the water, and review St. Exupéry's drawings and what they discussed in the past. St. Exupéry feels sad and a little frightened because with his heart he sees termination in this final review. St. Exupéry sees the snake that will bring death, the symbolic death of termination. But this is also the reality of death that is worked and reworked in the play of analysis, play deaths, banishments, separations and losses, explorations of the reversibility and irreversibility of play, the irreversibility of life. In play it seems as if there is no tangible change in reality. At the same time in play there is the exploration of the frightening aspects of chance and helplessness in life, the efforts at mastery through repetition emphasized by Waelder (1933). As the end approaches, St. Exupéry has repaired his engine and he tells the little prince, "my work has been successful, beyond anything that I had dared to hope" (p. 102). St. Exupéry describes his grief, "Once again I felt myself frozen by the sense of something irreparable. And I knew that I could not bear the thought of never hearing that laughter any more. For me, it was like a spring of fresh water in the desert" (p. 102f.).

Six years later St. Exupéry thinks about the little prince, "But there is one extraordinary thing . . . When I drew the muzzle for the little prince, I forgot to add the leather strap to it. He will never have been able to fasten it on his sheep. So now I keep wondering: what is happening on his planet? Perhaps the sheep has eaten the flower" (p. 109). In this way the analytic work continues after termination. Mysteries continue to be explored. In *The Little Prince* perhaps there is St. Exupéry's grieving for many things, including aspects of himself as a child, as the little prince. In the analytic process as in the possibilities of separation from the mother, the possibilities of the transitional object (Winnicott, 1971b), there is the grief that makes possible the transitional space. In this way play and analysis are an expanding of this transitional space making for a kind of creativity that is powerfully felt in *The Little Prince*. This is a life task because, as Winnicott (1971b) wrote, "the task of reality-acceptance is never completed, that no human being is free from the strain of relating inner and outer reality, and that relief from this strain is provided by an intermediate area of experience" (p. 15). I hope St. Exupéry would not mind if I said that analysts, too, travel in the African desert. Then when analysts write to, and talk with, each other, it has the possibility of communicating something unique but seen with the heart, "And, if you should come upon this spot, please do not hurry on. Wait for a time, exactly under the star. Then, if a little man appears who laughs, who has golden hair and who refuses to answer questions, you will know who he is. If this should

happen, please comfort me. Send me word that he has come back"
(p. 113).

BIBLIOGRAPHY

BIBRING, E. (1954). Psychoanalysis and the dynamic psychotherapies. *J. Amer. Psychoanal. Assn.*, 2:745–770.

CHASSEGUET-SMIRGEL, J. (1984). *The Ego Ideal.* New York: Norton.

FREUD, S. (1914). On narcissism. *S.E.*, 14:69–102.

———— (1927). The future of an illusion. *S. E.*, 21:3–56.

SAINT EXUPÉRY, A. (1943). *The Little Prince.* New York: Harcourt Brace Jovanovich.

SANTOSTEFANO, S. (1989). Coordinating outer space with inner self. In *Constructivist Perspectives on Developmental Psychopathology and Atypical Development,* ed. D. P. Keating & M. Rosen. Hillsdale, N.J.: Lawrence Erlbaum (in press).

STERN, D. (1985). *The Interpersonal World of the Infant.* New York: Basic Books.

STONE, L. (1981). Notes on the noninterpretive elements in the psychoanalytic situation and process. *J. Amer. Psychoanal. Assn.*, 29:89–118.

TOMPKINS, S. S. (1962–63). *Affect/Imagery/Consciousness,* 2 vols. New York: Springer.

———— (1981). The quest for primary motives. *J. Pers. Soc. Psychol.*, 41:306–329.

WINNICOTT, D. W. (1958). The capacity to be alone. *Int. J. Psychoanal.*, 39:416–420.

————(1971a). *Therapeutic Consultations in Child Psychiatry.* New York. Basic Books.

———— (1971b). *Playing and Reality.* New York: Basic Books.

WAELDER, R. (1933). The psychoanalytic theory of play. *Psychoanal. Q.*, 2:54–61.

Psychological Change in Jane Austen's *Pride and Prejudice*

RICHARD ALMOND, M.D.

JANE AUSTEN WAS AN ASTUTE OBSERVER OF HUMAN NATURE. HER BEST known novel, *Pride and Prejudice,* has as a major theme the process of psychological change. I will compare Austen's depiction with the psychoanalytic process to help identify universal features of how people change. This approach can be seen as the inverse of that of Spence (1982), who suggests that psychoanalysis can be understood as a process in which analyst and patient strive to interpret the "text" of the analytic dialogue in the manner of literary criticism.

As they develop their romantic bond, the novel's lovers, Elizabeth Bennet and Fitzwilliam Darcy, move from one psychological position to another. They each have some difficulties; they encounter traits and attitudes in themselves that prevent their development. To become partners each must change. This change does not occur in isolation; one serves as a foil for the other, like parent and child or patient and therapist.

In psychoanalysis we observe and participate in a powerful and change-inducing experience. Analysts differ significantly in their opinions about how change comes about (Freud, 1911–15; Frank, 1973; Kohut, 1987; Loewald, 1960; Panel, 1979). There are several reasons for this. The clinical situation is remarkably complex. The analyst, as a participant, has a vision influenced by being "inside" the process. Training leaves the analyst with preconceptions about how change occurs; the patient's resistance obscures much; and the ana-

Clinical associate professor, Department of Psychiatry and Behavioral Sciences, Stanford University School of Medicine. San Francisco Psychoanalytic Institute.

I would like to thank the following for their reviews of the manuscript: the members of the Palo Alto Writers Group; also Drs. Jerome Oremland, Alan Skolnikoff, Stanley Goodman, Kathrine MacVicar, and Michael Zimmerman.

lyst's countertransference may prevent awareness of the full process of change. Finally, agreement between analysts may be obscured by their differing theoretical dialects.

I have found a comparative approach useful in a study of individual change in psychiatric therapeutic communities (Almond, 1974). By comparing cross-cultural examples of a variety of healing groups, cults, and medicine fraternities, I could elucidate a common social organization and individual change process in such an organization. Here I shall use a literary case as a basis for examining how people change in a dyadic relationship. I assume that Jane Austen, an author who spent her life observing and writing about people, can tell us a great deal about how people change (Hardy, 1985; Paris, 1978; Rinaker, 1936). She comments on this interest herself, through the words of her central character:

> "I did not know before," continued Bingley immediately, "that you were a studier of character. It must be an amusing study."
> [Elizabeth:] "Yes, but intricate characters are the most amusing. They have at least that advantage."
> "The country," said Darcy, "can in general supply but few subjects for such study. In a country neighborhood you move in a very confined and unvarying society."
> [Elizabeth:] *"But people themselves alter so much, that there is something new to be observed in them for ever"* [p. 45, my italics].

An author has an interest in the general—that which will touch every reader. Jane Austen wrote about courtship; the difficulties of two young people coming together. The obstacles often seem represented in terms of status and individual reputation, but Austen leaves no doubts about the underlying psychological counterparts.

Pride and Prejudice is primarily about the evolution of Elizabeth Bennet. Every other character remains relatively static, with the exception of Darcy. Darcy's development is largely off stage. In emphasizing Elizabeth, I am taking the orientation of the therapist, who focuses largely on the patient. I shall look primarily at change in Elizabeth, because her mental state is in the foreground. But we must also consider how Darcy alters, and how the juxtaposition of their two states creates the dynamic of change: Darcy's shyness is protected by haughtiness. His disdain provokes Elizabeth. Elizabeth's injured feelings lead her, in turn, to tease and ignore Darcy. Darcy, accustomed to flattery, looks at Elizabeth with new interest. Her unselfconscious devotion to her sister, Jane, and her beautiful eyes complete the conquest of his heart.

This positive valence in Darcy allows the story to progress. Left to herself Elizabeth might remain cool, protecting herself from further slights. Now Darcy's interest provides a tug toward an attachment. When Darcy proposes, she responds with rage at his disdain for her status and family. This encounter is the stimulus for dramatic changes in both. It is the particulars of this mutual influence that I want to examine more closely, and then to compare to change in psychoanalytic process.

THE PSYCHOLOGICAL STORY

Elizabeth Bennet must get from her starting point—unmarried, with few prospects, the second of five daughters, with almost no dowry—to her end point as wife of Fitzwilliam Darcy. For Elizabeth leaving home is particularly difficult. She is in a central position in her family. Her father trusts her judgment above that of her mother and her sisters. He is more attached to her than to her sisters, and respects her more than he does his wife.

Elizabeth begins the novel with a set of intrapsychic conflicts and associated beliefs and feelings about herself and others. She puzzles over her worth. She is valued more than her sisters and her mother by Mr. Bennet, but this is an ambiguous preference. Elizabeth cannot replace Mrs. Bennet. Further, she is her mother's least favorite. In turn, she quietly scorns her mother's embarrassing behavior. Elizabeth's style is teasing and bantering. In this she is identified with her father. Her image of a mature, married woman is a negative one. The marital relationship is one that damages both parties, it makes women blithering and men cynical. Father disparages all women, certainly mother, and only Elizabeth's identification/alliance with him seems to protect her from the same fate.

At 20 Elizabeth faces a developmental task of early adulthood in her time or ours—leaving home. In her society this can only be done successfully through marriage. The task requires sufficient prior resolution of certain development issues. Deficiencies in Elizabeth's experience have interfered. Her identity as a woman is shaky. Attraction to a man, and the sexuality, ambition, and wishes for intimacy it implies are conflicted. These impulses must be denied—Elizabeth spends almost the entire novel oblivious to her attraction to Darcy—or dealt with vicariously as her sisters and friends enter romantic relationships. A narcissistic defense, based on an identification with her father, protects her from awareness of these conflicts.

A wealthy young man, Bingley, leases a nearby estate. At a ball he falls in love with Elizabeth's older sister, Jane. At the same ball Elizabeth is slighted when Bingley's friend, Darcy, comments in her hearing, "She is tolerable, but not handsome enough to tempt me; and I am in no humor at present to give consequence to young ladies who are slighted by other men" (p. 10). Elizabeth quickly copes with this insult by taking a disdainful attitude toward Darcy—the "prejudice" of the novel's title.

Elizabeth's first contact with Darcy is an evocation of earlier defeats, a verification of her worst fear: that she is unworthy. Darcy's disapproval may represent the idea that her wishes for a man are bad and should lead to her being shunned. The rejection resonates with her identification with her mother and her parents' unhappy marriage.

Darcy's insult makes him important in Elizabeth's life, though negatively. The rejecting nature of Darcy's first attention helps Elizabeth hide from herself her real interest in a man of status and property. From this point the psychological story is a series of ups and downs in her perception of Darcy and her feelings and attitude toward him.

Her concerns are the interpersonal, social counterparts to issues that Elizabeth must struggle with internally. To examine the intrapsychic issues, we must look first at Elizabeth's family situation. Mr. Bennet married, out of physical attraction, a woman he does not respect. He uses her and their daughters as the butt of his sarcasm and irony. Only Elizabeth, his favorite, is spared.

While it is flattering for Elizabeth to be the one person in the family whom Mr. Bennet treats with some respect, she is in a dilemma. She can be important in her family of origin, but she cannot move forward to establish a family of her own. Her identification with her mother is a problem, as is her image of marriage. She may know better about couples and relationships, but what she believes is what she has experienced. Early in the story Elizabeth deals with the dilemma by ignoring the issues of marriage and sexuality for herself, while altruistically supporting Jane's hopes for Bingley.

Jane falls ill while on a visit to Bingley's sisters. When Elizabeth rushes on foot across muddy fields to care for her, Darcy's interest is confirmed. He sees her beauty and her capacity for sincere, intense, loving concern. Darcy realizes, half-aware, that Elizabeth is capable of a love he would like to receive! During the visit we discover another element of connection. Darcy himself has an intense affectionate bond with his sister. Here is the having-in-common that is missing in the Bennets senior.

The visit softens the attitudes of both. Darcy realizes that he is in danger of falling in love. Elizabeth observes Darcy's interest, banters and flirts with him, but is less aware of any shift in herself. One way to understand this discrepancy is in terms of the social conventions regarding love to which Austen's characters subscribe. The man is to experience the initial intensity of attraction, while the woman's attraction is to be stimulated and inspired by the man's. But the conventions do what Elizabeth defensively needs to do—deny her interest in Darcy. After all, did Elizabeth need to rush *so* fervently to Jane's side? To whom was she rushing?

Elizabeth's denial is facilitated by meeting George Wickham, a man with grievances against Darcy. And when Darcy prompts Bingley to depart without a word to Jane, her mistrust is further confirmed.

Elizabeth and Darcy are next thrown together for six weeks as neighbors both visiting at Hunsford. Darcy's behavior makes it clear—to the reader, but not to the guarded Elizabeth—that he is in love with her. He stays on at Rosings because she is nearby. When they are together, he stares at her. Elizabeth is faced with a cognitive dissonance: her senses must tell her that Darcy is interested, her mind insists that he does not take her seriously. It is easiest for her to remain convinced that his attitude is condescending, that he is amusing himself at her expense. When Darcy unexpectedly declares his love and proposes, Elizabeth can still maintain her aversion because in the same breath he tells Elizabeth he loves her despite her family's low status and ungenteel behavior.

Although she has acted with polite reserve to Darcy previously, Elizabeth is not disinterested when he proposes. She gives vent to all her injured feelings and indignation. Her attack on Darcy is fortunate for the momentum of the relationship. Her tirade to Darcy contains three important elements. She makes an accusation that is justified—that Darcy has interfered in the relation between Jane and Bingley, and done Jane harm. She makes an accusation that is unfounded—she cites Wickham's grievances against Darcy. She makes Darcy aware of the discrepancy between his behavior and his self-concept—his insulting attitude toward her family and her status is not the behavior of a gentleman.

Darcy hands Elizabeth a letter the following morning. In it he is defensive and self-justifying, but also sincerely concerned, especially in the instance of his effect on Jane. His continuing respect for Elizabeth is indicated by his revealing a family secret: his sister had recently almost been seduced into an elopement by Wickham. This revelation is for Elizabeth the bolt from the blue. Her preconception that Wickham is good and Darcy bad is upset. The underlying psychological structure is upset as well. Elizabeth's self-protecting style of ironic detachment and pride is overturned by her discovering how wrong she has been about both men. She can now begin to entertain a positive interest in Darcy.

If she can consider loving Darcy, then Elizabeth can rehabilitate her attitude toward herself as a woman. While this is externally represented by the honor of a proposal from someone of his rank, it is internally represented by the possibility that the proposal and letter come from someone whom she can respect, someone who will value her.

The reader now feels, "Why can't they talk it over?" But the psychological evolution is not complete. Both Darcy and Elizabeth have much to learn. Elizabeth now knows that Darcy is good, but not that she loves him. Time is needed. Elizabeth returns home to all the relationships and patterns of her past, while questioning herself profoundly. She now feels separate from her parents—by possessing scandalous information about Darcy's sister, by knowledge of Darcy's love for her, and by her internal reevaluation. She now looks at her family with new eyes, from Darcy's critical point of view. This gives her pain.

Austen introduces here a long comment, clearly a reverie of Elizabeth's, on the flaws in her parents' marriage. That she can think about this now is the result of the fantasy stimulated by Darcy's proposal. If Darcy is, in fact, good and worthy, then she can think about marriage, but will it have the outcome of her parents'?

The next meeting between Elizabeth and Darcy is the most romantic. A new understanding of Darcy has broken through her defensive denial of interest. Visiting his large and attractive estate as a tourist, Elizabeth hears affectionate praise for him from the housekeeper. When Darcy appears, unexpectedly, Elizabeth is overcome. Her usual poise is gone—the power of her pull toward him overwhelms her defensive pride and its social expression, her capacity for playful teasing.

Why does the story not end here? It is plain that Darcy and Elizabeth love one another—plain now to *them* as well as to the reader. What interrupts the development of intimacy that follows the meeting at Pemberly? In the events of the story it is the news of her sister Lydia's flight with Wickham. Psychologically, it is the intrusion of impulsive sexuality. For Elizabeth this is a devastating setback. If Lydia's behavior represents Elizabeth's intrapsychic experience, it is the experience of a breakthrough of erotic ideas and impulses, propelled by the sudden rush of love. Elizabeth's reaction is shock, anxiety, and shame. She tells Darcy of Lydia's elopement, while at the same moment assuming that this will be the confirmation of his earlier rejection of her for her family's crassness. It is as though in her sudden realization of love for Darcy, she were loving a forbidden object, so that the next step in love—the erotic urge—has a forbidden meaning. Telling Darcy of Lydia is a confession to the forbidden object.

Elizabeth returns home, preoccupied with restitution of the sexual scandal, and with the well-being of the devastated family. It would seem—at least to the conscious Elizabeth—that she is returning to her psychological state at the outset. Yet she knows that Darcy loves her and that she loves him. It is this knowledge that leads her, when pressed to renounce Darcy by Lady Catherine, to refuse angrily. In doing this she is also proclaiming her autonomy, and asserting that the shame and guilt represented by Lydia do not apply to her. Having mastered the emergence of love and of sexual feeling, she no longer feels guilty and unworthy. She can choose Darcy as a psychological equal.

THE FICTIONAL RELATIONSHIP AND THERAPEUTIC PROCESS

My thesis is that the evolving relationship between the protagonists of *Pride and Prejudice* is comparable to a psychoanalytic process, and that we can learn from the parallel. To pursue this argument requires a framework for comparison. There are many different models and discussions of analytic process (e.g., Abrams, 1987; Freud, 1911–15; Kohut, 1984; Loewald, 1960; Schafer, 1983; Weinshel, 1984; Weiss and Sampson, 1987). Each of them speaks to some significant aspect of the complex interaction that occurs in the analytic relationship. For purposes of comparing the novel with the therapeutic process I propose a simple framework involving three elements: the *engagement* of the parties to change; the *mutual influence* they have upon one another; the source of *directionality* in the impact of one upon another.

One assumption should be made clear. It concerns whether the change process is viewed as *intrapsychic* in the *patient*, as *intrapsychic* within *both patient and analyst*, or as involving the system of *both psyches and their interaction* (Abrams, 1987). For my purposes only the last view is reasonable. The idea that the analytic process goes on *only* within the patient is a convenient, simplifying fiction that allows the practicing analyst to think about the patient's psyche as it evolves. But individual process cannot be isolated from its interpersonal context. The Heisenberg uncertainty phenomenon is frequently cited to support this view. I would argue from sciences that are closer to the data of psychoanalysis—ethology and anthropology—that humans are by nature interactive. The capacity for transference, in the broadest sense of the tendency to project personalized meanings out of past experience, is universal and constantly at play (Bird, 1972; Kohut, 1971). In the analytic situation we maximize the likelihood of the patient expressing these internally dominated meanings.

The analyst's style of involvement has a significant impact on the patient. Intervening infrequently and unpredictably increases the effect of the intervention on the patient. While the analyst seeks to intervene in relation to the most salient resistance to free association, the patient frequently reacts in terms of the subjective transference meaning of the intervention.

The reaction of the patient to the analyst's interventions in turn has an impact on the analyst, who seeks to deal with it in an ego-dominated manner. But as the extensive literature on countertransference indicates, the dispassionate analyst is neither real nor desirable. The working analyst allows for his or her emotional reaction to the patient and uses this to formulate the next intervention. While the analyst tries to make the internal process ego-dominated, the subsequent reaction to the patient (in the form of the next intervention) will reflect the composite of the analyst's emotional and cognitive response.

This more complex view of the analytic relationship makes it possible to view Elizabeth and Darcy in comparison with the analytic process. Elizabeth is in the foreground, but her behavior has a crucial impact on Darcy, an impact in turn that influences him and the subsequent effect he has upon her.

ENGAGEMENT

Darcy has Elizabeth's interest implicitly at the outset, since he is eligible. The first sentence of the novel is: "It is a truth *universally* acknowledged, that a single man in possession of a good fortune must be in want of a wife" (my italics).

In other words, Austen tells us, Darcy is of interest by definition. He has great wealth and noble connections. In our words, Darcy's status instantly evokes a powerful, but nonspecific transference. How does Darcy respond? Like a therapist, Darcy does not gratify this interest. In fact, he does something that hurts: he slights her. While the analyst at the outset of treatment does not intend to slight the patient, his initial role behavior has a similar effect—expected social responses are withheld, the patient is frustrated.

More specifically Darcy's initial "intervention" reevokes in Elizabeth the entire set of issues we have examined: her poor self-image, her ambivalence toward men and marriage. While the seeming effect of Darcy's behavior is to alienate her, she is involved. Her defensive response of derision acknowledges this: "Elizabeth remained with no very cordial feelings toward him. She told the story, however, with great spirit among her friends; for she had a lively, playful disposition, which delighted in anything ridiculous" (p. 11).

At their next meeting Darcy puzzles Elizabeth by his intense presence, his steady nonverbal attentiveness to her. Curiosity is added to her pique. The psychoanalyst can point out that Darcy has inadvertently created an ambiguity that allows Elizabeth to project onto Darcy meanings associated with fundamental issues, including the form of her oedipal romance. This powerful, attractive man disdains her, yet remains interested, perhaps to enjoy his superiority, like her father. The ambiguity of Darcy's behavior serves Elizabeth much as does the analyst's: interest without clear definition of attitude and involvement.

A wide variety of terms is used to describe the elements of the engagement aspect of the clinical situation. Just as Elizabeth is involved by a combination of hurt and interest, the elements of engagement in therapy are complex. They include positively tinged qualities of the special situation of therapy—positive transference, trust, holding, unconditional positive regard, empathic listening—as well as more neutrally intended aspects of the relationship—therapeutic alliance. As in *Pride and Prejudice*, there are initially negative and more primitive feelings that patients find so frightening. There is the anxious expectation that these impulses, desires, and action patterns will emerge more clearly under these conditions.

The wide variety of terms to describe this aspect of treatment is reflective, I believe, not so much of irreconcilable differences in theories, but of the complexity of the patient-therapist engagement, along with the variety of characteristics each party may bring to it.

The therapist's initial responses must form a "match" with the patient that the patient will experience as recognizable, but challenging. We do not respond to the patient's words in a conventional social manner. In the face of highly emotional material we may remain reflective; when emotion is missing, we may ask about it. We are looking constantly for that which social rules conspire to keep out of conversation.

Within this initial engagement are the seeds of the two other aspects of the process. The participants do not know what form the process will take. Elizabeth would deny well into her story that she is involved in a powerful attachment. And patients, while they have entered into treatment, will resist an awareness of both the feelings they have about the therapist and knowing that they are resisting this awareness (Gill, 1982).

In *Pride and Prejudice* engagement has a largely built-in propellant—the developmental press to bond in marriage. Property and status are powerful, both as external signifiers and as counterparts to internal issues of self-concept. Darcy is of interest to Elizabeth because he is wealthy and important, though she could not admit it. These traits initially correspond to her internal concept of herself as the oedipal victor, the most important woman in her family.

It is, in fact, the slap in the face of Darcy's initial disdain that provokes her interest. She will prove her worth—by showing him the same sort of indifference! This intrigues Darcy. At the novel's end Elizabeth reviews his attraction to her:

> [Elizabeth to Darcy:] "Now, be sincere; did you admire me for my impertinence?"
>
> "For the liveliness of your mind, I did."
>
> "You may as well call it impertinence at once. It was very little less. The fact is, that you were sick of civility, of deference, of officious attention. You were disgusted with the women who were always speaking and looking and thinking for your approbation alone. I roused and interested you, because I was so unlike them" [p. 420].

But there is attraction as well, and soon love on Darcy's side. This leads to his (for Elizabeth) puzzling show of interest. Both parties are caught in a tension of interest, denial, and underlying intense engagement. This engagement involves the very personality elements and conflicts that are preventing their further psychological development.

MUTUAL INFLUENCE

Engagement must be followed by a continuing pattern of interaction that both maintains involvement and steers toward change. Change is a much less likely psychological event than stasis. The ego strives for equilibrium (Hartmann, 1939). Even developmental change occurs in the face of resistance. In a sense, the psyche must be misled into change. In the novel as well as in treatment change occurs through an extensive series of interactions, whether these are conceptualized as interactions around resistances (Weinshel, 1984), tests (Weiss and Sampson, 1987), corrections in developmental disturbances (Settlage, 1985), or explorations of empathic failure (Kohut, 1971).

I subsume all these in the general category of mutual influence. Engagement sets the stage; mutual influence requires that a drama take place upon it. It also refers to the attunement of the two partners in the process of change. Engagement must be followed by a continuing pattern of interaction that both maintains involvement and promotes change. The effect of Darcy's initial snub of Elizabeth is to begin a series of interactions. Each action by one of the two has a particular impact upon the other. The impact, in turn, evokes a further counter-reaction. Darcy insults; Elizabeth is angry, but affected. Darcy shows interest; Elizabeth is cool and reserved, but curious. Darcy proposes; Elizabeth is enraged, but flattered. Darcy writes her; she is abashed and self-critical. Each step has its intrapsychic counterpart. Moving from one state to another provides Elizabeth with the opportunity of recognizing certain habitual modes of perceiving and judging, and ultimately these provide the impetus for change.

The process that brings about the possibility of internal change has an external, behavioral component. In this way mutual influences occur. Darcy is changed as well as Elizabeth. From the point of view of Elizabeth's process Darcy's changes bring out different and conflicting aspects of her psychology. By becoming an admirer, Darcy appeals to the high self-esteem side of Elizabeth, but evokes conflicts having to do with sexuality and competition. By being critical, Darcy impels Elizabeth to look at her defensive character style and ultimately to pass a test of self-scrutiny. In the symmetry of the novel Darcy is changed and improved correspondingly. He attests to it clearly in a reflection near the end of the novel:

> Painful recollections will intrude, which cannot, which ought not, to be repelled. I have been a selfish being all my life, in practice, though not in principle. As a child, I was taught what was right; but I was not taught to correct my temper. I was given good principles, but left to follow them in pride and conceit. Unfortunately, an only son (for many years an only child), I was spoiled by my parents, who though good themselves . . . allowed, encouraged, almost taught me to be selfish and overbearing—to care for none beyond my own family circle, to think meanly of all the rest of the world, to wish at least to think meanly of their sense of worth compared with my own. Such I was, from eight to eight and twenty; and *such I might still have been but for you*, dearest, loveliest Elizabeth! *What do I not owe you? You taught me a lesson, hard indeed at first, but most advantageous.* By you I was properly humbled [p. 408; my italics].

Elizabeth's stay at Netherfield to care for Jane provides occasion for several important internal developments. One concerns attitudes toward female rivals. Elizabeth demonstrates her love and devotion toward a loved sister, while withstanding courageously the barbs of Bingley's sisters. Protected by her desexualized role as nurse and sister, Elizabeth shows herself equal to her social superiors. All this occurs in front of Darcy, though Elizabeth would deny that it is for his benefit. She is working out concerns having to do with control over rivalrous situations. Unlike Miss Bingley, who openly fawns over Darcy, Elizabeth can keep cool in Darcy's presence and not slip into sycophancy or jealous anger.

This visit also gives Elizabeth opportunities to deal with Darcy on a daily basis. She musters her characteristic style of teasing, quick-wittedness, and irony to banter with him. In her transference Elizabeth is standing up to the father who scorns women. Darcy's interest must flatter her, but she protects herself from positive feelings. In many therapies, the positive side of the relationship is the most frightening for the patient. It is safer for Elizabeth to split her transference and feel the positive interest in Wickham. With him there is less conflict, even while there is no love. He is flattering and satisfies the wish for easy recognition and preference. He validates Elizabeth's feelings of past injury. She does not have to modify the resentment that Darcy has stirred and the older issues it represents—whether oedipal defeat, maternal rejection, or displacement by younger sisters.

At this point in an analysis we would say that Elizabeth has developed a transference neurosis. She is experiencing in her current relations a new version of earlier, inner experiences and conflicts and the associated defenses. Darcy, Wickham, Bingley's sisters, and other characters in lesser degree represent significant prior objects. Elizabeth has wrapped herself in a protective mantle of critical, teasing, ironic attitudes that make her safe from the feelings these figures arouse. Anxieties about her female identifications are allayed by transferring her concern from herself to Jane. Others might enlighten her and bring her projections in line with reality, but they do not: Darcy could let her know the truth about Wickham and about his feelings. Like the analyst, he lets things develop further, though inadvertently.

The period of Elizabeth's visit at Hunsford intensifies internal tensions and then brings them to a head in the climactic proposal episode. Darcy's steady, silent show of interest, his visits to the parsonage, his explanation of his earlier behavior to her—Elizabeth absorbs the meaning of none of these actions consciously. If anything, since she must be sensing his attitude unconsciously, she heightens her defensive view. When Darcy proposes, Elizabeth explodes in indignation. Her reaction *has* a basis in reality: Darcy is setting his pride above his gentleman's manners; Jane *was* mistreated; Elizabeth is being condemned for a family that she cannot help. But the true source of her feeling is in her neurotic conflicts.

At this moment Elizabeth's initial psychological position is confirmed in each respect. Her latent negative self-view is confirmed by Darcy's criticism; her idea of marriage is confirmed by the idea of wedding a man who loves, but cannot respect; her anger at men for depreciating women is provoked; and her narcissistic defensive stance is strengthened. All of this also serves to control sexual impulses that Darcy has implicitly called forth by proposing. It is far safer to return to the family home and its substitutive satisfactions.

In terms of analytic process this phase of the fictional relationship can be seen as the intensification of the transference neurosis, which often occurs unconsciously or preconsciously. The analyst's interpretation of elements of the transference neurosis are often greeted with the same sort of surprise, denial, and indignation as Elizabeth's, and for similar reasons. Consciousness of the emergence of conflicted issues intensifies defenses and resistance increases, at least temporarily.

Then comes Darcy's letter. Austen portrays the sequence of Elizabeth's inner states vividly. Initially she reads only for confirmation of her convictions. Then when she absorbs the significance of the revelations about Wickham, she is shaken; the whole structure of attitudes and feelings she has developed is invalid.

> She grew absolutely ashamed of herself. Of neither Darcy nor Wickham could she think without feeling that she had been blind, partial, prejudiced, absurd.
>
> "How despicably have I acted!" she cried; "I, who have prided myself on my discernment! I, who have valued myself on my abilities! who have often disdained the generous candor of my sister, and gratified my vanity in useless or blamable distrust. How humiliating is this discovery! yet, how just a humiliation! Had I been in love, I could not have been more wretchedly blind. But vanity, not love, has been my folly. Pleased with the preference of one, and offended by the neglect of the other, on the very beginning of our acquaintance, I have courted prepossession and ignorance, and driven reason away, where either were concerned. *Till this moment I never knew myself*" [p. 229; my italics].

This is the sort of self-recognition that we mean by "insight." Elizabeth has a sudden new picture of herself, one obtained in an intensely charged situation. Elizabeth does not alter instantaneously. Her assumptions have been shaken. She needs time to assimilate the implications of the new information and what it tells her about herself and about Darcy. Darcy, too, needs time. He has been shaken himself by Elizabeth's reaction. Since he knows that he loves, it is somewhat easier for him to readjust his view of her and himself. Viewing Darcy for our purposes as the therapist, his adjustment at this point involves his altering in a way that will reach Elizabeth effectively. He must account for her resistances.

The resolution of Elizabeth's issues is not simple. Darcy's letter has a different impact on various aspects of her conflict. She is enhanced by Darcy's regard, but at the same time her negative identifications are reinforced, for Darcy's judgment cannot now be lightly dismissed. Elizabeth's resentment of men has been vented, but then shown to be subjectively based. Most important, her narcissistic defenses are shaken, though the hysterical ones remain largely intact. It is also important that Elizabeth is separated from her family by these events. She thinks, "How much I shall have to conceal!"

A reverie on her parents' relationship is from Elizabeth's point of view. While it seems to focus on her father's permissiveness and her mother's vicarious infatuation with army officers, it is also about Elizabeth's new concern—that she be upright enough in self and family to satisfy Darcy's values. Though she banters with Jane about Darcy and denies to herself interest in him, the reverie indicates that she is moving away from her identification with Mr. Bennet's ironic detachment to a new attitude closer to Darcy's: a concern about principles and an acknowledgment that other people are truly important to her.

Mutual influence is an important component of working through. The analyst responds out of a combination of reactivity and reserve. The analyst is not disinterested, but his interests are different from the patient's. His responses provide psychologically new experiences for the patient. New perspectives on oneself require repeated iterations to become established. Because the patient will discount automatic, uninvolved responses quickly, the therapist must remain personally involved in his responses to the patient.

The lovers of *Pride and Prejudice* have an easier time than most therapist-patient dyads. They are propelled by a normal developmental impulse to bond, rather than by a wish to relieve troubling, established symptoms. Each presents the other with challenges and encouragements, and thus they succeed. All therapists have had experiences of brief consultations where the relief of a few impediments has led to a rapid improvement. In long-term therapy the therapist has a more difficult task because the patient is less interested in change. Because of the reluctance to change, the mutual influence process must have a bias.

DIRECTIONALITY

In analysis directionality is created by the analyst's remaining true to the values of the analytic process. Gradually the patient gives increasing weight to these values, which become merged with elements of the patient's ego ideal. This is what we mean, I believe, by ego dominance and identification with the analyst late in analysis. In *Pride and Prejudice* a major issue in the circular process between the two lovers is whether better values will predominate. Will Elizabeth's need for superficial admiration lead to her preferring Wickham over Darcy? Will her identification with her father prevent her from loving? Will Darcy's pride ruin not only *his* chance for love but Bingley's and Jane's as well?

In the circular process of mutual influence there is a tension which tests and at the same time pulls toward the ideal. Elizabeth's rejection is, as Darcy eventually acknowledges, the jolt he needed to repair a distorted view of himself and his world. She has brought him up to her level. He does not say, or feel, that she had some pride-swallowing to do herself.

After Darcy's letter Elizabeth is self-critical. She sees that Darcy is well-intentioned, and she strives now to be worthy of him. Part of this pull for Elizabeth is represented in terms of manners and so-cial/economic status. Various characters represent flagrant economic or social ambition. On the one hand, Elizabeth is above these, and Darcy admires this. On the other, Elizabeth experiences her family's crassness as a measure of herself, especially when Lydia runs off. She is convinced that Darcy will not have her now; he is too good for her. What Elizabeth is struggling with is the adequacy of her defenses once ironic detachment and hysterical denial have been stripped away. In effect she is thinking, "Without these do I have the ability to restrain the impulses to be (inappropriately) sexual, excessively aggressive? Am I capable of being the kind of person whom Darcy would respect?"

In other words, the directional pull of their influence on each other is toward that which each esteems. Each aspires and is pulled by love and painful self-examination toward the standard that the other comes to represent.

The role of the housekeeper, as of Jane earlier, speaks to another aspect of Elizabeth's conflict—the transfer of attachment from women to men. Because of the difficulties with identification and her view of marriage, Elizabeth fears and denies interest in men and associated sexuality. Here the feminine voices of encouragement give her the push she needs to overcome her hysterical unawareness. She can move from her unambivalent, close bond with her sister to one with a man.

Having mobilized the most central tendencies of the patient through the process of mutual influence, the therapist proposes a way out. He says, "Look, you are feeling like a child, and acting like one. You could try looking at all this from another point of view—mine, an adult one. As you do so, you may be able to see more clearly what you are involved in, and how you stay with it instead of moving ahead." Loewald (1960) suggests that the analyst, like the good mother, has in mind expectations that are just "ahead" of the patient developmentally.

I believe that the mechanism of directionality involves self-esteem. Self-concept lies at the interface of the intrapsychic and the interpersonal. Internally our egos are engaged in maintaining a complex homeostasis in which stability is balanced against change. In the context of treatment we speak of these two tendencies as the repetition compulsion and the wish for mastery. Every interaction puts this balance in play. Contact with someone who is perceived as having higher status creates the possibility of our acquiring the power we attribute to that status. With it we hope that we can improve self-esteem. Usually such changes are short-lived, because homeostatic mechanisms are not disturbed. But in treatment, and in the novel here, the relationship allows the impulse toward mastery to predominate.

Elizabeth begins with a conflicted sense of her worth. Prized by her father, and identified with him, she is superior to others; but for this relation she must be guilty and anxious, which makes her superiority brittle. Her identification with her mother further weakens her self-esteem. Seen in this way Darcy is, alternately, the father imago who arouses interest but bad self-feelings, and then the therapeutic good parent, who encourages her that she can rise above her prejudices. In the sense of Weiss and Sampson (1987) both Elizabeth herself and Darcy as seen by Elizabeth must pass "tests"—the shedding of old defenses, the capacity for change, and the adequacy of remaining defenses.

Darcy by his own admission has a similar problem. He holds to an old, but brittle superiority, which prevents attachments outside a family that consists now only of an adoring younger sister. By teasing him Elizabeth puts into play his wish for real, contemporary love and approbation. When he states his love in a superior, insulting way, she upbraids and rejects him. To win her he must aspire to a higher ideal, the gentleman. When he does, she can love him.

Austen sees the limitations of the capacity for change. Thus she recognizes what Kohut (1971) refers to as the need for properly attuned selfobjects. Elizabeth cannot solve the dilemma of sexuality on her own. It takes Darcy's active intervention to do this, when he rectifies the uncontrolled behavior of Lydia. Also important in the critical transition of their relationship is Darcy's capacity to identify his empathic failure in disrupting Bingley's relationship with Jane. His correction of his error extends to aiding the Bennets in the rescue of Lydia, symbolically participating in the development of Elizabeth's internal defensive capacities. Kohut would call this development of Elizabeth the product of transmuting internalization.

Both major characters experience moments of insight, intense awareness concerning contradictions in how they interpret their experience and a more objective reality. These flashes of insight have what Rothenberg (1988) calls Janusian quality, when two seemingly contradictory motivations or perceptions are entertained at the same moment, allowing a creative, new solution to develop. As Elizabeth reads and re-reads Darcy's letter of explanation the morning following his proposal, she sets side by side her earlier, neurotic transference images of him, herself, and others with a new set of images of each. Rather than simply abandoning one for another, she sees and gradually can make full use of the knowledge about herself that the realization provides.

SUMMARY

In the spirit of Jerome Frank's (1973) pioneering studies of universal characteristics in psychotherapeutic change, I have tried to demonstrate that character development in *Pride and Prejudice* can be understood in terms of psychoanalytic process. In the course of this thesis certain observations have emerged. Change occurs in the context of a relationship intense enough to disturb the tendency of personality to homeostasis (engagement). The change-inducing relationship is composed of a sequence of effects and countereffects (mutual influence). For these influences to be salutory (therapeutic) there must be a directional pull provided by the attitude of the primary agent of change, a pull that resonates with important motivations of the object of change (directionality).

In *Pride and Prejudice* we recurrently found self-concept, and particularly the question of worth, to be an important interface of these phenomena. As therapists we are familiar with this as a clinical issue. Study of the novel suggests that self-esteem may play a central role in motivating therapeutic change. This observation raises intriguing unanswered questions regarding the conceptualization of self-esteem in psychoanalytic thinking.

BIBLIOGRAPHY

ABRAMS, S. (1987). The psychoanalytic process. *Int. J. Psychoanal.*, 68:441–452.
ALMOND, R. (1974). *The Healing Community.* New York: Jason Aronson.
AUSTEN, J. (1813). *Pride and Prejudice.* New York: Washington Square Press, 1982.
BIRD, B. (1972). Notes on transference. *J. Amer. Psychoanal. Assn.*, 20:267–301.

FRANK, J. (1973). *Persuasion and Healing*, 2nd ed. Baltimore: Johns Hopkins Univ. Press.

FREUD, S. (1911–15). Papers on technique. *S.E.*, 12:89–171.

GARIS, R. (1968). Learning experiences and change. In *Critical Essays on Jane Austen*, ed. B. Southam. London: Routledge & Kegan Paul.

GILL, M. M. (1982). *The Analysis of Transference*. New York: Int. Univ. Press.

HARDY, J. (1985). *Jane Austen's Heroines*. Boston: Methuen.

HARTMANN, H. (1939). *The Ego and the Problem of Adaptation*. New York: Int. Univ. Press, 1958.

KOHUT, H. (1971). *The Analysis of the Self*. New York: Int. Univ. Press.

———(1984). *How Does Analysis Cure?* Chicago: Univ. Chicago Press.

Loewald, H. W. (1960). On the therapeutic action of psychoanalysis. *Int. J. Psychoanal.*, 41:16–33.

PANEL (1979). Conceptualizing the nature of therapeutic action of psychoanalysis. M. Scharfman, reporter. *J. Amer. Psychoanal. Assn.*, 27:627–642.

PARIS, B. (1978). *Character and Conflict in Jane Austen's Novels*. Detroit: Wayne State Univ. Press.

RINAKER, C. (1936). A psychoanalytic note on Jane Austen. *Psychoanal. Q.*, 5:108–115.

ROTHENBERG, A. (1988). *The Creative Process of Psychotherapy*. New York: Norton.

SCHAFER, R. (1983). *The Analytic Attitude*. New York: Basic Books.

SETTLAGE, C. F. (1985). Adult development and therapeutic process. Read at the Edward G. Billings' Lectureship on Clinical Implications of Adult Development, Denver, Colorado.

SPENCE, D. P. (1982). *Narrative Truth and Historical Truth*. New York: Norton.

WEINSHEL, E. M. (1984). Some observations on the psychoanalytic process. *Psychoanal. Q.*, 53:63–92.

WEISS, J. & SAMPSON, H. (1987). *The Psychoanalytic Process*. New York: Guilford Press.

A Note on "The Theme of the Three Caskets"

EUGENE J. MAHON, M.D.

SIGMUND FREUD HAD THE CAPACITY OF A GENIUS FOR DIPPING HIS MIND IN Shakespeare and running off with insights no one else would have noticed. In "The Theme of the Three Caskets" his attention was captured by a minor theme in *The Merchant of Venice*. Why he focused on this theme to the neglect of others is the subject matter of this brief speculative communication.

When one thinks of *The Merchant of Venice,* certain themes rush to mind more rapidly than others, given their gripping emotional intensity:

1. Shylock demanding a pound of flesh from Antonio for failure to repay the loan on time;

2. Shylock's poignant speech against prejudice;

> I am a Jew. Hath not a Jew eyes? Hath not a Jew hands, organs, dimensions, senses, affections, passions? fed with the same food, hurt with the same weapons, subject to the same diseases, healed by the same means, warmed and cooled by the same winter and summer, as a Christian is? If you prick us, do we not bleed? if you tickle us, do we not laugh? if you poison us, do we not die? and if you wrong us, shall we not revenge? If we are like you in the rest, we will resemble you in that. If a Jew wrong a Christian, what is his humility? Revenge. If a Christian wrong a Jew, what should his sufferance be by Christian example? Why, revenge. The villany you teach me I will execute, and it shall go hard but I will better the instruction.

3. Portia's remarkable speech about the quality of mercy;

Faculty, Columbia University Psychoanalytic Center for Training and Research; assistant clinical professor of psychiatry, College of Physicians and Surgeons, Columbia University, New York.

The quality of mercy is not strain'd,
It droppeth as the gentle rain from heaven
Upon the place beneath: it is twice bless'd;
It blesseth him that gives and him that takes:
'Tis mightiest in the mightiest; it becomes
The throned monarch better than his crown;
His sceptre shows the force of temporal power,
The attribute to awe and majesty,
Wherein doth sit the dread and fear of kings;
But mercy is above this sceptred sway,
It is enthroned in the hearts of kings,
It is an attribute to God himself,
And earthly power doth then show likest God's
When mercy seasons justice.

4. Her clever defeat of Shylock granting him his right to take a pound of Antonio's flesh but warning him that he is not entitled to any of Antonio's blood, so he must take flesh only and shed no drop of blood or he will forfeit all his holdings to the state. Shylock cannot comply with such an interpretation of the letter of the law. The villain is thwarted and the rest of the cast lives happily ever after.

5. The theme of the three caskets: Portia's choice of a husband will be decided by a primitive type of lottery. Her portrait is hidden in one of three caskets. The suitor must choose among gold, silver, and lead caskets. Her portrait is hidden in the lead casket. Bassanio, less opinionated than the Prince of Morocco or the Prince of Arragon who choose gold and silver, wins Portia's hand in marriage by choosing lead.

It is this theme of the three caskets which captures Freud's interest. He argues that the three caskets are a disguised representation of the Three Sisters, "the Fates, the Moerae, the Parcae or the Norns, the third of whom is called Atropos, the inexorable" (p. 296).

Freud uses *King Lear* as a further confirmation of his theory. If Freud needed far-fetched intuitive gymnastics to pull the Fates out of the three caskets,[1] in *Lear* the proof he was seeking was more obvious: an aged king at death's door, so to speak, plans to divide his kingdom between his three daughters. The youngest daughter refuses to flatter

---

1. Freud traced the "lead casket" through many disguises before he finally identified it as a representation of the third "fatal" sister. Casket, as he had already argued in the interpretation of dreams, is a symbol of woman. In *The Merchant of Venice*, Bassanio addressed the leaden casket, saying, "Thy paleness moves me more than eloquence" (p. 294). This "dumbness" of the lead and the dumbness of the third sister in many fairy tales (Cinderella comes immediately to mind) Freud equates with death.

him after the sycophantic manner of her elder sisters. She is disowned
for her lack of guile. At the end of the play, he carries her dead body on
stage, but not before he realizes her true if quieter virtue and his own
folly for being duped by clever speeches. Freud argues that though the
play has a wise lesson to offer: "one should not give up one's posses-
sions and rights during one's lifetime, and that one must guard against
accepting flattery at its face value" (p. 300), the profound effect of the
play lies in a deeper level of tragic meaning.

> Lear is an old man. It is for this reason, as we have already said, that the
> three sisters appear as his daughters. The relationship of a father to his
> children, which might be a fruitful source of many dramatic situations,
> is not turned to further account in the play. But Lear is not only an old
> man: he is a dying man. In this way the extraordinary premiss of the
> division of his inheritance loses all its strangeness. But the doomed man
> is not willing to renounce the love of women; he insists on hearing how
> much he is loved. Let us now recall the moving final scene, one of the
> culminating points of tragedy in modern drama. Lear carries Cordelia's
> dead body on to the stage. Cordelia is Death. If we reverse the situation it
> becomes intelligible and familiar to us. She is the Death-goddess who,
> like the Valkyrie in German mythology, carries away the dead hero from
> the battlefield. Eternal wisdom, clothed in the primaeval myth, bids the
> old man renounce love, choose death and make friends with the necessi-
> ty of dying [p. 301].

Freud's argument in an existential nutshell seems to be that man faced
with the realization of death softens the blow with aesthetic reversals of
reality in which the inevitable (death) rather than being suffered pas-
sively is chosen actively and turned into its opposite (romantic love).
This paper was written years before the appearance of Eros and
Thanatos in Freud's publications, but the seeds of "beyond the pleasure principle" had already begun to sprout, it would seem.

Freud's tone is decidedly modest at the beginning of his paper, even
though he will later, as we have seen, drag the reader into some dark
corridors of the mind. "Two scenes from Shakespeare, one from a
comedy and the other from a tragedy, have lately given me occasion for
posing and solving a small problem" (p. 289). The small problem, so
modestly introduced, seems to lead him inexorably toward the riddle
of death and man's ambivalence in accepting it or denying it. Given all
this insistence on death symbolism in *The Merchant of Venice* and *King
Lear,* one wonders why Freud did not seek *confirmatory associations for his
theory in the text under consideration.* He would have found a convincing
associative proof of his hypothesis in Shylock's wish to kill Antonio,

especially so given the manner of revenge Shylock had in mind for him.[2]

> If I should catch him once upon the hip
> I will feed fat the ancient grudge I bear him.

Shylock plans to cut a pound of flesh from Antonio's body. When Portia foils Shylock by insisting he take no blood, only flesh, surely all thinkable reversals have crystallized in this devilish denouement that Shakespeare presents us. Portia (the third sister of the Fates signifying death) disguises herself as a male judge whose mission it is to trick Shylock, thereby fooling Death, so to speak. The image of taking flesh without spilling blood can be seen as a macabre symbol of natural death: the body decays losing flesh, pound after pound taken away without bloodshed.[3] One is reminded of Robert Frost's arresting image of death in nature in general: "the slow smokeless burning of decay."

Is it not a puzzle therefore that Freud, whose intellect seemed to thrive on finding associations where others might miss the tributaries of meaning completely, neglected a seemingly obvious one? While it is impossible to reach into the creative ferment of the mind of a genius three quarters of a century after the fact and get hold of the gestational process *in statu nascendi*, the scanty historical evidence in our possession does excite some wild psychoanalytic speculations.

In *Freud: Living and Dying* Max Schur (1972) informs us:

> The conception of the paper on the "Three Caskets" took shape, according to Freud's correspondence, in the space of a few day in June, 1912, just after Freud's visit to Binswanger in Kreuzlingen when his young friend in the prime of life was facing a dim prognosis after surgery. Binswanger's crisis had in turn been preceded by an illness of Freud's mother, who was then 77 years old [p. 274].

This may not seem like too momentous a stimulus for the conception of a paper, unless one examines the visit to Kreuzlingen a little more deeply.

Here is a longer excerpt from Schur's work which supplies a highly conflictual context to the visit to Kreuzlingen:

> Jung did not know why Freud had gone to visit Binswanger in Kreuzlingen (which is not far from Zürich), and he felt jealous and slighted because Freud had not visited him during the same trip or at least arranged for a meeting. Actually, as it turned out later, Freud had notified Jung in time, but the latter had been out of town and had not

---

2. Freud makes no mention of Shylock or the "pound of flesh" throughout the paper!

3. If one were a riddle-maker, an arresting one would be: Question: What steals all flesh without spilling blood? Answer: Death by natural causes.

checked the date of arrival of Freud's letter. Jung kept referring in his increasingly irritable correspondence to the "Kreuzlingen gesture." Freud wrote Binswanger on July 29, 1912 that he was trying to separate scientific from personal problems with Jung in an effort to avoid a break, but that he was in any case not really pained by Jung's behavior.

> I am completely indifferent. Warned by earlier experiences, and proud of my elasticity, I withdrew my libido from him months ago, at the first signs, and I miss nothing now. Also, this time things are easier for me, for I can redistribute the quantity of libido that has been set free in new places, such as with you, Ferenczi, Rank, Sachs, Abraham, Jones, Brill, and others [p. 264].

It would seem that Freud had "withdrawn his libido" from Jung not long before the conception of "The Theme of the Three Caskets." The success of this "withdrawal" can be called in question by subsequent events months later in Munich when Freud and Jung argued about the Kreuzlingen incident and tried to bury the hatchet, so to speak. Freud had a fainting spell. This was not Freud's first "indirect expression" of ambivalence toward Jung, as has been well documented by Jones and Schur. (In fact, the fainting spells can be traced back to their genetic origins in "death wishes" against Freud's fated brother Julius.)

It is not necessary to trace the ambivalent ups and downs of the Freud-Jung alliance or misalliance any further. This has been well documented elsewhere. The only conjecture being entertained in that context refers to Freud's unconscious dispositions as he set pen to paper in June 1912, to write about the theme of the three caskets. I would propose the following formulation. The representation of death as a Jewish villain (Shylock) tearing a pound of flesh from a Christian (Antonio) would have strengthened Freud's thesis that a subplot (death in mythology, the theme of three caskets) was intimately connected to the main plot (death by revenge). This obvious association did not occur to the father of the associative method because it would have dragged other undesirables with it into consciousness: Binswanger's impending death (in point of fact, Binswanger lived on for 50 more years); but more significantly, death wishes against Jung, Binswanger's colleague. When one considers how fervently Freud wished to make psychoanalysis a cosmopolitan ecumenical discipline rather than a "local" science which could be disparaged or diminished by referring to it as "a Jewish enterprise," the demise of the Jung-Freud alliance must have been a bitter disappointment, as if a genuine bond between Christian and Jew had suddenly deteriorated into a Shylock-Antonio travesty. As with Antonio, this sadness may have been too much for Freud.

In sooth, I know not why I am so sad:
It wearies me; you say it wearies you;
But how I caught it, found it, or came by it,
What stuff 'tis made of, whereof it is born,
I am to learn;
And such a want-wit sadness makes of me,
That I have much ado to know myself.

No one can accuse Freud of not knowing himself or averting his eyes from the truth, however painful, but if the thesis of this paper is correct, it is reassuringly human to note that once in a while he flinched.

BIBLIOGRAPHY

FREUD, S. (1913). The theme of the three caskets. *S.E.*, 12:289–301.
SCHUR, M. (1972). *Freud: Living and Dying.* New York: Int. Univ. Press.

Winnicott and Freud

PETER L. RUDNYTSKY, Ph.D.

All this while you have been steadily doing psychoanalysis, not chopping from case to case, but 'bearing it
out even to the edge of doom.'
WINNICOTT TO ROGER MONEY-KYRLE, FEB. 2, 1968

AS ANDRÉ GREEN HAS OBSERVED, "WINNICOTT'S ORIGINALITY OF
thought and his originality as a person were inseparable" (Clancier and
Kalmanovitch, 1984, p. 139); and, in this essay, I approach the connections between Freud and Winnicott in both biographical and intellectual terms. I begin by taking the contrast between the attitudes toward
religion held by Freud and Winnicott as a point of departure for a
selective, but I hope suggestive, comparison of their personal histories.
I then turn to the domain of ideas and show how Winnicott's medita-
tion on the mother-child bond leads not only to a recasting of psychoanalytic theory but also to an account of culture as a whole. A brief
conclusion juxtaposes Winnicott's optimism and Freud's pessimism to
draw together the biographical and the theoretical threads of this
discussion.

I

Clare Winnicott told of one Sunday when Donald as a boy walked
home with his father from church and asked him about religion. Frederick Winnicott replied: "Listen, my boy. You read the Bible—what
you find there. And you decide for yourself what you want, you know.
It's free. You don't have to believe what I think. Make up your own

Assistant professor of English and comparative literature, Columbia University, and
1988-89 Fulbright Western European Regional Research Scholar. A German version of
this paper was read at the Sigmund Freud Gesellschaft in Vienna in March 1989.

mind about it. Just read the Bible."[1] In its fusion of liberal Christian values with an encouragement of freethinking, this parable of Winnicott and religion at once poses the paradox of his posture as a *believing skeptic*.[2]

Thus, on the one hand, as Clare Winnicott insisted, Donald "was *never* anti-religion" and "he was only too *thankful* if anybody could believe in anything." In "Children Learning," Winnicott asserted that "what is commonly called religion arises out of human nature" (1971, p. 143), though for him religion had nothing to do with miracles or the afterlife. This argument extended that of "Morals and Education," where Winnicott explained that by "religion" he meant that capacity for "such things as trust and 'belief in', and ideas of right and wrong" (1965b, p. 94), which evolves spontaneously in the child who is reared in an atmosphere of reliability and love.

On the other hand, in several late letters (to H. J. Howe, April 25, 1966; to Ian Rodger, June 3, 1969) Winnicott proudly identified himself as a modern-day Lollard who would once have been burned for his heretical views; and he wrote to the London *Times* on December 22, 1969 that "I would not describe myself as a practicing Christian, having reached a degree of maturity appropriate to age." Clare Winnicott recorded that Winnicott's discovery of Darwin "changed his attitude toward religion" and prompted his allegiance to "a scientific way of working." In "Psychoanalysis and Science," Winnicott stressed that "when a gap in knowledge turns up, the scientist does not flee to a supernatural explanation," though he gave this positivistic tenet a characteristically paradoxical twist when he added that this ability to tolerate uncertainty entails "a capacity for faith," a faith "perhaps in nothing" or else in "the inexorable laws that govern phenomena" (1986, p. 14).

1. Unless otherwise noted, quotations from Clare Winnicott are taken from a tape-recorded interview conducted by Dr. Michael Neve of the Wellcome Institute, University of London, in June 1983, less than a year before Mrs. Winnicott's death. A complete transcript will appear in my book, *The Psychoanalytic Vocation: Rank, Winnicott, and the Legacy of Freud*, to be published by Yale University Press. I thank Dr. Neve for permission to use this material. Letters to and from Winnicott without bibliographical documentation are quoted courtesy of the Archives of Psychiatry, The New York Hospital-Cornell Medical Center.

2. Clancier and Kalmanovitch (1984) use the concept of paradox as a guiding thread in their assessment of Winnicott. The only other comprehensive study of Winnicott available to date is that of Davis and Wallbridge (1981), though a book by Adam Phillips is forthcoming in the Modern Masters series. For further discussion of Winnicott's relationship to Freud, see Davis (1985). I am grateful to Madeleine Davis for reading this paper in manuscript.

Winnicott's benevolent attitude toward religion contrasts markedly with the militant atheism of Freud. How is this tension to be accommodated within a psychoanalytic *Weltanschauung*? In part, it is a healthy one, for surely every person oscillates between doubt and faith of some kind. In my judgment, however, Winnicott does not always draw a sufficiently clear distinction between his theses concerning the constructive role of illusion in human experience and children's "innate tendencies toward morality" (1964, p. 96)—both of which are highly compelling—and assertions of the existence of a transcendental God. Thus, when Winnicott declared in "Some Thoughts on the Meaning of the Word 'Democracy,'" "It is certainly helpful when the reigning monarch quite easily and sincerely . . . proclaims a belief in God" (1986, p. 255), he seemed to go beyond upholding the capacity for "belief in" to invest that belief with a positive supernatural content.[3]

To readers of Freud, Winnicott's youthful conversation with his father will inevitably recall a similar walk taken by Freud with *his* father. I refer to the story recounted in *The Interpretation of Dreams* (1900) of how Sigmund, then 10 or 12 years of age, was told by his father of the anti-Semitic abuse he had endured in his youth when his cap had been knocked off his head and he had been ordered off the pavement. Disillusioned by learning of his father's "unheroic" conduct on that occasion, Freud consolidated his identification with the warlike Semitic general Hannibal.

Both these incidents show the future psychoanalysts coming to terms simultaneously with their filial legacies and religious identities. Clare Winnicott noted that accompanying his father home from church was Donald's "privilege," and Freud wrote with evident feeling of what it meant to him "when my father began to take me with him on his walks and reveal to me in his talk his views upon things in the world we live in" (1900, p. 197). But the psychological impact of the episodes on the two boys could not have been more antithetical. Whereas Winnicott's walk had the positive effects of facilitating his maturation and deepening his respect for his father, that of Freud was correspondingly traumatic.

Freud's long-standing inhibition against visiting Rome, which provided the context for his discussion of this childhood memory, bore out his rueful statement that its shattering impact "was still being shown in all these emotions and dreams" (1900, p. 197). Indeed, Freud's bond-

---

3. See Meissner (1984) who, in discussing faith as a "transitional experience," sidestepped the question of "the truth value of the believer's faith" (p. 178) and termed the clash between supernatural and natural perspectives "perhaps the most significant and least resolvable" (p. 216) point of divergence between religion and psychoanalysis.

age to the repetition compulsion and his ambivalent struggles with male figures throughout his life confirmed the arrest in his emotional development due to his unresolved sense of disappointment in his father. The antinomy between these parallel events in the childhoods of Winnicott and Freud may be taken as emblematic of Clare Winnicott's generalization that "there aren't *disasters* in the Winnicott home; there are just funny episodes." And whereas Winnicott's ready assimilation of his father's Protestantism left him a believing skeptic, Freud's coming to terms with his religious patrimony made him into that more fiercely paradoxical being—a godless Jew, who very actively fought anti-Semitism.

As the walks of both Freud and Winnicott with their fathers were signs of "privilege," so in complementary ways both boys occupied favorable positions within their family constellations. Winnicott was the youngest of three children: his two siblings, 6 and 7 years older than he, were both girls. Freud, conversely, was the oldest of 7 surviving children of his parents' marriage (the eighth, Julius, died in infancy), the next five of whom were girls. At the same time, however, Freud was the offspring of his father's second (or third) marriage and thus for a time also the youngest in his family unit.

Freud (1917) wrote memorably that if a son "has been his mother's undisputed darling he retains throughout his life the triumphant feeling, the confidence in success, which not seldom brings actual success along with it" (p. 156). Alluding to the special problems posed by twins, Winnicott (1964) observed that the mother's task "is not to treat each child alike, but to treat each child as if that one were the only one" (p. 139).[4] Both men, it is fair to assume, received during their earliest years that special feeling of having been an "only child," which gave rise to their indomitable self-confidence. Freud, as is well known, openly viewed his life in heroic terms and identified with Hannibal and numerous other figures from history, literature, and myth. As Clare Winnicott told Michael Neve, Winnicott did not resemble Freud in this respect, but in a quieter way he did share something of Freud's sense of destiny. We can discern this conviction in a letter of September 23, 1966 to Inês Besouchet, a Brazilian analyst; Winnicott explained that he somehow found himself specializing "in that part of paediatrics which my colleagues were not so much interested in, namely the area covered by the words the emotional development of the child."

4. Compare Little's (1985) description of the outcome of her analysis with Winnicott: "I became aware that the D. W. whom I knew was different from the D. W. known to anyone else, even though others might know some of the same aspects of him. I 'created' him imaginatively for myself" (p. 36).

Both Freud and Winnicott were reared in extended family households: the family of Winnicott's father's elder brother, Richard, including five children, lived just across the road in Plymouth. In Freud's case, as I have argued elsewhere (1987, pp. 3–17), the involutions of kinship structure resulting from the disparity between the ages of his father and mother and from the fact that his father already had two grown sons from his first marriage predisposed Freud from his birth to the solving of riddles and eventual discovery of the Oedipus complex. Frederick Winnicott's family, in addition to being much better off materially than Jakob Freud's, was much less complicated. Clare Winnicott wrote in her memoir (1978) that the large household left "plenty of chances for many kinds of relationships, and there was scope for the inevitable tensions to be isolated and resolved within the total framework" (p. 21). Both Freud and Winnicott had the opportunity to play multiple roles within their family units, but once again, as in the walks with their fathers, Winnicott's came in more benign fashion.

One further difference between the upbringings of Winnicott and Freud is that Winnicott was reared in a far more female-dominated environment. Clare Winnicott listed all the women—including mother, sisters, an aunt, a governess, and a nanny—by whom Donald was surrounded, whereas his father was rarely at home, and reported his comment: "I was left too much to all my mothers. Thank goodness I was sent away at thirteen." He was dispatched to the Leys School in Cambridge by his father after he met a new friend at the age of 12 and one day uttered the word "drat" at the dinner table. Clare Winnicott (1978) quoted from Winnicott's notebook, which she read only after his death, that it meant a great deal to him to discover that his father "was there to kill and be killed" (p. 24).

But though this rearing in a feminine ambience doubtless sensitized Winnicott to the importance of the role of the mother, it did not lead him to sentimentalize it.[5] On the contrary, it was Freud who even in his final years naïvely claimed that a mother's relation to her son "is altogether the most perfect, the most free from ambivalence of all human relationships" (1933, p. 133). Winnicott (1964) wrote with far greater realism that "it may easily happen" that a woman "resents" the "terrible interference" with her life that comes with being pregnant and that "babies are a lot of trouble, and a positive nuisance unless they are wanted" (p. 19). Unlike Winnicott's mother, Freud's mother did in fact have more children after Sigmund, the next one (Julius) less than

5. Clare Winnicott's report that Winnicott read "the whole of Meredith" while serving as a medical officer on a destroyer during World War I helps to place his distrust of sentimentality in a literary context (Rodman, 1987, p. xxiv).

1½ years later. It is plausible to speculate that Freud idealized the mother-son relationship partly in order to deny his resentment at having been so soon displaced from his mother's lap and attentions. In two crucial letters to Fliess (October 3 and 15, 1897), Freud related an incident from his early childhood in which either he or his nanny stole coins from his mother. Winnicott (1964) addressed the causes of stealing in children: "A two-year child who is stealing pennies from his mother's handbag is playing at being a hungry infant who thought he created his mother, and who assumed that he had rights over her contents. Disillusionment can come only too quickly. The birth of a new baby, for instance, can be a terrible shock in just this particular way" (p. 164). Winnicott did not mention Freud, and may perhaps even have been unaware that his analysis bore on Freud's personal history, but it is no less pertinent for that reason.

Undoubtedly, Winnicott did have a happy childhood. But this good fortune was fraught with its own developmental perils. In his introduction to Winnicott's selected letters, Rodman (1987) suggested that "probably a study of his life would reveal the conditions under which 'being himself' had become a continuing issue" (p. xxix). Winnicott (1965a) himself remarked, in autobiographically resonant passages, that "children find in security a sort of challenge, a challenge to them to prove that they can break out," and that what is needed for the healthy development of the individual is "a well-graduated series of defiant iconoclastic actions, each of the series being compatible with the retention of an unconscious bond with the central figures or figure, the parents or the mother" (pp. 30, 92).

Clare Winnicott mentioned two such notorious "iconoclastic actions" in her interview with Michael Neve. In one instance Donald smacked a doll belonging to his sister with a croquet mallet because his father had teased him about it. But though he was "frightfully pleased" at this expression of defiance, he was likewise "quite glad when his father melted the wax of the doll's face and put it together again." Clare Winnicott (1978) quoted Winnicott's own interpretation of this event: "This early demonstration of the restitutive and reparative act certainly made an impression on me, and perhaps made me able to accept the fact that I myself, dear innocent child, had actually become violent directly with a doll, but indirectly with my good-tempered father, who was just then entering my conscious life" (p. 23).

The closest equivalent in Freud's life to this incident may be found in his analysis of the "botanical monograph" dream: "It had once amused my father to hand over a book with *coloured plates* . . . for me and my eldest sister to destroy. . . . I had been five years old at the time and my sister not yet three; and the picture of us blissfully pulling the book to pieces (leaf by leaf, like an *artichoke*, I found myself saying) was almost the only plastic memory I retained from that period of my life" (1900, p. 172).

Both Freud and Winnicott took pleasure in engaging in destructive acts. But whereas Freud's pulling apart of the book with his sister has been shown to be primarily a veiled allusion to child ...od sexual play and masturbation (Swales, 1982, p. 9), Winnicott's smashing of the doll's face and its repair by his father illustrated Melanie Klein's (1937) themes of love, guilt, and reparation.

Winnicott's second instance of rebelliousness came when he looked at himself in the mirror, decided he was "too nice," then started blotting his copybook, doing poorly in school, torturing flies, and so forth. As Clare Winnicott put it, the universally liked child needed to find the "other dimension" of "nastiness" in himself. In Winnicott's (1965b) own terms, it is not difficult to understand this compulsion to misbehave as the protest of his own suppressed True Self, including its destructive urges, against an outwardly compliant, but inauthentic, False Self. Winnicott often made the point that expressions of "the antisocial tendency"—from bed wetting in early childhood to stealing and more violent criminal behavior in adolescence and beyond—actually represent signs of hope in a deprived individual (1958, pp. 306–15; 1986, pp. 90–100). (Delinquency for Winnicott was the antisocial tendency compounded by secondary gains.) He wrote: "The child knows in his bones that it is *hope* that is locked up in wicked behaviour, and that *despair* is linked with compliance and false socialization" (1965b, p. 104).

A crucial moment in Winnicott's ongoing struggle to "be himself" came with his decision to become a doctor at 15 after he broke his collarbone during sports at school and chafed under the need to be treated in the infirmary (Clancier and Kalmanovitch, 1984, p. 100). (This decision entailed the disappointment of his father's hopes that Donald would succeed him in the family's wholesale hardware business.) Clare Winnicott (1978) quoted him as saying: "I could see that for the rest of my life I should have to depend on doctors if I became ill, and the only way out of this position was to become a doctor myself" (p. 25).

In December 1968 Winnicott suffered a grievous heart attack—one of a series during his later years—while on a lecture tour in New York. After returning to London, he wrote on January 31, 1969 to Dr. Crampton, the physician who had treated him in the cardiac care unit at Lenox Hill Hospital: "I recognise that I was in a rather peculiar state of mind during that illness and I am sure that you and your colleagues found me at times rather trying as a patient. As you did say to my wife, and this was helpful, you knew that the dependence of a patient who is very ill is a difficult thing, especially for a doctor who has at any rate some knowledge of what is going on." More than any other analyst, Winnicott stressed the primacy of dependence both in human development and in the analytic process. But this extraordinary sensitivity was undergirded by Winnicott's own difficulties in acknowledging his dependence on others.

In *On the History of the Psycho-Analytic Movement* (1914), Freud related a series of anecdotes designed to explain the "bad reception" accorded to his views on the "sexual aetiology of the neuroses" (p. 12). From his early encounters with three eminent senior physicians—Breuer, Charcot, and the Viennese gynecologist Chrobak—he took away a single lesson condensed in the memorable phrase of Charcot: "*C'est toujours la chose génitale*" (p. 14). Freud's epiphanies concerning sexuality found a counterpart in the way that Winnicott during his medical training learned—both by precept and example—from his mentor Dr. Thomas Horder the importance of practicing a nondirective technique with patients. According to Clare Winnicott, Horder exhorted him: "Listen to your patient. Don't you go in with your wonderful knowledge and apply it all. Just listen. They'll tell you quite a lot of things. You'll learn a lot if you listen."

Winnicott looked upon psychoanalysis as "a vast extension of history-taking, with therapeutics as a by-product" (1965b, p. 199); and in "Psychoanalysis and Science," he noted that the discovery of the free association technique enabled Freud to shift his attention from the removal of symptoms to a "more important" task: "to enable the patient to reveal himself to himself" (1986, p. 13). As he grew older Winnicott strove increasingly to hold in check what in "The Use of an Object" (1971) he called his "personal need to interpret." He distilled a lifetime of clinical wisdom: "I think I interpret mainly to let the patient know the limits of my understanding" (p. 86).

Freud, it must be admitted, did not always restrain his own "personal need to interpret" and, during his discovery of the phenomenon of transference in the Dora case, even exemplified Winnicott's (1965b) general description of "a bad analyst making good interpretations" (p. 252). Nonetheless, as Clare Winnicott put it, Winnicott "admired tremendously" not only Freud's "clear thinking" but above all his ability to "*change his mind*." Winnicott himself (1965b) averred that Freud "was easy to criticize because he was always critical of himself" (p. 177). Clare Winnicott brought out the depth of Winnicott's conviction that "once you're defending your position, you've lost sight of science." Characteristically, Winnicott (1965a) traced the capacity for "a scientific approach to phenomena" back to the baby at the breast, to the mother's successful introduction of the external world "in small doses, accurately graded to the infant's or child's understanding" (p. 28; see also 1958, p. 153). And though, as he admitted, "most of us, alas, have put at least some of human nature outside the realm of scientific inquiry," by his own lack of defensiveness he held up an ideal not only for psychoanalytic work but also for the conduct of our daily life.

II

That Winnicott should have grounded the capacity for a scientific *Weltanschauung* in the baby's experience at the breast is scarcely surprising. For, as Clare Winnicott (1978) remarked, although Winnicott's writings span a wide range of topics, including delinquency and adolescence, "his main contribution is likely to be in the study of the earliest relationships, and its application to the etiology of psychosis and the psychotic mechanisms in all of us" (p. 18). Whereas for Freud, in the sweeping peroration of *Totem and Taboo* (1913b), "the beginnings of religion, morals, society and art converge in the Oedipus complex" (p. 156), for Winnicott these "beginnings" lay even earlier in the child's bond with the "ordinary devoted mother."

Deservedly Winnicott's most famous concept, and that by which he elaborated his theoretical understanding of the mother-child relationship, is the transitional object, which, as Anna Freud wrote to him on October 30, 1968, "has conquered the analytic world." As he explained in his seminal paper, published in 1953, two essential features of this "first 'not-me' possession" are that it exists on the boundary between internal and external reality—in what he would term "potential space"—and that "it must survive instinctual loving, and also hating and, if it be a feature, pure aggression" (1971, pp. 1, 5).

The liminal status of the transitional object—the doll, blanket, or teddy bear to which the young child clings as he or she begins to separate from the mother—between fantasy and reality is integral to Winnicott's contention (1971, pp. 95–103) that art and cultural experience as a whole are located in this same intermediate realm of play. What is unique about Winnicott's approach to creativity is that he avoided treating works of art merely as products of instinctual sublimation, as is the case in classical Freudian theory, while yet insisting that their roots lay in infancy. The second aspect of the transitional object— its capacity to withstand instinctual loving and hating—gets to Winnicott's assumptions about human nature. Although he rejected Freud's hypothesis of the death instinct, which was championed by Melanie Klein, Winnicott took over from Klein the conviction that "the primitive love impulse has an aggressive aim; being ruthless, it carries with it a variable quantity of destructive ideas unaffected by concern" (Winnicott, 1965b, p. 22). Because the infant's aggression—in Winnicott's view, initially a diffused expression of the life force—comes to be focused on the mother's breast, as the first external object and in fantasy an *object of attack,* both it and its surrogates must continue to exist if the infant is to achieve the sense of guilt that heralds the *stage of concern* (1965b), as Winnicott renamed Klein's depressive position.

Winnicott's (1971) most important later development of the idea of transitional objects is to be found in "The Use of an Object." This paper is suffused by a tragic aura because of the fact that, when it was first read to the New York Psychoanalytic Society, on November 12, 1968, it was sharply criticized by its three discussants—Edith Jacobson, Samuel Ritvo, and Bernard D. Fine—and Winnicott suffered the heart attack to which I have already alluded shortly thereafter. None of these individuals, of course, is in any way responsible for what ensued, and indeed the record shows that the tone of the meeting was one of spirited intellectual exchange untainted by any personal rancor.[6] But Winnicott, who is quoted as having responded "in a charming and whimsical fashion" that "his concept was torn to pieces and that he would be happy to give it up," regarded the evening as a failure; and it is impossible wholly to disentangle the theme of the paper—the survival of the analyst—from the circumstances of its presentation.

The American analysts were troubled in part by Winnicott's terminology—his definition of "relating" to an object as a purely subjective phenomenon that precedes its objective "use." Above all, however, they took issue with what I have identified as the Kleinian component of Winnicott's paper, namely, the thesis that all object relationships have a destructive root, and that the object's survival of its fantasied destruction is thus the precondition for its assuming of an independent existence: "Essentially Dr. Jacobson could not understand Dr. Winnicott's meaning of 'destructive attack' and 'survival'; and she described as an extreme statement his summary comment—that 'the

6. The library of the New York Psychoanalytic Institute contains, in addition to the original version of Winnicott's paper, which differs slightly from that eventually published, a summary of the entire proceedings prepared by David Milrod, as well as the complete texts of the responses by Jacobson and Fine. The ensuing quotations are from Milrod's summary. I am grateful to Mr. David Ross, librarian of the Institute, for making these materials available to me.

object is always being destroyed,' a destruction which becomes the unconscious back-cloth for love of a real object." "Dr. Ritvo could not understand the statement that acceptance of the object outside the subject's omnipotent control meant the destruction of the object." "Dr. Fine found it unclear and not at all proven that in the process of developing from what Dr. Winnicott calls object-relating to object use that the subject destroys the object."

The proposition that the primitive love impulse contains an irreducible core of aggressiveness is admittedly not subject to empirical verification. But a compelling argument in its favor is offered by Milner (1957), who pointed to the "double fact that what one loves most, because one needs it most, is necessarily separate from oneself; and yet the primitive urge of loving is to make what one loves part of oneself. So that in loving it one has, in one's primitive wish, destroyed it as something separate and outside and having an identity of its own" (p. 66). She added: "The cannibal may be prompted to eat his enemy by love for his courage and strength and the wish to preserve these, but it is a love which certainly does not preserve the loved enemy in his original form" (p. 58).

As the responses of the New York analysts show, "The Use of an Object" is incomprehensible without some appreciation of this line of reasoning; and this paper, which Winnicott said belonged to "the direct line of development that is particularly mine" (1971, p. 86), is important precisely because it disclosed the connection between his twin themes of ruthlessness and the shift from a subjective to an objective mode of experiencing reality. When the mother has failed to do so, the analyst of the borderline patient must be placed "outside the area of omnipotent control" by bearing the brunt of the "maximum destructiveness" of which the patient is capable; and this "capacity to survive" means specifically "not retaliate" (p. 91).

An extension of Winnicott's ideas concerning transitional objects to the political sphere may be seen in "The Place of the Monarchy." Indeed, the title of this paper in manuscript was "Applied Theory," and it began with the following words omitted from the posthumously published version: "An application of theory provides a test, a test of its validity and its usefulness. As an exercise in the application of the theory of what I call 'transitional phenomena'. . . ." Winnicott built on his view of what it means to "use" an object to argue that "*what is good is always being destroyed*," and that the continued survival of the monarchy despite popular unconscious desires for its destruction therefore helps to make England "a place to live in" rather than merely "to fear or be complied with or to be lost in" (1986, pp. 262, 264). Whatever "sentimental or scandalous" stories may be invented, he observed, the monarch retains a collective "dream-significance" by refusing to divulge the details of his or her personal life; and "in the centre of it all is a woman (or man) who has or has not the capacity to survive, to exist without reacting to provocation or to seduction, until at death a successor determined by heredity takes over this tremendous responsibility" (p. 266).

As this characterization makes clear, Winnicott envisioned, as it were, a metonymic chain, in which the nonretaliating monarch takes the place of the analyst, who in turn substitutes for the transitional object of infancy. But the transitional object itself is a surrogate for the breast of the mother as well as a "symbol of the union" (1971, p. 114) between the infant and the "environment-mother" who knows when to minister to the infant's needs. Winnicott (1964, pp. 45–49) described in wonderfully evocative detail the feeding process between mother and baby: In some unpredictable way, the breast of the mother, who holds her baby lovingly and without anxiety, comes into contact with the baby's mouth and saliva begins to flow.[7] The saliva is a sign of ideas in the baby's mind, and "Gradually the mother enables the baby to build up in imagination the very thing she has to offer." After nursing for a time, the baby turns away, having "finished with the idea" of the breast, and the nipple disappears. A few minutes later, the process recommences. The baby turns again toward the nipple, which the mother willingly offers, and "a new contact is made, just at the right moment." As Winnicott emphasized, it is especially in the second phase of the experience, "where she takes the nipple away from the baby as the baby ceases to want it or to believe in it, that she establishes herself as the mother."

This prototypical encounter of the infant with the breast, which is repeated until it becomes part of a regular and reliable feeding schedule, was pivotal to Winnicott's thought because it suggested the possibility of discovering in the external world what one has imagined, thus preparing the way for the ontological paradox of the transitional object—its simultaneous existence in fantasy and reality—and making

---

7. For a theoretical elaboration of the issues underlying the dynamic of the feeding situation, see the 1941 paper on "The Observation of Infants in a Set Situation" (1958). This paper was singled out by Clare Winnicott as one of the best examples of Winnicott's scientific technique. A forerunner to the theory of the transitional object, it includes a commentary on the *fort-da* episode in *Beyond the Pleasure Principle* (1920), which has attracted so much attention in French psychoanalytic circles.

creativity in general possible.[8] Of course, the breast will not always be available, and Winnicott (1971, pp. 1–25) insisted that a gradual process of disillusionment must follow the infant's acquisition of the capacity for illusion. But unlike Lacan (1949), who viewed the ego's relation to the world as constituted by an insurmountable *"méconnaissance,"* Winnicott offered a far more benign vision of the power of language and other vehicles of the imagination to give access to a reality which they themselves help to create.

I believe that this progression from "Transitional Objects and Transitional Phenomena" through "The Use of an Object" to "The Place of the Monarchy" illuminates not only how Winnicott enriched psychoanalytic theory by complementing Freud's paradigm of the oedipus complex with a powerful model of the relationship between mother and child, but also how this model gave him a tool with which to investigate apparently remote cultural problems. Indeed, whereas Lacan elevated the oedipus complex into a linguistic Name-of-the-Father, Winnicott (1964) may be said to have spoken of an equally universal Name-of-the-Mother: "there is a separated-out phenomenon that we can call WOMAN which dominates the whole scene, and affects all our arguments. WOMAN is the unacknowledged mother of the first stages of life of every man and woman" (p. 192).[9] In a moment of candor, he pointed to the autobiographical roots of his work on devotion: "to make a fully informed and fully felt acknowledgement to my own mother" (1986, p. 126).

Although Winnicott differed from Freud in emphasizing not the father but the mother as the prototype for later transference relationships, the two analysts were in accord in approaching political questions from the standpoint of individual development. As Winnicott (1965b) wrote: "Cultural influences are of course important, vitally important; but these cultural influences can themselves be studied as an overlap of innumerable personal patterns. In other words, the clue to social and group psychology is in the psychology of the

8. "Ought we not to say that by fitting in with the infant's impulse the mother allows the baby the *illusion* that what is there is the thing created by the baby; as a result there is not only the physical experience of instinctual satisfaction, but also an emotional union, and the belief in reality as something about which one can have illusions" (Winnicott, 1958, p. 163).

9. The Lacanian Name-of-the-Father contains in French a play on the words *Nom-du-Père* ("name of the father") and *Non-du-Père* ("no of the father"), which is lost in English translation, and for which what I call Winnicott's Name-of-the-Mother possesses no equivalent.

individual" (p. 15). Despite being derided by fashionable Marxist thought as a form of "bourgeois individualism,"[10] and although there are times when it is preferable to adopt a more global perspective, this reliance on individual experience as a touchstone of truth remains at the heart of psychoanalysis.

Even those who disagree with him must admire Winnicott for having recognized that his allegiance to psychoanalysis had political implications, and for seeking to make these explicit. In "Some Thoughts on the Meaning of the Word 'Democracy,'" he openly argued that democracy is the most "mature" form of social organization. Winnicott defined maturity in individual terms as "an appropriate degree of emotional development" for a person's "chronological age and social setting" (1986, p. 241). Thus, since this conviction coexisted with his reverence for the queen as a collective transitional object, as in matters of religion he was a believing skeptic, so in the political sphere he was no less paradoxically a *democratic monarchist*.

Indeed, precisely by virtue of being Winnicott's boldest venture into "applied theory," the paper on democracy highlighted the questionable features of his outlook with utmost clarity. For example, Winnicott ascribed the importance of the secret ballot to the fact that "it ensures the freedom of the people to express deep feelings, *apart from conscious thoughts*" (1986, p. 241). Although this analysis shed unexpected light on the vagaries of the democratic process, it overlooked the point that the secret ballot is above all intended to secure freedom from political oppression. Similarly, when Winnicott explained the phenomenon of dictatorship in terms of a collective need to seek domination at the hands of a leader who takes on "the magical qualities of the all-powerful woman of fantasy" (p. 253), the insight was at once constructive and compelling. But he prefaced it by saying that "there is no relation to the father which has such a quality" of absolute dependence as that to the mother, "and for this reason a man who in a political sense is at the top can be appreciated much more objectively by the group than a woman can be if she is in a similar position" (p. 253). With this remark, he at once underestimated the degree of ambivalence that disturbs people's perceptions of fathers and disparaged the capacity of women to assume positions of authority.

But just as it is possible to uphold Winnicott's concept of "belief in"

---

10. For a forceful exposition of this Althusserian Marxist position, see Jameson (1981): "the need to transcend individualistic categories of interpretation is in many ways the fundamental issue for any doctrine of the political unconscious" (p. 68).

without using it to justify the existence of God, so I would maintain that his assertion of a link between biological and social processes remains valid despite occasional lapses into sexist stereotypes.[11] In any event, when confronted by his less enlightened pronouncements on social or religious issues, one may recall Winnicott's own admonition that if the student "must read instead of making observations let him read descriptions by many different authors, not looking to one or another as the purveyor of the truth" (1964, p. 147).

III

Prompted by a question from Michael Neve, Clare Winnicott agreed that there was an "enormous difference" between the optimism of Winnicott and the pessimism of Freud. Citing the statistic that Winnicott saw 60,000 parents with their children during nearly 40 years of practice at Paddington Green and his other clinics, she observed that, because of his training in pediatrics and extensive "experience of normal family-working," his outlook "comes with something positive. It comes at psychoanalysis from health, rather than from illness." Winnicott himself went even further: "It is of first importance for us to acknowledge openly that absence of psychoneurotic illness may be health, but it is not life" (1971, p. 100).

This opposition between the optimism of Winnicott and pessimism of Freud inheres in their religious attitudes, and if Freud's preoccupation with the sense of guilt identifies him as an heir of St. Augustine, the playfulness and paradoxicality of Winnicott make him akin rather to Erasmus. Between them, Freud and Winnicott reincarnate a perennial dichotomy in the history of ideas. On the one hand, there are those thinkers who emphasize the innate depravity of human nature; on the other, there are those who see people as basically good and accentuate the influence of the environment in shaping them for better or worse.

Winnicott, who affirmed in "Morals and Education" that "Religions have made much of original sin, but have not all come round to the idea of original goodness" (1965b, p. 94), was well aware of the theological resonances of his recasting of psychoanalytic theory. Indeed, he expressly rejected the concept of the death instinct because it "could be described as a reassertion of the principle of original sin. I have tried to

11. Winnicott (1971, pp. 72–85) differentiated the "female elements" and "male elements" in people of both sexes in terms of a distinction between *being* and *doing*. For a searching critique of his assumptions concerning masculinity and femininity, see Chodorow (1978).

develop the theme that what both Freud and Klein avoided in so doing
was the full implication of dependence and therefore of the environmental factor" (1971, p. 70). And yet, as we have seen, Winnicott
concurred with Klein that "it is necessary to retain the idea of the attack
on the mother's body which is ruthless and which only gradually
gathers to itself guilt feeling" (Rodman, 1987, p. 109). Thus, Winnicott's temperament was in no sense utopian, and his comic vision was
one that had transmuted—without betraying—the tragic wisdom of
Freud.

Winnicott's revision of Freud's libido theory provides a case in point.
Whereas in Freud's scheme (1905) development was seen as passing
through a series of foreordained psychosexual stages, any one of which
might become a fixation point for later regressions, Winnicott was
concerned "not merely with regression to good and bad points in the
instinct experiences of the individual, but also to good and bad points
in the environmental adaptation to ego needs and id needs in the
individual's history" (1958, p. 283). Thus, he spoke not of "regression"
but of *"regression to dependence,"* which communicates the deprived individual's hope that "certain aspects of the environment which failed
originally may be relived, with the environment this time succeeding
instead of failing in its function of facilitating the inherited tendency in
the individual to develop and to mature" (1965b, p. 128).

Winnicott's revision of the libido theory in turn has a direct bearing
on the practice of psychoanalytic therapy. Within a traditional Freudian perspective, therapeutic action is attributed to the "breaking up and
reorganizing of existing pathological structures" (Atwood and
Stolorow, 1984, p. 61). If the past exerts a determining influence on a
person's behavior, and is itself unalterable, then all that can be hoped
for is that, through becoming aware of one's compulsions to repeat, a
feedback loop of consciousness, as it were, may be introduced which
somewhat diminishes their tyrannical sway. But this is a limited aim at
best, especially since psychoanalysis sees the intellect as relatively helpless against the power of unconscious forces; and Freud, as is well
known, came by 1937 to espouse an attitude of therapeutic pessimism.

From a Winnicottian standpoint, however, the objective of psychoanalytic therapy, with the borderline patient, is not so much to *undo* the
past, or even to understand it intellectually—though this has its
place—but rather to facilitate "growth of psychical structure that is
missing or deficient as a consequence of developmental voids and
interferences" (Atwood and Stolorow, 1984, p. 61). In other words, an
arrested maturational process is brought to completion: *"The patient
needs to reach back through the transference trauma to the state of affairs before*

the original trauma. . . . Reproduction in the treatment of examples as they arise of the original environmental failure, along with the patient's experience of anger that is appropriate, frees the patient's maturational processes; . . . and the next phase needs to be a period of emotional growth in which the character builds up positively and loses its distortions" (Winnicott, 1965b, p. 209). Like his modification of the libido theory in order to take into account the role of the environment, Winnicott's reconceptualization of the dynamics of treatment provided a more hopeful version of psychoanalysis while yet remaining true to Freud's fundamental principles.

It is a fitting testament to Winnicott's comic spirit that his last words, spoken to his wife after watching a televised film about old cars, should have been: "What a happy-making film." Clare Winnicott likewise reported to Michael Neve that Winnicott died in his sleep on the floor, and that the two of them "*always* sat on the floor—him on the one side, me on the other." This detail takes on symbolic significance in light of Winnicott's challenge to the "armchair philosopher" to "come out of his chair and sit on the floor with his patient" (1971, p. 90) to discover what it means for someone to *use* an object. No armchair psychoanalyst he, Winnicott was not afraid to meet his patients—young and old—on even ground.

Many of those who knew Winnicott have mentioned how deeply they were impressed by his physical presence. Masud Khan (1975) wrote that "what stands out vividly is his relaxed physicality and a lambent concentration in his person" (p. xi). Marion Milner (1978) compared him to a clown in a troop of acrobats, who occasionally "made a fruitless attempt to jump up and reach the bar. Then, suddenly, he made a great leap and there he was, whirling around on the bar, all his clothes flying out, like a huge Catherine wheel, to roars of delight from the crowd" (p. 37). Clare Winnicott vividly recalled Winnicott's bodily energy in her interview with Michael Neve—whether in the image of him climbing a tree to chop down a branch in the last year of his life, or riding a bicycle down Hammersmith Hill with his feet on the handlebars, or driving a car with his head through the roof and his walking stick on the accelerator.[12] This vitality was integral to Winnicott's genius as a therapist and helped to make him truly, in his wife's words, "the *most* spontaneous thing that ever lived."

12. Winnicott's files contain amusing documentation of the bicycle incident. After receiving a letter of warning on April 29, 1967 from the Metropolitan Police, Winnicott—ever the indefatigable correspondent—replied on May 5 acknowledging "the infringement of an important traffic regulation" and taking due notice of the injunction "to avoid danger or annoyance to other people or danger to yourself."

Nor can his exceptional talents in the fields of art and music be overlooked. Clare Winnicott reported that he would "*rush* up and play the piano between patients," and end the day with "a musical outburst fortissimo." He often played Brahms and Bach, and near the end of his life "was permanently listening to late Beethoven quartets." Winnicott profited analytically from his gifts as a visual artist through his use of the "squiggle technique" with children. Hand-painted Christmas cards prepared with Clare were an annual event, and even his signature could be fashioned into a captivating squiggle (see Davis, 1987, p. 500)! These creative powers are in marked contrast to Freud, who was notoriously insensible to music and likewise gave no evidence of artistic endowment. It was perhaps for this reason that Freud wrote brilliant criticism of both literature and plastic art, whereas Winnicott—whose theory of art as inhabiting the same "potential space" as childhood play is the most satisfactory psychoanalytic account—had virtually nothing to say about specific works of any kind. Alone among psychoanalysts, however, Winnicott approached Freud as a master of expository prose.

For Winnicott (1965a), the moment at which the infant begins to feel a sense of integration was one of extreme vulnerability: "Only if someone has her arms round the infant at this time can the I AM moment be endured, or rather, perhaps, risked" (p. 148). Elsewhere, Winnicott appealed to the memory of having been held by "everlasting arms" as an experiential basis for religious belief: "We may use that word 'God,' we can make a specific link with the Christian church and doctrine, but it is a series of steps" (1971, p. 149). But this invocation of a mother's love may be contrasted with Freud's stoical resignation in the final sentence of "The Theme of the Three Caskets" (1913a): "it is in vain that an old man yearns for the love of woman as he had it first from his mother; the third of the Fates alone, the silent Goddess of Death, will take him into her arms" (p. 301). Between these antipodes of faith and doubt, the psychoanalytic thinker must continue to steer.

BIBLIOGRAPHY

Atwood, G. E. & Stolorow, R. D. (1984). *Structures of Subjectivity.* Hillsdale, N.J.: Analytic Press.

Chodorow, N. (1978). *The Reproduction of Mothering.* Berkeley: Univ. California Press, 1979.

Clancier, A. & Kalmanovitch, J. (1984). *Winnicott and Paradox,* tr. A. Sheridan. London: Tavistock Publications, 1987.

Davis, M. (1985). Some thoughts on Winnicott and Freud. *Bull. Brit. Assn. Psychother.,* pp. 57–71.

———(1987). The writing of D. W. Winnicott. *Int. Rev. Psychoanal.*, 14:491–501.

———& WALLBRIDGE, D. (1981). *Boundary and Space*. Harmondsworth: Penguin Books, 1983.

FREUD, S. (1900). The interpretation of dreams. *S.E.*, 4 & 5.

———(1905). Three essays on the theory of sexuality. *S.E.*, 7:125–245.

———(1913a). The theme of the three caskets. *S.E.*, 12:291–301.

———(1913b). Totem and taboo. *S.E.*, 13:1–161.

———(1914). On the history of the psycho-analytic movement. *S.E.*, 14:7–66.

———(1917). A childhood recollection from *Dichtung und Wahrheit. S.E.*, 17:147–156.

———(1920). Beyond the pleasure principle. *S.E.*, 18:7–64.

———(1933). New introductory lectures on psycho-analysis. *S.E.*, 22:7–182.

———(1937). Analysis terminable and interminable. *S.E.*, 23:216–253.

GROLNICK, S., BARKIN, L., & MUENSTERBERGER, W., eds. (1978). *Between Reality and Fantasy*. New York: Jason Aronson.

JAMESON, F. (1981). *The Political Unconscious*. Ithaca: Cornell Univ. Press.

KHAN, M. (1975). Introduction to Winnicott (1958), pp. xi-1.

KLEIN, M. (1937). Love, guilt, and reparation. In *The Writings of Melanie Klein*, 1:306–43. New York: Free Press, 1984.

LACAN, J. (1949). The mirror stage as formative of the function of the I as revealed in psychoanalytic experience. In *Écrits*, tr. A. Sheridan. New York: Norton, pp. 1–7.

LITTLE, M. I. (1985). Winnicott working in areas where psychotic anxieties predominate. *Free Associations*, 3:9–42.

MEISSNER, W. W. (1984). *Psychoanalysis and Religious Experience*. New Haven: Yale Univ. Press.

MILNER, M. (1957). *On Not Being Able to Paint*. New York: Int. Univ. Press, 1979.

———(1978). D. W. Winnicott and the two-way journey. In Grolnick et al. (1978), pp. 37–42.

MILROD, D. (1968). Summary of D. W. Winnicott, "The Use of an Object" and Discussions by Edith Jacobson, Bernard D. Fine, and Samuel Ritvo. The New York Psychoanalytic Society, November 12.

RODMAN, F. R., ed. (1987). *The Spontaneous Gesture*. Cambridge, Mass.: Harvard Univ. Press.

RUDNYTSKY, P. L. (1987). *Freud and Oedipus*. New York: Columbia Univ. Press.

SWALES, P. J. (1982). Freud, Minna Bernays, and the language of flowers. Privately published.

WINNICOTT, C. (1978). D. W. W.: A reflection. In Grolnick et al. (1978), pp. 17–33.

WINNICOTT, D. W. (1958). *Through Paediatrics to Psycho-Analysis*. New York: Basic Books, 1975.

———(1964). *The Child, the Family, and the Outside World*. Harmondsworth: Penguin Books, 1985.

———(1965a). *The Family and Individual Development*. London: Tavistock Publications, 1984.

————(1965b). *The Maturational Processes and the Facilitating Environment.* New York: Int. Univ. Press, 1966.

————(1971). *Playing and Reality.* London: Tavistock Publications, 1984.

————(1986). *Home Is Where We Start From,* ed. C. Winnicott, R. Shepherd, & M. Davis. New York: Norton.

Primary Art Objects

Psychoanalytic Reflections on Picturebooks for Children

ELLEN HANDLER SPITZ, Ph.D.

It has long since become common knowledge that the experiences of a person's first five years exercise a determining effect on his life, which nothing later can withstand. Much that deserves knowing might be said about the way in which these early impressions maintain themselves against any influences in more mature periods of life.

FREUD (1939, p. 125)

RECENT SCHOLARSHIP IN THE HUMANITIES HAS QUESTIONED THE NARROW range of cultural objects that fall under serious interpretive scrutiny. This paper responds to that critique by examining a relatively neglected category of such objects, namely, the picturebook. In addition, psychoanalysis, in postulating such universal constructs as drive, ego, and early object relations as primary influences on the child's psyche, wrestles only intermittently and marginally with the impact of cultural context. This interdisciplinary study aims to address that gap by demonstrating the impact of artifacts such as the picturebook on the developing child's mind and to urge the need for interpreting them. Highly

Visiting lecturer of aesthetics in psychiatry, Cornell University Medical College.

Versions of this paper were given as Child Psychiatry Grand Rounds at New York Hospital-Cornell Medical Center, Westchester Division and at the Gardiner program in Psychoanalysis and the Humanities, Yale University. I wish to thank Drs. Albert Solnit and Paulina Kernberg and the members of their respective groups for stimulating discussions that led to revisions of this paper.

Also, I wish to acknowledge the support of the National Endowment for the Humanities Summer Institute on "Image and Text" (1988) under the direction of Profs. Michael Fried and Ronald Paulson of the Johns Hopkins University.

charged and subtly coded, reprinted and experienced by generations of children, the classic texts discussed here are worthy of consideration by researchers and educators in the field of early childhood, clinicians, and scholars interested in image-text relations.

I

A tradition for such exploration was established by the pioneering work of Anna Freud, who advocated the application of psychoanalytic insights into early childhood to realms that extend beyond the clinic but, in turn, impinge on it. More proximally, however, the questions that have motivated my work stem from suggestive papers by Winnicott (1966) and Greenacre (1957). Both of these papers address the child's initial experiences with the arts and culture but in highly speculative modes. Like theirs, my own work is principally interpretive rather than empirical, yet it differs in attempting to ground theory by the use of concrete examples. Drawn from the repertoire of picturebooks currently available in the United States, these examples have been chosen for their longevity (lasting in one case over a half century). Such longevity speaks to the ongoing capacity of these and similar artifacts to enthrall not only children but adults and to stimulate the latter to recapture and share their own earliest moments of fantasy and illusion.

My topic, precisely, is the initiation of young children into the arts and culture by means of artifacts designed expressly for their use. Among the spectrum of such artifacts, I have chosen the picturebook because of its hybrid form: it combines the two great sign systems of image and text in a physical object (i.e., book) that carries enormous cultural signification; its temporal and spatial coordinates allow it to be perceived and handled intimately and repetitively and thus to be preserved and cherished or mutilated and destroyed. It serves as a prototype for various highly differentiated aesthetic objects that the child will encounter as he or she matures.

Parallel to the psychoanalytic construct of advancing from primary to secondary process is the notion, deeply implanted in our cultural heritage, of a necessary turning from (pictured) images to (written) words. While programmatically (in our educational system, for example) we have valued words over images and elevated reason above imagination, we know that to deny our daydreams and fantasies altogether would be to lose touch with complementary aspects of our human nature. Parenthetically, it is interesting to note that the prevalence of television and other visual media seems in our time to be effecting an alteration in, or perhaps even a reversal of, this accepted direction.

Nevertheless, the movement away from images and toward the pre-eminence of words (reflected in some religious as well as developmental and historical contexts) can be interpreted, psychoanalytically speaking, partly in terms of a fear of regression—a viewpoint paralleled by the twin notion that when we do value the *imagery* of art, the *spectacle* of theater, and the *illusions* conjured up by poetic texts, we do so in no small part because they foster and permit a pleasurable, safe, and limited regression. To employ this model is to comprehend in part the fascination of the picturebook. Enjoyed by children from under a year to about five years of age, it is an object designed to span the border between image and word at precisely that juncture in the life-span when intrapsychic bridges between these realms are being constructed. In negotiating the gap between experience, perception, and the written word, children use picturebooks as a transitional form—but a form that is, in its own right, quintessentially an art.

In addition, it is essential to stress the role of the reading adult whose own engagement over time with both artifact and child is fundamental. As in the Suzuki approach to learning violin (McDonald, 1970), it is human relationship that must initially contextualize cultural object, infusing it with richness and layered meanings that resonate with a lasting vibrato, empowering young minds to take the next step, which is toward rewarding solitary experiences with cultural objects.

II

Piping into inner fantasy life often at very deep levels, the picturebook simultaneously transmits ethical values, aesthetic values (tastes), and basic cultural knowledge. Many of its most enduring messages are, as I shall endeavor to show, subliminally conveyed (for a fascinating recent discussion of subliminal visual stimulation, see Fisher, 1988). It assists children in forming concrete and symbolic connections between space and time, nature and culture, inside and outside, and self and other. Partaking in a mini-tradition, namely, an iconographic and literary tradition with interconnecting references, the genre establishes modes of pictorial and verbal citation; in so doing, it initiates young minds into the realm of cultural cross-reference and builds a foundation for future interpretive activity.

One of the finest picturebooks, *Goodnight Moon* (by Margaret Wise Brown and Clement Hurd, originally published in 1947), for example, begins with visual references to both a favorite nursery rhyme, "The

Cow Jumped over the Moon," and a beloved nursery tale, "The Three Bears." These pictorial quotes (given as framed decorations on the wall of a bunny-child's bedroom, the frames serving as emblematic equivalents of quotation marks) are anchored later in the text with verbal labels. When, however, a direct address is made to the cow ("Goodnight cow jumping over the moon"), the image is released from its frame and liberated to become a signifier for more than the words of the rhyme. Flying through the air with a page all to herself, the leaping cow is free to evoke associations for the child as an image. Yet, importantly among these associations, whether available to consciousness or not, are the child's previous experiences of having heard, shared, and repeated the rhyme. Thus, encounters with one picturebook may call up, through such citation, encounters with other cultural objects, and connections among books, imagery, poetry, and shared good feelings are established and reinforced. (The three bears, incidentally, who are at least potentially frightening at bedtime, remain, *unlike* the friendly cow, confined *within* their frame: they are bid "good night" while securely contained within clearly bounded limits.)

In an essay devoted principally to a detailed interpretation of one picturebook (Spitz, 1988), I have discussed the ways in which this genre simultaneously urges children toward words, language, and secondary process while at the same time validating and privileging their inner worlds of fantasy. I have also used a theatrical metaphor to emphasize its performance aspect. The child, unable as yet to read, listens to the voice of an adult who serves rather like a violinist translating the notes of a score into audible sound and whose accuracy, interpretive skill, enthusiasm, timing, and contact with the listener all affect the reception of the music. Like a musical (or mother theatrical) performer, the mother (or other adult) must mediate between child and cultural object. She is, of course, also a listener herself and not unaffected by the "music." (Note, for a description of this, Plato's Ion, whose eyes fill with tears, hair stands on end, and heart throbs when he is called upon to speak certain lines.) Further, just as the musician "holds" her audience, so also the picturebook reader sits comfortably close to and often holds the child in her lap.

We may theorize about the role of the adult reader by evoking another concept of Winnicott's, namely the "holding environment." Our knowledge of the course of cognitive and psychosexual development teaches us that young children can only gradually separate fantasy from reality and that, in the years when picturebooks are used, representations are not yet easily distinguished from objects of representation. (The fact that small children believe, for instance, that persons visible to them on the television screen actually exist inside the set and can be directly addressed has been exploited to great effect by such programs as *Mister Rogers' Neighborhood,* where the host Fred Rogers engages in "dialogue" with his youthful audience.)

Thus, we must expect that picturebooks may occasionally elicit anxiety, regressive fantasy, or hostile impulses. Both because of the immaturity of their audience and because, like other works of art, they do, necessarily, call forth vivid moments of identification and projection, picturebooks require a containment which their given formal elements may not always prove adequate to provide. This additional contextualization must come from the reading adult who creates precisely what can be called an extended "holding environment." Reading adults serve as editors and improvisers—explaining vocabulary, pointing out pictorial details, elaborating a theme, or occasionally censoring the text by substitution or omission; they expand the boundaries of the object to include a legacy of shared experience. The significance of this role is manifest when we consider the fate of children who suffer its absence. Left to experience cultural artifacts on their own, such children miss an essential step in the initiation process. They may experience motivational difficulties in learning to read or, in some cases, fail to develop a deep love for books. Each time, however, a small child is helped by an adult (or older child) to undergo the rising and falling of narrative tension and the stunning immediate effects of color and graphics, his or her heightened achievement of mastery and pleasure marks a way-station on the path of initiation into the realm of arts and culture.

In a recent lecture to a group of first-time mothers, I asked them to try and remember frightening images from books that were read to them in their own early childhoods. With gentle prodding, many divulged such memories—often of oral aggression (e.g., the toothy disembodied grin of the Cheshire cat; the huge, gaping mouth of Monstro the Whale from *Pinocchio*), or the death of a parent (e.g., the page in *Babar* where a "wicked hunter" has shot the young elephant's mother). A propos of this last example, however, I have discovered that many adults, while fondly recalling the Babar of their childhood, fail utterly to remember his mother's violent death at the start of the story. However, in recalling their own anxiety, often readily accessible despite the passage of years, many of these mothers were sensitized, at least momentarily, to the powerful impact of pictorial imagery on the psyches of their own children.

Asked to recall what techniques they had invented to cope with their fear, several remembered anticipating the offending page and turning it over quickly. Others reported having closed their eyes while peeking furtively. In general, avoidance was the most frequently reported defense. None could remember (or admit) tearing or mutilating a disturbing page or scribbling over an especially troubling picture. These other, more extreme, iconoclastic measures, when resorted to, signal a conversion of terror into rage and, by provoking parental response, may serve to bring a child's secret fear into the open. In so serving, such destructive nonverbal responses to imagery may be counted as communication in the sense that Winnicott (1956) described it.

Just as parents (or other caretaking adults) in their mediating and interpreting roles respond according to vicissitudes of their own, as well as their assessment of the child's needs, so it is with the child. Different developmental stages, for example, dictate new agendas or altered patterns of response to well-loved picturebooks. In one case, a boy aged 2, searched obsessively for the moons in *Where the Wild Things Are* (by Maurice Sendak, originally published in 1963) and asked for the moon on each page where it is not represented. Later, at 4 years of age, loving the book still, the same boy had no interest in moons, but expressed anxiety during the wild orgy depicted in the center pages where pictures completely supersede written text (Spitz, 1988). In the absence of further data, one might speculate on the basis of developmental stage theory that whereas separation had preoccupied him at the time of his initial encounter with the book, the control of sexual and aggressive impulses had, by age 4, come into prominence as a theme of greater moment. Of special interest here is that the desire to see the image of the *moon* may also be linked with the child's relationship to a specific pictorial convention (as I shall show) as well as the salient fact that, in spite of all the changes that had occurred in his life between the ages of 2 and 4, one picturebook remained capable of sustaining his interest, keeping up with him, so to speak, and symbolizing the major motifs of his ongoing development—a testament to the power of the genre.

III

Oldest historically, and among the earliest developmentally, among different types of picturebooks, is the alphabet primer. Juxtaposing a picture with its name and initial letter in expectable sequence, primers afford a model of language acquisition based on the priority of noun or name. As an imitative, static model of learning, the primer locks into nonreversible hierarchical order not only its terms, i.e., image and text, but the relative positions of reader and listener. Even here, however, the message may be amplified and/or subverted. Bright pictures (of wild animals, for instance) can leap out of pages to haunt young minds and spark extended fantasy. This tendency on the part of images to escape being controlled by words, like the unruly tendency of primary process to erupt into reasoned discourse, crops up, therefore, even in this most predictable of formats. Its best examples are those like *Brian Wildsmith's ABC* (winner of the Kate Greenaway award, 1963) that openly strive to extract aesthetic response and carry children—by innovative color, scale, gesture, and design—far beyond the fixedness of prescribed arrangement. In such cases, each noun seems to engender a verb, every picture gives birth to story, and staid primers blossom into works of art.

IV

Even prior to the primer, children still in the crawling stage may encounter picturebooks like *Pat the Bunny*, which conjoin the perceptual and verbal with kinaesthetic, olfactory, and tactile experience, strongly prioritizing the latter. Such objects emphasize the physicality, the materiality of art—qualities which, as adults acculturated into a universe of abstract codes, we learn early on to decathect. Yet, touching, holding, loving, all intimately related for the small child, are transferrable, displaceable, by means of these transitional forms, to physically more remote encounters later on with sophisticated cultural objects.

Pat the Bunny (by Dorothy Kunhardt, originally published in 1942) conveys cultural myths and values of enduring significance to children often too young either to walk or to speak in complete sentences. The first page addresses its naïve spectator in the second person and explicitly invites him or her to identify with its characters. Two blond children, the boy taller than the girl, are pictured on the facing page. Without placing undue emphasis on this particular image, it is worthwhile to consider how many girls feel ashamed and embarrassed years later if they grow taller than boys and to consider the beauty ethic innocently implicit in this picture. The final page is a repetition of this one with variations. Paul and Judy wave good-bye, and the boy protects or restrains the girl in a gesture that indicates a certain element of control.

Explicitly, the imagery of this simple book sets up for the preoedipal child the positive oedipal situation as a paradigm: the mother encourages her son to insert his finger into the hole of her ring; while the father, holding his daughter against his body, invites her to touch his unshaven face. Like the children, the mother is blond. Thus, pictorially, the book conveys that little girls can stay the way they are and grow up to resemble mother; whereas boys, resembling the mother at this stage, must radically differentiate themselves from her if they are (later on) to resemble the dark father. In terms of the performance metaphor I have evoked above, the child in relation to this tactile-type book becomes an actor in the drama and participates directly with the reading adult.

A slightly more advanced and complex version of this tactile-type picturebook is entitled *Is This the House of Mistress Mouse?* (by Richard Scarry, originally published in 1964) in which the child repeatedly inserts his or her forefinger into a hole to feel a furry substance that turns out to be the hide of several different (frightening) animals before it can be interpreted as belonging to the house of the (friendly and maternal) title character and being, in fact, the fur of her new baby. Here, libidinal, ego, and object-related issues call forth a gamut of emotions ranging from anticipation to pleasurable satisfaction by way of anxiety, dread, surprise, bewilderment, and delight.

Repetitive encounters with the book confer a sense of mastery: the child's wish for a happy ending is threatened but always finally achieved. The happy ending, however, involves not merely fulfillment of the original wish (Mister Mouse finds Mistress Mouse) but the surprise appearance of their new baby. Entirely unheralded in the text, a complete mystery to its parents, this baby is greeted with unmitigated joy and then the book abruptly ends. Thus, image and text collaborate here to foreclose the intense curiosity and ambivalence stirred up by this event. This is an excellent example of a case in which additional parental contextualization seems warranted. Parenthetically, the book closes with the baby's crib placed under a window through which a moon shines—an image that is gradually building in its associative value for the child-reader. This picture also encodes gender difference by depicting the mother dressed in the same color as the baby and as rushing toward the crib with arms extended toward the child; father mouse admires baby from a distance, his hands behind his back.

V

Some picturebooks seem targeted at specific developmental themes. I shall mention four currently available examples. *Goodnight Moon* (see above) ranks supreme and was eulogized in a *New York Times* editorial (Feb. 14, 1988) when its gifted illustrator died earlier this year. Speaking directly to every small child's fear of the dark and the recurrent anxieties surrounding bedtime separation from primary objects, this book, with elegance and simplicity, offers itself to sleepy toddlers as a primary art object. In visual terms, it soothes and comforts by creating a solid and cosy space that, as its pages are rhythmically turned, grows progressively darker, while, instead of disappearing, all the child's familiar things—comb, brush, mittens, doll house—remain securely in place, and, with unwavering constancy, a moon shines in through the window.

Noodle (published originally in 1937, reissued in 1965, now available in paperback) is a book for upper age-range toddlers who can later on read it to themselves. Its 50-year-long record is a tribute to the inspired collaboration of author Munro Leaf (famous for his *Story of Ferdinand* the bull of 1936) and artist Ludwig Bemelmans (originator of *Madeline,* 1939). Noodle is a dachshund whose short front legs make it hard for him to dig holes because the dirt flies up and hits him in the tummy. One day, after much labor, he digs up a wishbone and expresses the desire to be some other size and shape than he presently is. Visited by an unforgettable dog fairy (who arrives onomatopoetically in "a whirr and a buzz and a flip-flap of wings"), Noodle learns that he will be granted his wish but must choose the new size and shape in just a few hours. After visiting the nearby zoo and interviewing other animals concerning their size and shape, Noodle returns home to eat and nap. When the dog fairy returns to grant his wish, he tells her he has decided to remain "Just exactly the size and shape [he is] *right now.*"

In her classic paper "Early Physical Determinants in the Development of a Sense of Identity," Phyllis Greenacre (1958) persuasively argues that children's awareness of and acceptance of their own bodies must serve as a basis for all future identity formation and reality testing. *Noodle* symbolically digs up this *bedrock* issue and the inevitable disappointments, longings, and conflicts surrounding it. Adumbrated here are wishes to be the sex one is not (to have both male and female genitalia) as well as to alter the details of, and changes in, one's body image. Digging down into the earth (at the cost of considerable discomfort), the little dachshund comes up with, of all things, a *wishbone* (with protuberances and hollow that are repeated in various guises throughout the book and convey a vague bisexuality). Even without a detailed analysis of format and style, we can note the occasional strategic matching of the shape of the printed text on the left-hand page with that of the image on the right—a schema that underscores the theme of bodily size and shape. Stylistically, the drawings convey a spontaneous whimsy associated often with children's own linear art. Psychosexual innuendoes abound (such as the picture of Noodle poking his nose into the hollow earth to smell the bone), and older children can readily associate to other tales involving wishes and fairies. Poetic devices such as onomatopoeia and alliteration reinforce the impact of theme and variations as Noodle visits in turn a male zebra, a married female hippopotamus, an unmarried female ostrich, and finally a male giraffe.

Where's Wallace? (by Hilary Knight, author of *Eloise,* dated originally 1965 and recently reissued in paperback) concerns a mischievous orangutan who repeatedly escapes from his cage in a zoo and thus forces his keeper (and the child-reader) to find him. Because the fumbling keeper (aptly named Mr. Frumbee) absent-mindedly leaves Wallace's cage door ajar, the child can perceive the adult as a collaborator in his thrillingly dangerous game of running away, hiding, and being found. The terror of actually being lost is mitigated even further because, in addition to rigging the cage, the keeper (and child-reader) always have advance knowledge of the limited milieu (page-space) in which the creature is bound to be hiding and thus found. In this way, the format of the book provides multiple roles for the child—who can identify simultaneously and serially with hider, seeker, finder, and the one found.

Each locale into which Wallace disappears (e.g., department store, museum of natural history, circus, ocean beach, amusement park) is delineated in minute graphic detail and carefully includes repeated unnamed figures—a runner, a baby, a knitting lady, a man with a bass viol, and a naughty little girl with pigtails whose mother is always depicted with frantic gestures—who provide a thread of visual continuity in locales which are, in any case, never entirely foreign to the child-reader. Thus, while directly addressing the themes of separation anxiety and object constancy, *Where's Wallace?* concurrently explores a number of environments of cultural significance for the child. Parenthetically, this is also the case with another brilliant picturebook, *Madeline,* where the narrative is set against backgrounds that depict Notre Dame, Sacré Coeur, Place Vendôme, the Eiffel tower, etc., so that the child who loves this story becomes visually acquainted with the city of Paris.

My last example in this series is *Harold and the Purple Crayon* (by Crockett Johnson, originally published in 1955). This physically minute book of purple line drawings calls upon children to identify directly with its creator, to become, as it were, artists and authors of their own invented worlds. It valorizes the realm of make-believe and models the creation of bedtime fantasies: little Harold draws one himself before our eyes with his purple crayon. After giving it form and projecting into it his private wishes and danger situations, after pleasing, exciting, scaring, and rescuing himself, he ingeniously finds his way back to the safety of his bedroom. In the last picture, he lies snugly in bed with the moon shining through his window. After drawing (*sic*) the covers up, his purple crayon drops to the floor, and Harold drops (*sic*) off to sleep—these verbal puns serving as analogues for the visual puns that have carried the story along from page to page in a witty and wonderful secondary elaboration of the unpredictable associative links of the primary process.

Again in this book, the moon plays a central role. In fact, it is Harold's memory of the moon shining through his bedroom window that enables him, when lost, to find his way back to familiar surroundings. I wish to underline the potent effect of *quotation* here—the point that young children preconsciously associate to Harold's empowering memory their own prior experiences with picturebooks such as *Goodnight Moon*. In this way, a repertoire of cultural reference is gradually accumulated. To sharpen my point, the referent for "moon" is never simply the one out there in the sky, but importantly all the *pictured moons* the child has known and loved. Parenthetically, the most brilliant children's book to deploy this symbol is probably James Thurber's *Many Moons* (1943), a masterpiece that deserves a separate paper of its own.

I would like at this point, before going on, to address the possible meanings to the young child of the repetitive symbolism of moon shining through window, a visual trope consistent in the picturebooks discussed here thus far. Clearly, the moon figures in part as a maternal symbol, not only because of its roundness, suggestive of the breast, but perhaps also because of its repetitive cycles: like the mother, the moon disappears gradually and predictably reappears—changing shape but always recognizable. Illuminating the darkness, it, again like the mother, serves as a beacon in the frightening realm of the unknown. Associated by the child with time for bed and thus separation, its predictable presence stands as a constant, a bulwark against the fear of strangeness and boundlessness that loss of parental objects betokens. In this sense, the moon shining through the window may be seen as a pictorial representation of the very "holding environment" instantiated by the reading of the picturebook itself in the company of the caretaking adult.

Furthermore, as depicted in these texts, the moon, shining in through a window, can be seen as mirroring the child's own face as he or she looks at the pictured scene from the other side. A fine example may be found in Ungerer's *Moon Man* (1967), where the beholder is meant to identify with the soft, round-faced title character whose envious narrative ends in a peaceful return to familiar surroundings. Thus, in keeping with Paulina Kernberg's (1987) studies of the young child's conflation of self and maternal object in the mirror, we might interpret the presence of the moon as representing not only the maternal object per se but perhaps a form of transitional or self object. According to this interpretation, the window through which the moon is visible figures both the door through which the mother appears and disappears and, likewise, the frame of a mirror.

VI

Now, I shall turn to a unique artifact: a small collection of picturebooks originally published by Maurice Sendak in 1962 entitled *The Nutshell Library*.[1] After a glance at its general format, I shall conclude this essay by focusing on one of its four volumes. Compact enough in size to turn even the smallest child into a giant, this novel work can be taken as paradigmatic of the primary art object in all the senses I have attempted to convey. Moving zestfully in two directions, it fosters fantasy while turning inexorably toward secondary process, ego autonomy, mastery, and object permanence. Metaphorically it focuses on oral themes: growing up (it teaches) means filling up, nourishing the self, with good things for both mouth and stomach, eye and mind. It conveys the message that growing *up* entails growing *into* a culture; that, in order to achieve this, one must both eat and read, activities that confer comfort and pleasure as well as genuine power and mastery.

The slipcase of *The Nutshell Library* contains four tiny volumes that measure less than 3 x 4 inches. These volumes are not packed in any foreordained sequence, as the end leaf of each lists the order differently. They are as follows: a counting book, *One Was Johnny;* a book of months, *Chicken Soup with Rice;* an alphabet primer, *Alligators All Around;* and an ethical tract, *Pierre.* Thus, each conveys a different kind of knowledge to the young mind and, because their order is unfixed, they subtly teach that no one kind of knowledge may be prized or prioritized over any other. All are important, all equally valid.

The slipcase instantiates the very nutshell that is imprinted upon its every side, its contents, the volumes themselves, thus being its nourishing and delicious nutmeats. (One thinks, parenthetically, of the collegiate expression: "to crack a book.") Each of the three sides of the slipcover is designed like a miniature stage set with a small white curtain overhead inscribed with the name of author-artist Maurice Sendak. Thus, they participate in the metaphor of theater, spectacle, and performance established earlier in this essay. However, whereas I spoke earlier of the reading adult as a performer-artist with respect to a child-audience, *The Nutshell Library* dramatizes its themes somewhat

1. I am indebted to the perceptive literary insights of Prof. Cheryl Torsney (1986) and gratefully acknowledge her permission to draw on them.

differently: here, the metaphor shifts to a direct, unmediated relationship between child and book: *the book will stage itself for the child.*
Masquerading characters in each of the volumes serve to underscore
this trope and assert that imagination (make-believe) is central to all
learning.

Each miniature stage depicted on the slipcover is flanked by columns
decorated with oak leaves and topped by fluted acorn capitals. Supporting these columns are blocks with smiling faces that suggest traditional masks of comedy (no tragedy). An acorn and silver crown adorn
the top of the slipcase. Joining the anonymous Latin quotation that
translates "Tall oaks from little acorns grow" with Francis Bacon's
"Knowledge is power" ("Nam et ipsa scientia potestas est"), we may
interpret the iconography as saying that small children, like acorns, can
become powerful like oak trees through the acquisition of knowledge,
the imbibing of culture.

This theme is graphically portrayed on the back of the slipcase,
where, onstage face to face, sit two characters from the books inside:
the little boy from *Chicken Soup* licks his lips and spoons up steaming
liquid from his bowl, while a happy alligator from *Alligators All Around*
reads from an open book. The parallelism here equates these two kinds
of consumption and depicts them both as deeply satisfying. Interestingly, these figures are upstaged by a cat and rat (characters from
One Was Johnny) whose story of hunt and chase seems ready to begin—
the cat looking smug with back arched, the mouse poised sniffing,
about to run. Thus, suspense links the theatrical metaphor with the
acts of reading and taking in.

Other characters from the books inhabit stages on slipcover front
and binding. Pierre reads face to face with his lion (who is also reading),
and, on the binding, the monkey from *One Was Johnny* reads peacefully
under the chandelier from which he swings wildly in his book. All these
characters, if interpreted as reading about themselves in their own
books, express by analogy the pleasure of children who can relive (and
eventually sublimate) their own silliness, naughtiness, disorder, and
disobedience through symbolic representation in cultural objects.

In addition to their visual elements, all four books build ingenious
bridges between a toddler's joy in experimenting with sound, early
language play, and sophisticated devices of poetic diction. Simple repetition is used not only pictorially but in refrains. In *Chicken Soup with
Rice* the refrain is reiterated on every page of the text, as is very nearly
the case in *Pierre*, where the title character continually chants, "I don't
care!" *Alligators All Around* features alliteration, a form of repetition
used not only by masters of poetic language but by infants practicing

with word-sounds. Thus, this alphabet primer strengthens a child's grasp of the sound of letters by offering phrases such as "B bursting balloons," "G getting giggles," "M making macaroni," and "Y yackety-yacking." In *Chicken Soup with Rice*, alliteration is unforgettably the major trope for the month of January: "In January / it's so nice / while slipping / on the sliding ice / to sip hot chicken soup / with rice. / Sipping once / sipping twice / sipping chicken soup / with rice."

Celebrated throughout the year, chicken soup is symbolic of basic oral comfort, a restorative to which the child can repair in every kind of weather—weather standing here as a metaphor for the child's varied and mercurial inner states. A figure for love, it is analogized by image and text with cultural experience. As pointed out above, the book of months and counting book, whose protagonists are visually inter-changeable, suggest that being alone with a book, like having a bowl of hot chicken soup, can enable one to feel loved, nourished, sustained.

With regard to the theme of quotation, the counting book offers a nose-pecking blackbird, undoubtedly one of the four-and-twenty baked in a pie from the nursery rhyme "Sing a Song of Sixpence." This pecking blackbird also figures in Sendak's own self-reflexive iconography and appears, for example, in *Hector Protector* and *As I Went Over the Water* (1965). The tiger selling old clothes, also a character in the counting book, inescapably refers by reversal to the tale of "Little Black Sambo," where the tigers *take* the little boy's *new* clothes; furthermore, whereas those tigers threaten to eat the child up, here it is the little boy who tells the animals that if they don't leave him alone, he will devour them! A small white dog appears in *The Nutshell Library*, another Sendak creation, who stars in *Higglety Pigglety Pop!* (1967) and plays a walk-on (or, perhaps, a run-on) role in *Where the Wild Things Are*.

VII

Psychoanalytically speaking, the meatiest nut in the shell is *Pierre*, subtitled "a cautionary tale in five chapters and a prologue." Self-confessedly literary in its format, this book is the ethics primer of the set. Its deliberate stylization (the prologue is a limerick) serves not only to introduce formal elements but also, because the content is frightening (little boy eaten by a lion), to alienate and defend the child-reader from its impact. Likewise, the foreign name of its protagonist (Pierre as opposed to Peter) functions to distance the title character and forestall too immediate an identification (Torsney, 1988).

Pierre's drama is that of a little boy who responds to his mother's affection, offer of breakfast, etc., by repeating the words: "I don't care!" The mother soon leaves, and the father appears. To each of the latter's commands, threats, bribes, and entreaties, the child reiterates his response: "I don't care!" Mother and father now both depart, and a hungry lion arrives. To all the lion's questions, such as whether Pierre would like to die, whether he realizes that the lion can eat him up, and whether, finally, he has anything else to say, Pierre produces his classic retort. On the page following this interchange, we find a conspicuous gap: Pierre is missing! The lion, filling the entire space occupied previously by both figures, looks smug: the accompanying text is terse: "So the lion ate Pierre."

Arriving home, the mother and father find a lion sick in Pierre's bed. Suspecting the worse, they assault him and inquire about their son. Classically, the lion replies, "I don't care!" On the next page, a doctor shakes the lion upside down; whereupon Pierre falls out on the floor.[2] After being hugged by his mother and queried by his father, the little boy reassures them both, and together they all ride home astride the lion. Pierre, perched on the lion's head, finally shouts, "Yes, indeed I care!" The lion remains with them "as a weekend guest," and, as in all true fables, the last line informs us of the moral, which is: "CARE!"

A truly memorable creation, Pierre's lion condenses many aspects of a child's inner life. He represents previously disowned aggression turned now against the self, aggression for which the parents first serve as both willing and unwilling objects; in addition, he represents the parental introjects themselves combined into a punitive, primitive superego forerunner—an active version of the passive aggression expressed by the child's behavior. For Pierre does not attack the parents directly; in adopting a typically oppositional stance, he aggresses against them by contrarily *not* doing, *not* responding. He *won't* eat, *won't* go to town, in fact turns the milk pitcher, bowl, broom, and himself (quite literally) upside down.

This upside-down motif figures prominently in the drama. A small panel of drawings frames the book, ornamenting both the "Table of Contents" and the final page. In sequence, these drawings depict

2. The text says, curiously, that when Pierre fell out, he "laughed because he wasn't dead." In keeping with the Judaic motifs that interweave Sendak's works (e.g., the Yiddish expression "wilde chaye"—wild animal—which underlies his marvelous conception of the "wild things" and the stars of David in both *In the Night Kitchen* and *Dear Mili*, where Hebrew letters are engraved on the tombstones), Pierre's particular laughter at this moment of survival can be interpreted as evoking the Biblical Isaac (Yitzchak, "One who laughs"). Pierre, like Yitzchak in the Akedah (the binding, *Genesis* 22:1–19) survives what could only be experienced by a child as the extremity of parental aggression and abandonment.

Pierre performing a headstand; the last of them, however, in which he actually stands on his head, shows his right arm rising from the ground and right leg bending as if to indicate that he is about to flip over again and come right side up. Thus, a process is indicated: the drawings suggest that although a child may indeed turn himself upside down, he can right himself as well. This motif also signifies in the dramatic action: not only does Pierre infuriate his father by talking to him from a feet-up posture early on, but later the lion, having swallowed Pierre, must (in turn) be turned upside down in order to release him.

The lion, we note, comes onstage only after Pierre's parents leave. In abandoning their (dependent) young child, parents may become, in that child's fantasy, bad and threatening, for they display, as it were, their trump card: their ultimate power to desert. In this (Kleinian) sense, the lion represents also the projected badness of the abandoning parents. In addition, their absence leaves Pierre without external objects on whom to vent his aggression; thus, it now turns against him and must be confronted. In keeping with the oral theme of *The Nutshell Library* and the developmental imperatives of its young readers, the lion not only threatens (with words) but actually eats Pierre (Pierre disappears from the page). Before this, however, he is informed that, after being eaten, he will be *inside* the lion; in other words, things will be *inside out:* the child's projected aggression will consume him. Thus, the upside-down motif extends to encompass that of inside-out.

Significantly, when the parents return, they do not hesitate to aggress directly against the lion (mother pulls his hair and father lifts a chair to strike him). At no point in the story previously, however, did either parent attack Pierre. It is the child's triumphant aggression, his bad introject, they attack, not the child himself. This important distinction is made by both sign systems—image and text. It powerfully implies the ongoing love of these parents for their child and the survival of that love in the face of developmentally induced negativity.

Verbally and pictorially, both parents conform to conventional gender stereotypes: mother calls Pierre "darling," offers him food, cries and hugs him when he emerges from the lion; father disciplines him, criticizes, commands, reasons, bargains, and asks him if he is all right when he reappears. Thus, typical roles inscribed by our culture are reinforced by the picturebook. Mother wears high heels, fur-trimmed coat, and a whimsical hat; father sports a mustache, overcoat, and fedora.

In the end, not just Pierre but also the parents are shown riding home on the lion, thus indicating that mastery of aggression is an issue not only for children but for entire families. Riding—as a symbol for control and mastery—occurs again, parenthetically, in *Where the Wild Things Are,* where Max (a visual double for Pierre) rides one of his introjects in the wild orgy scene. (One also recalls Freud's 1923 metaphor of the ego riding the forces of the id.) Finally, it matters that Pierre's lion does not depart ignominiously but, rather, stays on with the family. Thus, aggression is portrayed as an ongoing theme that will not vanish but must be continually addressed.

VIII

My effort in this paper has been to indicate, with the aid of psychoanalytic developmental theory, the impact of the picturebook on young minds, its role in the process of acculturation, and its value for interdisciplinary studies.[3] Deceptively simple, this genre establishes—by means of image, text, performing adult, and attentive child—a liminal space in which fantasy blossoms, psychological issues are symbolically enacted, and the roots of cultural knowledge pleasurably implanted.

"Culture" derives from the Latin, "colo," which means "to till, to husband, to raise, to nurture." If we view culture in the light of this etymology—as a nurturing matrix for the growth of symbolic and semantic structures—it comes into sharp focus as a setting for early drive and object relations. Thus, while Greenacre (1957) has proposed the notion of "collective alternates" in the life of the gifted child, we may wish to extend her usage and accord a higher priority to significant artifacts in the lives of all children—especially to those artifacts uniquely designed to appeal to them, indoctrinate them, and expand their mental function. In closing, it is well to add that an essay such as this inevitably raises larger questions as to the deep impact of culture on psyche—its inextricability, perhaps, from biologically derived determinants.

BIBLIOGRAPHY

BEMELMANS, L. (1939). *Madeline.* New York: Simon & Schuster. (Most recent edition, Penguin Books, 1987.)

3. A propos of this impact, picturebooks designed with avowedly ideological aims deserve at least a mention here. In a recent lecture, Professor Yosef Yerushalmi (1988) presented repugnant examples of widely circulated Nazi picturebooks for children from the 1930s. These depict the Jew as a fox or, in one book, as a poisonous mushroom. In the latter book, blond German youngsters are shown distinguishing Jews from Aryans as noxious fungi that must be differentiated from safe, edible species. Sparks of bigotry and hatred, thus kindled, are not in later years easily extinguished.

BROWN, M. W. & HURD, C. (1947). *Goodnight Moon*. New York: Harper & Row.

FISHER, C. (1988). Further observations on the Poetzl phenomenon. *Psychoanal. Contemp. Thought*, 11:3–56.

FREUD, S. (1923). The ego and the id. *S.E.*, 19:3–66.

———(1939). Moses and monotheism. *S.E.*, 23:3–137.

GREENACRE, P. (1957). The childhood of the artist. In *Emotional Growth*. New York: Int. Univ. Press, 1971, vol. 2, pp. 479–504.

———(1958). Early physical determinants in the development of a sense of identity. In *Emotional Growth*. New York: Int. Univ. Press, 1971, vol. 1, pp. 113–127.

JOHNSON, C. (1955). *Harold and the Purple Crayon*. New York: Harper & Row.

KERNBERG, P. (1987). Mother-child interaction and mirror behavior. *Infant Mental Health Journal*, 8:4. Winter.

KNIGHT, H. (1964). *Where's Wallace?* New York: Harper & Row.

KUNHARDT, D. (1942). *Pat the Bunny*. Racine, Wisc.: Golden Press.

LEAF, M. (1937). *Noodle*. New York: Four Winds Press.

McDONALD, M. (1970). Transitional tunes and musical development. *Psychoanal. Study Child*, 25:503–520.

PLATO. *The Dialogues of Plato*, tr. B. Jowett. New York: Random House, 1937.

SCARRY, R. (1964). *Is This the House of Mistress Mouse?* Racine, Wisc.: Golden Press.

SENDAK, M. (1962). *The Nutshell Library*. New York: Harper & Row.

———(1963). *Where the Wild Things Are*. New York: Harper & Row.

SPITZ, E. H. (1988). Picturing the child's inner world of fantasy. *Psychoanal. Study Child*, 43:433–447.

THURBER, J. (1943). *Many Moons*. New York & London: Harcourt Brace Jovanovich.

Tools of Childhood. *The New York Times*, editorial. Feb. 14, 1988.

TORSNEY, C. B. (1986). *The Nutshell Library* as literary primer. Unpublished essay, read to the Modern Language Association.

UNGERER, T. (1967). *Moon Man*. New York: Harper & Row.

WILDSMITH, B. (1962). *Brian Wildsmith's ABC*. Oxford: Oxford Univ. Press.

WINNICOTT, D. W. (1956). The antisocial tendency. In *Collected Papers*. New York: Basic Books, 1958, pp. 306–315.

———(1966). The location of cultural experience. *Int. J. Psychoanal.*, 48:368–372.

YERUSHALMI, Y. (1988). Alisa in Wonderland: The book and the Jewish child. Lecture at the Jewish Theological Seminary, December 7.

Terror Writing by the Formerly Terrified

A Look at Stephen King

LENORE C. TERR, M.D.

EARLY IN 1987 I SAW ROB REINER'S FILM, *STAND BY ME*. WHAT SHOWED first and most obviously about this film was its marvelous presentation of a passage into adolescence theme. The movie *Stand by Me*, as a matter of fact, is a very American, very charming, and very accurate portrayal of what it means to be a 12-year-old boy at the brink of manhood. The moviegoer sees and enjoys four boys' overblown sense of "macho," their need to break off babyish ties with family, their intense concern about their own genital apparatus, their deep distrust of all adults, and their dawning realization of abstractions such as "intimacy" or "hypocrisy." The prepubertal dialogue in the film is great. Although I grew up as a girl and never heard any of my 12-year-old friends term one another "wet ends" or throw out invective such as "suck my fat one," the preadolescent in me still understands. The children of *Stand by Me* are speaking the language of American childhood.

This "passage into adolescence" theme may be what the reader wishes to think about when a film, as accurately evocative of preadolescent childhood as this one is, comes up for discussion. However, there was something else in *Stand by Me* to which I will devote this entire paper—and that is its mood of terror. Terror strikes the viewer of this film, I think, from the very beginning. A full-grown man sits in a pickup truck reading his newspaper. His best friend from childhood, Chris Chambers, has been killed trying to break up a knife fight in a fast food restaurant. How suddenly, how unexpectedly does a life end. How horrifying.

Clinical professor of psychiatry at the University of California, San Francisco School of Medicine.

But we have little time to reflect. We immediately meet the four boys from the truck-owner's past. First there is Teddy Duchamp whose psychotic father, a war veteran, has burned up the boy's ear and rendered Teddy partially deaf. Teddy is an abused child. A second boy, Vern Tessio, turns out to be fat, a little stupid, money-obsessed, and besieged at home by a frighteningly delinquent, older brother. The third and the leader of the small gang, Chris Chambers, a dead-man-to-be as we already know, has a dad who drinks himself stuporous but often comes home invigorated enough to beat the boy silly. And fourth, we meet Gordon Lachance, an author-to-be, the narrator. Gordon, too, it seems, is living a nightmare. His older brother, Dennis, has been killed a few months ago in an auto accident. Gordon is the "invisible man" at home. His parents are the benumbed survivors of a personal disaster. The young lads of the film are four extremely stressed youngsters—two sure-fire psychic trauma victims and two youngsters suffering the possible effects of horrible, ongoing, external events. Although in a small-town control study of 25 ordinary children, I found 10 who were psychically traumatized or severely frightened (Terr, 1983a), even *I* felt surprised to count 4 of 4 in this movie. This film would be no ordinary "passage into adolescence" film, I began to feel the first time that I watched it.

One settles into the movie, however, and begins feeling the plain, ordinary feelings of a journey into adolescence when—close to the middle—a scene develops that is so scary, so monsterous, so unexpected that it reproduces the feeling of childhood trauma right then and there. A train unexpectedly appears and almost runs down the four boys on a narrow trestle high above a gorge. I remember saying to myself during this scene, "Whoever wrote this movie is playing post-traumatic games with me." And I remember that suddenly my mind found channels other than the movie with which to occupy itself.

"The writer of this film," I said to myself, "obviously is a man because boy life is so accurately portrayed. He has been writing most of his life because the boy in this film is writing at age 12 and he already knows that he *will* be a writer." The author actually saw a dead mutilated child in his own childhood. I believe that this must have occurred in reality because the writer has set up such a strange goal for this "journey into adolescence" trek along the tracks—the goal of finding and viewing the dead, mutilated body of a boy hit by a train. And the author of this story has been traumatized himself in some way by a train. It happened when he was young—some time in the 1950s because this is the era so carefully portrayed on film, complete with striped, collared shirts, early rock tunes, hot rod cars, and several presently extinct species of comic book. "Brilliant," I said, "but is this true? Let's go look it up tomorrow."

We stayed on for the credits. The writer of the novella from which the film, *Stand by Me,* was taken, a story called "The Body" (in *Different Seasons*), is Stephen King. Stephen King is the most widely read, widely watched, widely interviewed, and widely followed writer of horror fiction alive today. By sensing the terror in *Stand by Me,* I had run into the master of terror himself.

The next day I visited a book store and checked out Stephen King's life. It only took one look to determine that my guesses about the writer had been right. I found this autobiographical quote in King's own nonfiction account of the recent history of horror writing, *Danse Macabre* (1981a) and I later found a duplicate in Douglas Winter's book (1986) on Stephen King. I have also added a point about urinary incontinence that I found later—from *Bare Bones,* Underwood and Miller's (1988) collection of Stephen King interviews. This is how Stephen King, himself, puts it:

> . . . the event occurred when I was barely four, so perhaps I can be excused for remembering [my mother's] story of it but not the actual event.
>
> According to Mom, I had gone off to play at a neighbor's house—a house that was near a railroad line. About an hour after I left I came back (she said), as white as a ghost. I would not speak for the rest of that day; I would not tell her why I'd not waited to be picked up or phoned that I wanted to come home; I would not tell her why my chum's mom hadn't walked me back but had allowed me to come alone. [In an interview from 1983, King says he had also "peed in my pants" before coming home.]
>
> It turned out that the kid I had been playing with had been run over by a freight train while playing on or crossing the tracks (years later, my mother told me that they had picked up the pieces in a wicker basket). My Mom never knew if I had been near him when it happened, or if it had occurred before I even arrived, or if I had wandered away after it happened. Perhaps she had her own ideas on the subject. But as I've said, I have no memory of the incident at all; only of having been told about it some years after the fact [p. 83f.].

Now that we have reviewed Stephen King's autobiographical statement about his 4-year-old traumatic experience with a train, let me propose how I will proceed. I wish to use Stephen King's horror writing as "a single case report" of posttraumatic play (Terr, 1981) in art. Posttraumatic play probably serves as a basis for a significant fraction of the world's artistic endeavor. In the past I have shown how childhood trauma drove Edgar Allan Poe, Edith Wharton, René Magritte, Alfred Hitchcock, and Ingmar Bergman to establish certain themes in their art (Terr, 1987a). Creative work may be inspired by external events that overwhelm and overpower the young psyche, forcing repeated attempts to discharge the "traumatic anxiety" that was originally stirred up. If trauma infects a very talented youngster, that child may hone his talents down to the purpose of lancing this ever-purulent abscess.

In considering Stephen King's horror writing, therefore, I will present five topics: (1) how Stephen King's life shows the ongoing influence of his childhood trauma; (2) how King's childhood experience and his posttraumatic symptoms are directly put into his fictional plots; (3) how King's story lines express his fear of psychiatry and psychoanalysis; (4) how King uses certain writing techniques to stir up the sense of trauma in his reader; and (5) how King inspires posttraumatic contagion and mass hysteria.

KING'S LIFE

> As to whether he was warped as a child or just born that way, the answer is as obvious as it is ultimately insignificant. Of course he was, and you better watch out.
>
> Tabitha King, Stephen King's wife,
> as quoted by Douglas Winter (p. 12)

How does what we know of King's life reflect his trauma at age 4? Much more happens in a lifetime than one trauma. I must caution myself about this point as well as cautioning you. We will only pick up glimmers of the early trauma—not the whole picture—in King's life and in his creations.

Despite his penchant for granting interviews, making appearances at horror and supernatural conferences, and writing short, semisarcastic autobiographical sketches, Stephen King is a very private kind of person. He lives in Bangor, Maine with his wife and his three children behind a gate that features two huge bats on posts that loom over a spider-web entrance. We have been given the skeleton of King's life but not the fleshed-out version. Stephen King was born in 1947 in Portland, Maine. His father left one plain day when King was 2. The elder Mr. King said he was going out to buy cigarettes and he never returned. Stephen King has no idea today if "the bastard" is alive or dead (Underwood and Miller, p. 35). He never supported the family. There was not contact after age 2 except for Stephen's discovery at around age 12 of a pile of science fiction paperbacks that his father had left in Aunt Ethelyn's attic (King, *Danse Macabre*, p. 94). This, of course, must in part have settled young King into the choice of writing as a career and even have helped to set his course toward fantasy fiction. But as a matter of fact Stephen King was writing horror stories from the time he was 7 years old (Winter, 1986). His first work was a tale of a run-amok dinosaur that eventually turned tail after a whiff of some belts and boots. Old dinosaurs were "allergic" to leather, according to the 7-year-old Stephen.

Stephen King's mother is consistently praised by the author as a woman who worked herself to the raw skin at menial jobs in order to support Stephen and his 2-year-older, adopted brother, David. Any possible criticism of King's mother is only implied, not stated by King. The trio, mother and two boys, drifted from place to place in New England and the Midwest until Stephen reached the age of 11 and the family settled in Durham, Maine with Mrs. King's aging parents. King's mother was a deeply religious Methodist. She insisted that the family attend church two to three times a week. Stephen's mother used the stories of the Bible to get her points across to her sons. She also confined the boys in an outhouse when they acted up, insisting that they pray while locked inside (Winter, 1986). Whether King's mother still lives as the Bible-spouting horror-of-a-mother depicted in *Carrie* is only a point for speculation. King never spoke of any such analogy in print or in interviews. But he *does* say that one cannot beat the Bible stories as horror literature (Underwood and Miller, p. 187).

Although we know only the barebone outlines of Stephen King's life, the train trauma and the loss of his father appear to be the two major external forces behind the character of the writer. Stephen suffered the fearful symptoms of psychic trauma as a child—bugs, monsters, fires, explosions, storms, the dark terrified him—and he is still a fearful man—bugs, elevators, planes ("I hate surrendering control of my life," he says), the dark, and choking (his mother died of cancer and that night, "practically the same minute actually [my] son had a terrible choking fit in bed at home") *still* terrify him (Underwood and Miller, pp. 24–56). As a boy Stephen King was lonely, fat, unathletic, unhappy, and fascinated with the supernatural. One cannot tell much about his relationship with his older brother. King says nothing that indicates particular closeness or intense rivalry. When he was a boy, Stephen King put together a secret scrapbook on the exploits of the mass murderer, Charles Starkweather. The Holocaust occupied his mind, too.

Stephen King may have repeatedly played "trains" posttraumatically during his latency years. He says that he liked to pretend by himself about Sodom and Gomorrah, ever-mindful of how Lot's wife had turned back to look at the two cities and had turned to salt. "I used to pretend," he says, "I was one of these guys running away [from Sodom and Gomorrah] and could hear the city burning behind me and the screams from the bolts of fire coming down from heaven—I could feel my head go 'Boooooom!' Scared the shit out of me" (Underwood and Miller, p. 187). This sounds very much like the type of activity one could expect from a child who, spending some time with a friend at the railway tracks, ran away from a quickly advancing train, not looking back until it was too late. "Boooooom!" King's stated response to his own game, as a matter of fact—feeling more scared than he felt before—is typical of what happens to children who play a posttraumatic game. Posttraumatic play does little to relieve the kind of anxiety stirred up by psychic trauma.

As a boy King began writing because he needed to. His stories flowed at their best when, he says, they were "unconsciously" done. Stephen King consistently wrote of horror and the supernatural. A sufferer—always—of terrible dreams and insomnia, he conveyed his nightmares to people through his writing. As he became more adept at writing, Stephen was able to substitute writing for that old, monstrous Sodom and Gomorrah game that he had played. King's writing became his posttraumatic play, in other words. As a character says in *It* (1986), "He sold nightmares to others—that was his trade." Like other childhood trauma victims, King has never believed in his own personal future (Terr, 1983b, 1984). Convinced until age 20 that "I'd never live to reach twenty," he now frets that one of his children will die in childhood. As for his own future, he says, "I go day by day" (Underwood and Miller, p. 19). His life goal is "to try and stay alive" (*ibid.*, p. 177). Or put in King's strident, metaphoric tone, "we know that sooner or later we're all going to be eating worms, whether it's fifty years or sixty. It might be tomorrow. It might happen today" (*ibid.*, p. 193).

Stephen King had a second chance to write a new, phony life biography when, between 1977 and 1982, as a successful novelist, he wrote the Richard Bachman books. (King needed to write the books under the pseudonym because he tended to write more than his publishers could allow him to publish.) The Bachman biography, like much of King's other writing, turned out to be playfully posttraumatic. Bachman was supposedly an isolate living alone with his wife on a New Hampshire farm. He had spent several years at sea before settling down, similar to what King's mother had told him of his father, a man who supposedly wandered about the world having love affairs and adopting various aliases—Spansky, Pollock, and finally King. Richard Bachman, the pretend writer, had had a brain tumor removed successfully with very delicate surgery. That sounds traumatic. But he had also experienced a permanent, absolutely uncorrectable disaster. Bachman's only child, a son, crashed through a closed well cover, fell in, and drowned. So Richard Bachman, Stephen King's phony self, also suffered from psychic trauma.

King, as a college student at the University of Maine, Orono, majored in English. He delved into abusive substances. He drank and still drinks prodigious amounts of beer ("Two quarts a day," he says in Underwood and Miller, p. 169). He took and still takes dozens of headache pills. (There is a chance that King's headaches started as psychophysiologic reenactments of his train trauma [Terr, 1983b]. The Sodom and Gomorrah game had included a "Boooooom" in Stephen's head.) King self-admittedly indulged in about 60 psychedelic "trips" in college (Underwood and Miller, p. 43), but he uses no street drugs to speak of now and says he never had a bad psychedelic experience or a residual effect from the drugs. One might insert a hypothetical question here: Was King's college drug experimentation (and perhaps that of others) a posttraumatic phenomenon, an attempt to recreate a traumatic state but under control? King does not give enough personal material on this subject to form any answer.

King taught high school in Maine for a short time in order to support his young family after he graduated from college—but by his mid-20s, *Carrie*, his first novel, was doing very well and had been sold as a movie. His success from that time on was a matter of spiraling fame and fortunes.

From this brief summary, I think it is clear that Stephen King currently suffers many of the symptoms and signs of posttraumatic stress disorder of childhood. He suffers nightmares, fears, headaches, insomnia, a sense of futurelessness, and very active denial. But he has never seen a psychiatrist or a psychoanalyst, as far as I can tell. King says he is afraid that psychoanalysis kills creativity. He uses Ray Bradbury as one example of an author whose writing was better when he was "totally-apparently-fucked up" than it has been since he was treated and became, according to King, "very boring" (Underwood and Miller, p. 163). King says he cannot remember his trauma from about age 4. But that age is slightly old for a total amnesia on the basis of developmental immaturity (from a study I did, age 28 to 36 months appeared to be the approximate cutoff point for verbal memory of documented traumatic events [Terr, 1988]). King's characters in fiction have slippable, "on again, off again" amnesias, by the way. We can see examples of this in *It* and *Pet Sematary*. One wonders if the partial memory of King's fictional protagonists is closer to the author's actual life experience than is his autobiographical claim to total amnesia.

Stephen King says he believes he could write, if he wanted to, non-horror fiction. But he does not. And he has not. His writing is devoted to one emotion—terror. It is this narrowing of theme that defines his art as a traumatic product.

I wish to point out one more posttraumatic and semi-auto-biographical note from the movie, *Stand by Me*, the film that first introduced me to King. Did the young King actually view the body in the basket that day at the railroad tracks, or did he see it solely in his mind's eye? I would guess the latter from King's latency-aged Sodom and Gomorrah game in which the object was to run away from a cataclysm without looking back. But we cannot tell for sure what of "The Body" the author did or did not see from his statements or from his film. There is no question, however, that corpses preoccupy King, and that the idea or the actual viewing of that body bothered him indeed. In his novella, "The Body," from which Rob Reiner took his movie, King spends 7 pages describing the boy's dead body. In his 7 pages, Stephen King sends in the ants, the maggots, a beetle, some ugly swellings, some bad smells, and a hail storm to attack the youthful cadaver at the railroad tracks. But Rob Reiner does not go for any "gross outs" in *Stand by Me*. A film director is able to correct for the overly zealous writer. Reiner showed his "body" in two segments lasting about two seconds apiece. The director had nothing to prove with his young cadaver. He went for the PG ratings, not for the audience's "shit-in-the-pants level." (This, by the way, is not how I talk. It is how Stephen King talks.) No matter how bland and likable Reiner makes it, however, we were seeing in this film the 4-year-old King's visualization, his re-membered or imagined "body." This visualization, the remnant of King's trauma, still had the power to create a shiver up the collective spine of the audience. King, as a matter of fact, points to "The Body" as an example of his flexibility as a novelist. He does not *have* to write horror stories, he says (Underwood and Miller, p. 124). But an instant later King states, "I haven't been able to get away from horror entirely, even here."

KING'S PLOTS

If you write a novel where the boogeyman gets some-body else's children, maybe they'll never get your own children.

Stephen King, as quoted in
Underwood and Miller (p. 3)

Stephen King puts his old, literal nemesis, the train, into his stories. A train kills Frank Dodd's father in *The Dead Zone,* smashing the man's body between two flat cars. Trains zoom by a switchman's severed head the beginning of *Cycle of the Werewolf.* Trains even participate in the climax of *Christine,* a novel about a car, as King opens a crucial chapter with a rock song quote from Mark Dinning: "That fateful night the car was stalled, Upon the railroad track, I pulled you out and you were safe, But you went running back" (p. 421). Trains whiz by in the night in several of King's stories. They whistle in the backgrounds. They help set his tone of terror.

But King's ancient trains become even more interesting when translated by him into their mechanical analogues, devices that can smash or grind up human beings at "will." In fact, the more I read the works of Stephen King, the more I realized that his mechanical monsters were, by far, his most appealing characters. King's machines have more personality than his humans. They have malicious souls—gamey, foxy ways about them. They like surprises. They share few values with humans—they have no morality, no wishes for money or success, no patriotism, no hope. These are POWER machines. And the human beings that they meet look like flies in their paths.

King gives us several killer automobiles (one starts out Bachman's *Thinner*). A murderous taxi-truck collision sets up the plot for *The Dead Zone,* a story in which a young man develops prescience because of the accident. We find an unrelenting, devilish pickup truck in "Uncle Otto's Truck" (*Skeleton Crew*), and ten wheelers come to take over the world in "Trucks" (*ibid.*). But King's machines do not necessarily need legs, wheels, or other propelling mechanisms to do their damage. Toy soldiers wipe out a Mafia killer in "Battleground" (*Night Shift*). Exploding oil tanks blow up much of the civilization that was not wiped out already by a plague in *The Stand.* A malicious ironing machine goes after people in "The Mangler"; King's short story expresses the same theme Nathaniel Hawthorne outlined to himself a hundred years before (King's *Night Shift,* and Hawthorne's *American Notebooks,* as quoted by Manguel, 1983, p. 950). The only difference between the two men's plots about a killer industrial machine is that whereas Hawthorne's people come to the mangler, King's mangler comes to the people. In order to be like King's ancient train, the machine, whether or not it has legs, must be the one to move.

King makes mechanical monsters primary to his plots. An exploding furnace destroys the Overlook Hotel in *The Shining.* Stanley Kubrick, who made the film from King's novel, vetoed King's screenplay and eliminated the explosion of the hotel. In an interview after the movie was made, King expressed dissatisfaction with Kubrick's interpretation. He didn't like the director's emphasis on the people who had lived in the Overlook Hotel. "The hotel was not evil," King said, "because those people [the bad ones in the hotel's history] had been there, but those people went there because the place was evil" (Underwood and Miller, p. 96f.).

King's latest mechanical monster is his runaway Coke machine in *The Tommyknockers*. He likes the beast. "Every now and then," he says, "it will find a pedestrian and run him down. One of the main characters is a wimp. I was glad to see him go . . . his car stalls. He's walking along and here comes this Coke machine. . . . So it hits the guy and he's like a bug on the windshield. He's just smashed on the front of this Coke machine and the glass panel is broken, and all of the money is coming out of the coin return. That was it for me. I could see it. It was just there and it was absurd, but at the same time it had weight and reality for me" (Underwood and Miller, p. 83f.). My own favorite character in all of Stephen King is *Christine*, a malicious, vindictive, sexy 1958 Plymouth.

King cannot escape his "trains" even when he sets up a plot that centers upon an animalistic horror—a vampire, a devil, or a chimera, for instance. In order "properly" to terrify his reader, King unconsciously reaches to the train metaphor. King's monster of *The Stand*, Flagg, a kind of devil, has a black visage, yellow beacon eyes, and legs that can move faster than a car. When Flagg unmasks himself to a woman, she sees "the searchlight of his face bear down upon her in the gloom." When a crowd, an instant before they are all vaporized in a nuclear explosion, sees Flagg unmasked, he is "something monstrous . . . something slumped and hunched almost without shape— something with enormous yellow eyes." For King, I think, the devil looks like a locomotive.

The train metaphor also permeates the climax of *It*. When Bill, the hero, spots "It," "It was perhaps fifteen feet high and as black as a moonless night. Each of its legs were as thick as a muscle-builder's thigh. It's eyes were bright, malevolent rubies" and "It's belly bulged grotesquely, almost dragging on the floor as It moved." When Bill at last glimpsed the "shape behind the shape," he saw "lights, saw an endless crawling hairy thing which was made of light and nothing else, orange light, dead light that mocked life." This sounds like a child's-eye view of an old, lumbering, Maine freight train, orange refrigerator cars and all.

One cannot escape the train in King. Monsters rush forward at "express train speed" (*It*). A dying person with terminal breathing problems (in *The Stand*) says, "Listen to me, I sound like a fuckin freight train goin up a hill." King's "Woman's Credo" begins, "Thank you,

Men, for the railroads" (*The Stand*). A man goes through a crisis and feels flattened by "a night-running train" (*The Dead Zone*). A pregnant woman is decapitated in a freak taxi-truck accident at the emergency entrance to a New York City hospital ("The Breathing Method" in *Different Seasons*). As her mouth puckers in the gutter where her severed head has landed, the pregnant woman's body on the sidewalk makes the huff-puff sounds and gestures of a train. The body delivers a normal infant—all because the woman had been taught in her Lamaze classes to "breath like a locomotive." This, of course, *is* King's "breathing method." Its trainlike origins are horrifying.

King knows—naturally, for the experience and the symptoms are his own—how to present posttraumatic symptoms in his plots. I will use *Stand by Me* as my only example here, not because there are no others, but because the symptoms were so clearly presented on film by Rob Reiner. First, King shows us posttraumatic play. Teddy Duchamp, for instance, cannot get enough of his "chicken" games at the railway track (with a locomotive). He is obsessed with war and insists upon hearing warlike endings to the most peaceable of tales. Teddy's father, a crazed war hero, burned off Teddy's ear. Since then Teddy cannot get enough of wars. He cannot play enough to suit himself. Teddy is playing posttraumatically, unconsciously, repetitively and dangerously inside of Stephen King's own posttraumatic play, his writing. It is "play within play."

In *Stand by Me* Teddy Duchamp insists upon finishing up Gordon Lachance's "Lard Ass Hogan" story, a Stephen King story within a story. Teddy says that Lard Ass will go home, shoot his father, and join the Texas Rangers. Teddy, in other words, must play with his own trauma every chance he gets, even if a story he is finishing belongs to somebody else.

Stephen King gives us several other posttraumatic symptoms in "The Body." He gives us intense visualizations. Gordie Lachance repeatedly sees, at his leisure I might add (Terr, 1979), scenes of his life with Dennis, his unexpectedly dead brother. Gordon, obviously traumatized, also experiences a posttraumatic dream. King recognizes both of these posttraumatic symptoms; they are not unfamiliar to him. Reiner picks them up for his film. They are extremely cinematic.

Gordon's parents exhibit extreme psychic numbing, another type of posttraumatic symptom. Gordon's friend, Teddy, is so habitually enraged that one suspects that he has gone through a massive personality change after his father's attack upon his ear. King gives us multiple reenactments (Teddy Duchamp's character) as well as single ones (Gordon Lachance's need to view a "body," some "body," any "body"). King also gives us a profound sense of futurelessness. As opposed to Rob Reiner who is satisfied with "killing" only Chris Chambers in his adulthood, King kills off each of the three young playmates of the writer-to-be in his novella.

King warns us of all these deaths-to-be with a retrospective rework-ing, an "omen" (Terr, 1979). King's "omen" comes when the four boys are flipping coins in a junkyard. They get "a goocher." Each lad comes up "tails." A "goocher" apparently means terrible luck. They may die, Vern says. King follows at this point in his novella with an explanation of the premature deaths of each one of his three friends. Reiner wisely omits this overkill. But there is little question for me at this point that we are viewing the obsessional retrospections of a child who has asked "Why me? Why me?" too many times to count—enough times, as a matter of fact, to have discovered an "omen."

KING'S FICTIONAL PSYCHOANALYSTS AND PSYCHIATRISTS

> "So nice," the boogeyman said as it shambled out [of the closet]. It still held its Dr. Harper mask in one rotted, spade-claw hand.
>
> Stephen King, "The Boogeyman"
> in *Night Shift* (p. 104)

Stephen King appears to be afraid of psychoanalysis and psychiatry. Neither was probably available to him shortly after his encounter with the train. After all, the family was hard up financially and King's moth-er believed in healing through religion, not science. King, I think, must have grown up thinking he would be able to write his way out of his trauma. He says now, for instance, "I think of getting all this [fear] out—you know, there are people who are full of fear in our society who pay psychiatrists $75 or $80 an hour and it's not even a full hour, it's about fifty minutes. And I get rid of all this stuff by writing and people pay *me*. It's great. I love it" (Underwood and Miller, p. 12). King cannot really get rid of his terror, however. If any "traumatic anxiety" at all is discharged by his writing, it leaks out so slowly that it would take forever to get it all out. King seems afraid of losing his fears. He thinks that he would become boring if he were to be deprived of his personal "hang-ups." King is so used to living with his horror that, when asked by Edwin Pouncey how he became interested in "that sort of stuff," he replied, "There's no answer to that question, particularly not a Freudi-an or Jungian one. . . . I think it's innate, sort of bred in the bone" (*ibid.*, p. 56).

It appears that childhood trauma victims, the longer they wait after an ordeal, come to feel that they can get by without professional intervention. As time goes on, victims come to feel afraid of reopening old wounds. They avoid the analyst. King appears to have done this throughout his life.

The most important factor that causes the avoidance of psychoanalysts and psychiatrists is the trauma victim's sense that nothing external should be able to change a normal person into a disordered one. A trauma victim will go to great lengths in order to prove to himself that he is still "normal," just as he was before. This means, of course, staying away from mental health professionals. And Stephen King does this on his own behalf and on his characters' behalf.

The two definitely traumatized boys of King's semiautobiographical *Stand by Me,* Teddy Duchamp and Gordon Lechance, appear not to have visited a psychiatrist. Nor have their two friends. Psychoanalysis and psychiatry lie outside, in other words, of Stephen King's own experience. These fictional boys could have benefited from some of the techniques that were available for psychic trauma even in the 1950s. David Levy (1939) had already developed his abreactive techniques for very young trauma victims. Anna Freud's child analytic techniques (1926) and Melanie Klein's play therapy (1932) had caught hold in the field at large.

But Stephen King developed his childhood hatred and fear of psychiatry despite the possibility that it very likely could have afforded him some relief. "They experiment with you," King implies in several of his books (see, in particular, *The Stand*). "They don't know what they're doing," he says in others (*The Dead Zone* and *Firestarter*). "Philosophy taken from psychoanalysis has ruined religion" (*'Salem's Lot*). King even tries to tell us in a tale or two that psychoanalysts and behavioral psychiatry specialists are evil ("The Boogeyman" and "Quitters, Inc.," *Night Shift*).

Stephen King gives us no psychiatric interventions to speak of in his semiautobiographical *Stand by Me*—just, as a matter of fact, a junkman's dirty allusion to Teddy Duchamp's father being locked up in the state hospital, the place for the criminally insane. *That* is all you can expect of psychiatry, King is telling us.

KING'S WRITING TECHNIQUE

> I recognize terror as the finest emotion . . . and so I
> will try to terrorize the reader. But if I find that I
> cannot terrify . . . I will try to horrify; and if I find that

> I cannot horrify, I'll go for the gross-out.
> Stephen King, *Danse Macabre* (p. 25)

How does the horrified writer transmit his horror to the nonhorrified reader? If he is talented enough, as Stephen King certainly is, he transmits his fear through a number of specific writing techniques which mimic the sensations of psychic trauma.

First of all, King "telescopes"—he tells what terrible things will happen before they happen. For example, on page 5 of the massive King novel, *It*, we read that cute, little Georgie Denbrough of Derry, Maine, yellow slicker and all, is going to die. He dies, all right—but not until pages 14, 15, and 16. We know it ahead of time, but we have to sweat through a packet of pages until we find out just how gruesome Georgie's death will be. King is doing with writing technique what the mind does after trauma. He creates a sense of futurelessness, of no tomorrow. The way in which he telescopes the future into the present, there *is* no future.

Second, King establishes absolute trust in his reader's (or viewer's) mind by forcing the audience to identify. King's protagonists play with the same Bicycle Playing Cards, listen to the same old Philco radios, eat the same hastily put-together hamburgers, lose food into the same campfires in the same sorts of silly ways, and secretly enjoy the same glimpses of nature that *we* do. King's homey details are authentic. The audience *must* identify. King forces us to. He gives us the comic books we used to love and the songs we used to sing; and then he blasts us out of our seats with something for which we were not prepared—something that was not supposed to happen at all; something unexpected, shocking, overwhelming. The idea of trauma is to feel plain, very normal, and then to be mowed down with something extraordinary. King gives us all-too-familiar brand names, songs, and characters, and then—with a sudden onslaught that knocks us off our chairs—he gives us his trauma.

Third and fourth, King uses masses of detail and slow-motion writing. He does not hesitate, for instance, to pull out an arm or to impale an eye. Slow motion and intense detailing are both typical of how psychic trauma hits the victim's perceptual apparatus at the moment of traumatic impact. King mimics these perceptions repeatedly.

In *Firestarter*, for instance, we have the death of an enemy, U.S. government agent that is witnessed in extraordinary detail by Andy, one of the two protagonists: "The stakes for the beans to climb on were still there, and one of them rammed through this fellow's throat and came out the other side with a wet punching sound that Andy never forgot. He twitched in the garden like a landed trout, the bean-pole protruding from his neck like the shaft on an arrow, blood gushing down the front of his shirt as he made weak gargling sounds" (p. 119). Or, we have the death of the preschooler protagonist, Gage, in *Pet Sematary:* "Gage seemed to realize that the game was over, that your parents didn't *scream* at you when it was just a game, and he had tried to put on the brakes, but by then the sound of the truck was *very* loud, the sound of it filled the world. It was thundering . . . and then Gage's forward motion had carried him out into the road, and the truck had been thunder, the truck had been sunlight on high chrome, the truck had been the deep-throated shrieking bellow of an air horn, and that had been Saturday, that had been three days ago" (p. 233).

Stephen King slows time way down when he comes to a traumatic death. His pacing forces Moochie Welsh to take four pages to die at the hands of *Christine,* the vengeful car. Gage's death in *Pet Sematary* is reviewed twice (on pp. 233, 238f.), but then Gage's ruined body is reviewed on at least 8 more pages (pp. 247f., 298, 312, 341ff., 350, 366). This time-slowing technique obviously makes the detailing absolutely "gross." But it also re-creates the sensation of sudden, intense, horrifying stimuli. It mimics the perception of trauma, in other words, as close as one can come to this in language. King may speed up the time it takes for the *aftermath* of a terrible external event ("that had been three days ago"), for instance, but he will highlight every detail of the event itself as slowly as he can go.

Fifth, if a King character dies, the dead person may be allowed to do the impossible, in other words, to leave a traumatically dying man's oral report, or a journal, of how it felt to die suddenly and unexpectedly. This "oral report," a blow-by-blow description of the traumatic dying process, is given by King to the reader in order to provide immediate, fresh detail. It forces the reader to identify. King also affords himself, in this way, a vehicle to go over his train trauma from his dead friend's point of view. Gage has left us a "journal" of this type in *Pet Sematary.* One hardly notices at the end of the paragraph I quoted above when the person King is telling us about becomes Gage's father, not the dying Gage himself.

Sixth, King frequently breaks what I think is a technical writing taboo—he kills off children and then does postmortems on their young bodies. This taboo against the death and mutilation of children extends to some extremely effective horror writers, Edgar Poe and Edith Wharton, for instance. Henry James did kill a child, in his *Turn of the Screw* (1898), but he never would have had his reader dwell upon the child's dead body. King forces this upon us again and again. In order to repeat his own particular trauma, he must subject his reader to this relatively unspeakable topic.

King is not always happy with his killings and mutilations of children. According to Douglas Winter (1986), King did not feel entirely comfortable with the death he wrote for Tad Trenton, age 4, of *Cujo*. Tad dies of dehydration, trapped for several days with his mother in a broken-down Pinto as a rabid dog attacks their car. Several people wrote King when *Cujo* came out, asking, "How could you let that happen?" They recognized that their beloved author had broken a taboo. King says, "My response was that sometimes children do die, by crib death, or they get hit by cars. God help us, they even get killed by dogs. . . . The only thing I could write back is, 'I'm not God. I just wrote the damn book. He died. I didn't want him to die'" (Underwood and Miller, p. 114). The director of the film, *Cujo*, Lewis Teague, made sure that Tad Trenton did not die in his film. Tad looks like he is dead in the movie, but his mother applies CPR and it works.

A seventh horror writing technique in Stephen King—and one that also bestows his books with the sense of trauma—is the technique of inserting supernatural effects into a story after a protagonist has been traumatized. King characters hallucinate visually (*It, The Shining,* and *The Stand*). But first they are psychically overwhelmed. They develop "powers"—for example, Danny (of *The Shining*), Johnny (of *The Dead Zone*), George (of "Gramma," *Skeleton Crew*), and *Carrie*. Each character appears to develop his powers from a trauma, even though King tends to make other excuses for it (genetics, LSD, witchcraft, congenital tendencies). King's power sensations are identical to the supernatural feelings some trauma victims report after terrible events (Terr, 1984, 1985). The particular powers King creates may be wilder ones than trauma victims actually say they experience. For instance, a King protagonist may experience telekinesis (*Carrie*), mutation into another being (*Christine* or "I Am a Doorway" in *Night Shift*), pyrokinesis (*Firestarter*), or even the ability to kill people by deleting their names from a computer tape ("Word Processor of the Gods" in *Skeleton Crew*). But almost every one of King's supernaturally gifted characters is traumatized first. It often seems coincidental, but in this way King's strange-sounding collection of "powers" rests upon an authentic psychological foundation, psychic trauma.

If one could write schizophrenic language into a book that made sense, the reader of the book would *feel* schizophrenic as he read. By writing traumatic and posttraumatic sensations into his books, Stephen King forces his reader to *feel* traumatized.

KING AND POSTTRAUMATIC CONTAGION

> "Matt, do you know what's going to happen to you if
> you even let out a whisper of what you've told me
> [about vampires in town]?"
>   Matt didn't answer.
>   "People are going to start tapping their foreheads
> behind your back when you go by in the street. Little
> kids are going to get out their Halloween wax teeth
> when they see you coming and jump out and yell *Boo!*
> when you walk by their hedge. Somebody will invent a
> rhyme like *One, two, three, four, I'm gonna suck your blood
> some more.* The high school kids will pick it up and you'll
> hear it in the halls when you pass. . . . They'll turn your
> life into a nightmare."
> Stephen King, *Salem's Lot* (p. 176)

Stephen King has an innate understanding of posttraumatic contagion. He knows mass hysteria. He has been a "trauma watcher," one
would say, since 1951 when he was 4 years old. King likes to scare
people because *he* was scared, and he was only 4. He likes people to feel
so scared that they might come close to dying ("I suppose the ultimate
triumph would be to have somebody drop dead of a heart attack,
literally scared to death. I'd say, 'Gee, that's a shame,' and I'd mean it,
but part of me would be thinking, Jesus, that really *worked!*" (Underwood and Miller, p. 50). King wants others to die of fright because *he*
was almost killed at 4. He wishes to turn the tables.

King understands trauma perfectly, but he does not perfectly understand his fans. Fans must be a little crazy, he implies. In his recent
novel, *Misery* (1987a), Annie Wilkes, a nurse and the writer-pro-
tagonist's "number one fan," holds the author captive in her house and
tries to force him—through drugs and the use of a hatchet—to write
the kind of story *she* wants him to write. The fan, King is saying here, is
an uncontrollable force.

King distrusts the psychics and fortune-tellers that one would guess
would be King's fierce advocates because of the stories he writes (*The
Dead Zone,* or "I Know What You Need" from *Night Shift*). He says that
most of these people are "fakes" (Underwood and Miller, p. 37). Of
teenagers—whom he likes and understands, by the way (see *Christine*
for a look at the lives and dreams of adolescents)—King says they feel
like monsters with their pimples and their awkward gaits, and that is
why they read his monster tales. But Offer et al. (1981), from their

large-scale studies of normal adolescents, tell us "no"—most teenagers do not feel like monsters; most of them feel pretty good.

Although Stephen King does not understand his fans very well, he knows how to worry them. King does not bother much with trying to stir up oedipal conflicts or guilt, both inner concerns. He is interested entirely in external concerns. He knows that threats in the direction of the loss of human control are a way to move his audience toward hysteria. King outlined in his Billerica Library lecture (Underwood and Miller) a list of what has worried most people during his lifetime. He includes nuclear war, radiation, Reds, cancer, plagues, terrorists, and machines. King is right. People *are* afraid of these. I would add to the list running out of food and water, the world population getting out of hand, and toxic contamination.

King writes almost his entire list into the novel, *The Stand,* but he has also figured out that he does not have to mention his list *out loud* to inspire the sensation of hysteria. His audience will become hysterical over the implications. King never explains in "Children of the Corn" (*Night Shift*), for instance, why, in order for corn to grow well, human sacrifice is required. Could it be radiation problems, toxic waste, or a long drought? King does not need to say anything. He is better off letting his reader think his own worst possible case scenario. We do not need to know exactly why vapors and monsters spread throughout New England in "The Mist" (*Skeleton Crew*). It scares us more not knowing.

Like all good politicians and demagogues, Stephen King has his hand to the pulse of his audience. He knows people feel terrified today of cancer. So he kills almost everybody in the world (*The Stand*) with a mysterious, in-dwelling plague. He knows they drive highways and cruise into drive-in restaurants, ever aware that they could die in a freak car accident or a fight. So King organizes his best "end of the world story" at a truck-stop restaurant, creating thinking trucks who decide to dominate the world of people once and for all ("Trucks," *Night Shift*). King knows that if one in the audience laughs, many will laugh—if one screams, everyone will scream. There are advantages to films, he says, because "the panic jumps from one person to the next" (Underwood and Miller, p. 206). He even knows, acknowledges, and brags that three real-life murders have been patterned after his stories (*ibid.,* p. 51f.). In a sense King likes this. He realizes that he can exert a contagious effect upon masses of people, choir boys and murderers alike. "Maybe there is a copycat syndrome at work here," he says, "as with the Tylenol poisonings" (*ibid.,* p. 52).

Stephen King gives us his "copycat syndrome" in the famous Lard

Ass Hogan scene from his story "The Body," the story that was made into the film, *Stand by Me,* that stands at the center of this essay. The story of Lard Ass Hogan shows how easily mass hysteria can be generated by an author who is in tune with the contagiousness of human discomfort. Lard Ass, an obese unhappy boy, swears revenge on his town. He enters the town's pie-eating contest, first drinking a bottle of castor oil. Lard Ass downs six blueberry pies faster than does anybody else, but then he vomits. The other pie-eating contestants immediately follow suit, disgorging themselves of massive amounts of blueberry. They do not *want* to, but they have to. King's characters are out of control. Then King has his fun. He writes statements like, "Puke was everywhere." He eventually "treats" his reader to the mass emesis of an entire town. We can tell from the almost hysterical sensation in our stomachs that King is getting to *us,* too. "I declare this contest a draw," Lard Ass announces into the town microphone. And we put the book down for an instant—relieved that Stephen King has temporarily stopped his "game."

King vacillates between saying that his audience is fearless—therefore they like him as a challenge to their macho-ness—or that they are terribly fearful and thus they rehearse with him for their own deaths. Like Alfred Hitchcock (Terr, 1987a), Stephen King says that he thinks his audience is reassured by his works—they looked in and they did not get destroyed (Underwood and Miller, p. 9). He says the audience likes that. But on other occasions King changes his mind. Perhaps horror novels are runs-through for death, for losing all control (*ibid.*, p. 203). King, when speaking of death, goes to his ancient and dreaded train as the metaphor. "We know it's going to happen," he says. "The electric train goes around and around and it goes under and around the tunnels and over the scenic mountains. But in the end it always goes off the end of the table. Crash" (*ibid.*, p. 10).

King's two inconsistent points about why he is so loved, so read, probably *do* correctly appraise how parts of his audience react to him. Both are probably correct. Some people in King's audience are probably reassured by his horror writing as they are by their own examination dreams (Freud, 1900), where the dreamer wakes up relieved to find everything to the opposite of the dream. (One of my patients, a depressed 35-year-old accountant, says she loves lingering over King's cadavers. She goes slowly, savoring every word.) Others in King's audience are hopped up—overexcited, "wired" after experiencing King. As in the "traumatic dream" where the dreamer wakes up feeling worse than he felt before, the reader catches a little of King's anxiety. He will have bad dreams. A woman once wrote to King after reading

Salem's Lot, King's rewrite of the "Dracula" story, complaining that he had given her three nights of terrible insomnia. King wrote back, "I'm *glad* you were awake for three nights. I wish it had been six" (Underwood and Miller, p. 4).

Children love Stephen King. A few, however, finish his books and leave his movies feeling scared. But why would an unscared kid expose himself to an awareness of trauma—to a knowledge of the loss of control, sudden death, and helplessness? And why would he like it? Because a child may feel that an awareness of trauma will grant him a modicum of control. I am reminded of a 13-year-old boy who came to me for brief psychotherapy simply because he had slept through a Northern California earthquake. "If I slept through it," he said to me, "I could die in my sleep in an earthquake. And then I'd never have a chance to do anything to save myself." *That* is a fear of loss of control— a normal fear, but an externally inspired, not an internally derived one. The fear of loss of control is probably what leads an audience to Stephen King. King knows all about psychic trauma and, perhaps, he can point out something new. If King introduces us to a monster, a truck, a chimera, or a killer train, for instance, we might learn something about traumas-to-be. Knowing is controlling, after all.

Before I close, I want to relate a final story about Stephen King, his audience, and the film, *Stand by Me* that inspired this little investigation. An eminent child psychiatrist from the state of Maine, Diane Schetky, was invited to the annual benefit dinner given by the Camden, Maine YMCA.[1] The benefactors partook of a banquet dinner and a few wines. Then the speaker of the evening came forward. It was Stephen King, a beer in each shirt pocket. He would do a "reading," not a speech, he said. So he picked up the "story within a story" from his novella, "The Body," the story I have just related, the tale of Lard Ass Hogan, the blueberry puker. King read the entire account to his satiated audience. He told it with great gusto. One person excused himself and moved, perhaps a little quickly, toward a restroom—then another—and another. The great audience manipulator was trying his own little experiment. He knew that what is gross, what is surprising, and what is beyond control might be contagious, even among a group of—how would *he* put it?—"fat cats."

Stephen King cannot stop playing with his trauma. You've seen him, the real him, on an American Express television ad staving off a flying bookcase and some swinging sconces. He likes to play. He wants to

---

1. Thanks to Diane Schetky for telling me this story and for allowing me to publish it.

play. Right now one of his games is to say that "The Body" and its film derivative, *Stand by Me,* has nothing at all to do with him. It is another boy's camp story, he says (Underwood and Miller, p. 17). But Stephen King is a trauma victim, struck terrified in his own childhood by a train. He cannot escape this train. The traumatized child still lives inside of the adult King. And that child wishes to play with us and with our children. King's immense popularity indicates that *we* want to play too.

BIBLIOGRAPHY

FREUD, A. (1926). *The Psychoanalytical Treatment of Children.* London: Imago Publishing, 1946.

FREUD, S. (1900). The interpretation of dreams. *S.E.,* 4 & 5.

JAMES, H. (1898). *The Turn of the Screw,* Avon, Conn.: Heritage, 1949.

KING, S. (1974). *Carrie.* New York: Doubleday.

———(1975). *Salem's Lot.* New York: Doubleday.

———(1977). *The Shining.* Garden City, N.Y.: Doubleday.

———(1978a). *Night Shift.* Garden City, N.Y.: Doubleday.

———(1978b). *The Stand.* Garden City, N.Y.: Doubleday.

———(1979). *The Dead Zone.* New York: Viking Press.

———(1980). *Firestarter.* New York: Viking Press. New York: New American Library, Signet, 1981.

———(1981a). *Danse Macabre.* New York: Everest House. New York: Berkeley, 1983.

———(1981b). *Cujo.* New York: Viking Press.

———(1982). *Different Seasons.* New York: Viking Press.

———(1983a). *Christine.* New York: Viking Press.

———(1983b). *Pet Sematary.* Garden City, N.Y.: Doubleday. New York: New American Library, Signet, 1984.

———(1984) (as Richard Bachman). *Thinner.* New York: New American Library, NAL Books.

———(1985a). *The Bachman Books.* New York: New American Library, NAL Books.

———(1985b). *Skeleton Crew.* New York: Putnam.

———(1985c). *Cycle of the Werewolf.* New York: New American Library, Plume.

———(1986). *It.* New York: Viking Press.

———(1987a). *Misery.* New York: Viking Press.

———(1987b). *The Tommyknockers.* New York: Putnam.

KLEIN, M. (1932). *The Psychoanalysis of Children.* London: Hogarth Press.

LEVY, D. (1939). Release therapy. *Amer. J. Orthopsychiat.,* 9:713–736.

MANGUEL, A. (1983). *Black Water.* New York: Potter.

OFFER, D., OSTROV, E., & HOWARD, K. (1981). The mental health professional's concept of the normal adolescent. *Arch. Gen. Psychiat.,* 38:149–152.

TERR, L. C. (1979). Children of Chowchilla. *Psychoanal. Study Child*, 34:547–623.

———(1981). "Forbidden games." *J. Amer. Acad. Child Psychiat.*, 20:741–760.

———(1983a). Life attitudes, dreams, and psychic trauma in a group of "normal" children. *J. Amer. Acad. Child Psychiat.*, 22:221–230.

———(1983b). Chowchilla revisited. *Amer. J. Psychiat.*, 140:1543–1550.

———(1984). Time and trauma. *Psychoanal. Study Child*, 39:633–666.

———(1985). Remembered images and trauma. *Psychoanal. Study Child*, 40:493–533.

———(1987a). Childhood trauma and the creative product. *Psychoanal. Study Child*, 42:545–572.

———(1987b). The trauma and extreme stress disorders. Samuel G. Hibbs award lecture, American Psychiatric Association, Annual Meeting, Chicago.

———(1988). What happens to the memories of early trauma? *J. Amer. Acad. Child Psychiat.*, 27:96–104.

UNDERWOOD, J. & MILLER, C., eds. (1988). *Bare Bones*. New York: McGraw-Hill.

WINTER, D. (1986). *Stephen King*. New York: New American Library, Plume.

Looking for Anna Freud's Mother

ELISABETH YOUNG-BRUEHL, Ph.D.

THE EVOLUTION OF SIGMUND FREUD'S VIEWS ON FEMALE PSYCHOLOGY IS directly and dramatically linked to his youngest daughter's psychology. In an essay he wrote in 1919 and then in another, written in 1925, he registered two crucial revisions of the general picture of female development presented in his *Three Essays on the Theory of Sexuality;* these steps prepared the way for his last and most influential statements, "Female Sexuality" (1931) and "Femininity" (1933). The 1919 and 1925 essays both depend heavily on the insights Freud gained as he analyzed his daughter. The confidentiality of the analytic situation is protected in the essays, but they nonetheless report Anna Freud's analysis as he conducted it in two phases, between 1918 and 1922, and then between 1924 and 1925.

In my biography of Anna Freud, I was able to track in great detail the course of her analysis by weaving Freud's reports in "'A Child Is Being Beaten'" (1919) and "Some Psychical Consequences of the Anatomical Distinction between the Sexes" (1925) together with three types of material written by Anna Freud herself. She left in her literary estate both a series of poems and prose pieces dating from the period of the first analysis, and her early correspondences, chiefly with Lou Andreas Salomé and Max Eitingon, the two of her father's colleagues and friends with whom Anna Freud was closest. In the public domain, she left her first clinical paper, "Beating Fantasies and Daydreams," published in 1922, which is both a commentary on "'A Child Is Being Beaten'" and a thinly disguised report on her own case.

The richness of this documentation, the detail it yielded, presented me with a big temptation: to go on and find Anna Freud's story continued in "Female Sexuality" and "Femininity," the essays in which Freud stressed the role of the mother in a girl's early development. The

Professor of Letters at Wesleyan University; author of *Hannah Arendt: For Love of the World* (1982) and *Anna Freud: A Biography* (1988).

further possibility that was offered by constructing Freud's late essays on female psychology as episodes in his daughter's story was alluring: that I would also find Anna Freud's mother, who had eluded many another type of biographical detective work and remained as a shadowy figure in my family album. Such historical and biographical neatness! The story of Freud's views on female psychology and the story of Anna Freud's analysis are the same story! I imagined myself showing in Freud's theory and in Anna Freud's analysis the importance of the mother as not just a nurturer but a love object and also the importance of the preoedipal period as far more than just a stage of oral erotism. As these demonstrations proceeded in my fantasy, the very specific mother I had been unable to create in Anna Freud's biography— Martha Freud—came into view, like a painting under a palimpsest.

I am going to re-create this crossroads in my work, and show a biographer's dream interrupted by lack of information just as it was about to come true. Sympathy over my frustration would be appreciated, but I also have a larger purpose in reconstructing this path to a piece of "applied psychoanalysis." Walking to the end of it, I think I learned something, and I would like to share it.

I

Both Sigmund Freud's "'A Child Is Being Beaten'" and Anna Freud's "Beating Fantasies and Daydreams" are illustrations of Freud's dictum that the oedipus complex is the nucleus of the neuroses. Freud studied male patients whose beating fantasies reflected both the mother love/father rivalry familiar to him since the 1890s, and also the mother identification and "passive" or "homosexual" father love that had assumed more and more significance in Freud's work after *Three Essays on the Theory of Sexuality*. His four female patients had beating fantasies that clearly reflected the oedipal situation Freud had always emphasized for females: father love/mother rivalry—the converse of the male's configuration. But he also saw that the females he studied, who fended off incestuous wishes by assuming male disguises in their own fantasies, often ended up with powerful father identifications. The father identifications seemed to him defensive: they further protected the girls from incestuous wishes, and eventually protected them from any kind of sexual involvement—made them safely ascetic. There is no mention in the essay, however, of what should logically have been the corollary of the father identification: that is, daughterly mother love.

Anna Freud's case study, on the other hand, is not comparative. She concentrates on one subject—a girl who is very like herself—and takes

as her particular subject the role of sublimation in the girl's mental life. Her patient eventually gives up her beating fantasies and their climax, an act of masturbation, for what she calls "nice stories," a superstructure which has been relieved of the sexual content of the beating fantasy. Eventually, the nice stories are also transformed, into short stories. The desired gratification is no longer masturbation but praise from a reading audience. What becomes of the girl's desire for her father or of her sexual life in general is not clear; and the girl's mother is not even so much as mentioned.

Freud's essay, by contrast, does imply that the male fantasizers were more or less overtly homosexual (or mother-identified) and that the females were more or less asexual and able to overcome their father love only through father identification. Freud was impressed enough by the differences between the male and the female beating fantasies, despite the fact that all the fantasizers were in love with their fathers and in conflict over their intense masturbation activity, to be shaken in his conviction that males and females undergo analogous developments until they diverge at the oedipal crossroads. But the differences between the male and female fantasies were not pursued in the essay, which ends, rather, with a general reflection on repression that rejects two unsatisfactory theories: Adler's notion that both sexes repress "the feminine" and Fliess's idea that both sexes repress the mental sexual content opposite to their anatomical sexuality. Freud argued against the "sexualization of repression" because he was impressed by the variety of repression.

This same theme runs into the case study of a female homosexual, where Freud (1920a) concludes with a tabulation of three sets of characteristics that must be accounted for in any adequate understanding of homosexuality—or heterosexuality: physical sexual characteristics, mental sexual characteristics (masculine or feminine attitude), and kind of object choice. (Earlier, in *Three Essays,* he had also added a fourth: kind of aim, preference for type of sexual activity.) These characteristics, he notes, "up to a certain point, vary independently of one another, and are met with in different individuals in manifold permutations" (p. 170). Researchers who concentrate their attention on object choice will miss the fact that male homosexuals, although they chose male lovers, "have experienced a specially strong fixation on their mother" (p. 171). He does not make a similar general claim about female homosexuals, although the subject of the case study was a female homosexual. This young woman's attachment to her mother, Freud had noted, was important: but he viewed it as secondary, that is, as an attachment that assumed great importance for her when her love

for her father was bitterly disappointed. (The same can be said of the 1915 case of a female's paranoia "running counter to psychoanalytic theory.") Once again, daughterly mother love is invoked but not explored.

Freud made two important statements about infantile sexuality after the 1920 case, "The Infantile Genital Organization" (1923) and "The Dissolution of the Oedipus Complex" (1924), but both of these repeat the basic premise about female development that Freud had laid down in *The Interpretation of Dreams* and *Three Essays on the Theory of Sexuality:* the first love of the little girl is for her father, as the first love of the little boy is for his mother, and their developments are therefore analogous, mirror images. So, it was momentous when this premise, held for 30 years, was abandoned in "Some Psychical Consequences of the Anatomical Distinction between the Sexes" (1925).

Freud did not himself herald the shift in his views. He simply says of males and females that "In both cases the mother is the original object" (p. 251). Later he speaks vaguely of the girl's "affectionate relation to her mother." The purpose of the paper is not, really, to explore this relation; it is, rather, to ask how the relation comes to an end, how the girl comes to turn toward her father. Penis envy, which had always been a key ingredient of Freud's theory of female development, takes on a function in this paper that it had not had before: the girl turns away from her mother because she holds her mother responsible for the fact that she has come into the world so ill-equipped. The route of this turn can be complex and involve a displacement: the girl displaces her hostility toward her mother onto a sibling, claiming that the mother is fonder of the sibling. In general, penis envy converts easily into jealousy.

One would expect Freud biographers to wonder what brought about the realization that girls, like boys, first love their mothers—though it is very interesting to note that not one of Freud's male biographers, from Ernest Jones to Peter Gay, has found the matter worth puzzling over. What impresses Freud's male biographers is how little, despite the oedipus complex, mothers figure in Freud's case studies of males, and how Freud's attention to the oedipus complex seems to have kept him from exploring the preoedipal period *in males*. It is assumed that Freud's preoedipal relationship to his own mother somehow troubled his view of mothers in the case studies and obscured from his view the preoedipal period in males. This veil, of course, then extended to the preoedipal period in females as well. "Freud, it seems, had good reason to find the subject of woman somewhat mysterious, even a little threatening," says Peter Gay (1988) after making an argument of this sort.

Actually, the matter seems a bit more complex. But I want to pause here to note that the Freud biographers are participating in a trend that now dominates psychobiography. Psychobiography, as Freud and his immediate followers practiced it, focused on the oedipal period. But since the late 1940s, psychobiography, which always seems to follow trends within psychoanalysis—because it is, after all, "applied psychoanalysis"—has been more and more frequently conducted as a search for mother love in the first two to three years of life. There have been very few psychobiographies of women until quite recently, but the search for the preoedipal period is also a trend in them, and one augmented by feminist writings on female development such as Nancy Chodorow's *The Reproduction of Mothering* (1978).

Freud's preoedipal relationship to his mother—whatever that may have been—was not responsible for three facts that need to be taken into account. First, Freud's views on the importance of penis envy for women were articulated in the context of debates among his followers. They had been resoundingly seconded by Karl Abraham (1920) in a very influential article, "Manifestations of the Female Castration Complex." In this essay, Abraham, even though he had a special interest in oral erotism, did not, however, speak of daughterly mother love. Only shortly later, Karen Horney (1923) had come forth with a dissenting view: penis envy, she argued, is a secondary formation, something which develops after a little girl is disappointed in her love of her father; it does not turn her toward her father. This debate converged with another.

Melanie Klein arrived in Vienna six months before Freud wrote "Some Psychical Consequences of the Anatomical Distinction between the Sexes" to give a startling paper, one that sounded to Freud's circle like a replay in slightly different terms of Otto Rank's "birth trauma" theory, which had recently provoked such a split in the little psychoanalytic movement. The central trauma of infancy, Klein (1948) argued, is weaning. Babies of both sexes form their first object relation to their mother's breast—it is a "part object" for them—and this relation is the foundation of all others. Sexual differentiation does not take place along Freudian lines: the girl does not really turn to her father—for any reason, certainly not penis envy. Mother love was certainly the centerpiece of this paper, but the girl's love was not a specific topic.

Freud, in other words, had two oppositional views, very different from each other, to take into account in 1925. Both questioned his views on penis envy. At the same time a second factor came into play: Freud had in his own practice in Vienna a number of women who were, as patients, of a different sort than the women he had treated earlier in his career. These were professional women, psychoanalytic trainees. The "masculinity complex," as Freud understood it, was pronounced in them; they seemed living arguments for his claim that he had underestimated the effects on a woman's character of penis envy.

Anna Freud was one of these trainees. And I think that it is reasonable to argue—I did so in my biography—that a third fact that needs to be taken into account in considering Freud's change of viewpoint is that "Some Psychical Consequences of the Anatomical Distinction between the Sexes" contains another case study of Anna Freud. Freud himself links the essay to his earlier "'A Child Is Being Beaten'" with the following remark:

> Even after penis-envy has abandoned its true object, it continues to exist: by an easy displacement it persists in the character-trait of jealousy. . . . While I was still unaware of this source of jealousy and was considering the phantasy 'a child is being beaten', which occurs so commonly in girls, I constructed a first phase for it in which its meaning was that another child, a rival of whom the subject was jealous, was to be beaten. This phantasy seems to be a relic of the phallic period in girls. The peculiar rigidity which struck me so much in the monotonous formula 'a child is being beaten' can probably be interpreted in a special way. The child which is being beaten (or caressed) may ultimately be nothing more nor less than the clitoris itself, so that at its very lowest level the statement will contain a confession of masturbation, which has remained attached to the content of the formula from its beginning in the phallic phase till later life [p. 254].

The connection between intense masturbation, the beating fantasy, and jealousy of a sibling is palpable in Anna Freud's life, and it is important to note that the sibling who was her chief rival, her next older sister Sophie, had, in fact, always been her mother's favorite girl child and had secured her special place even more firmly when she became the first producer of grandchildren. After Sophie's death in the 1921 influenza epidemic, Anna Freud became a kind of surrogate mother to her sister's two little boys—in a sense, she took her sister's place.

Sophie Freud Halberstadt's boys were 3 and 8 years old in 1922, when Anna Freud, having finished the first of her analyses, took care of them for two months in their home in Hamburg. The youngest, Heinz, was her first toddler observational subject, while Ernst was the age of the elementary school children she had taught for five years in Vienna. Her letters home to her father from Hamburg are full of reports about the boys. And Anna Freud, 27 years old, in the role of the surrogate mother, seems to have identified with her own mother, whom she had almost always tended to present as a rival in all the documents preceding this Hamburg stay.

To note this mother identification without qualification, however, is inadequate. For Anna Freud had, as an infant, been cared for by a *Kinderfrau*, a woman named Josefine and called Jo by her charge. She had also had as another mother figure her aunt, Minna Bernays, her mother's maiden sister. When she was caring for her nephews, she had the assistance of a Hamburg relative of her brother-in-law's, and she called this woman a "good Minna," but that does not make clear whether she spoke from identification with her mother or with the *Kinderfrau*. What the day-to-day relationship of Martha Freud, Minna Bernays, and the *Kinderfrau* Josefine was is not determinable; how they existed in relation to each other in Anna Freud's memory is not evident in the surviving letters. There are only clues.

In 1922, Anna Freud visited several times in Göttingen with Lou Andreas-Salomé, who had spent a month with the Freuds in Vienna the previous December. Sigmund Freud had clearly brought his colleague into his household to befriend his daughter and to offer her a quasi-analytic relationship with a woman—a model woman of great intelligence and sensitivity, respected as an analyst and as a writer. Lou Andreas-Salomé referred to Anna Freud in letters to Sigmund Freud as "Daughter Anna," but this mother was like none of Anna Freud's other mothers.

It was to Lou Andreas-Salomé that Anna Freud confided her reaction to the surgery performed on her father's jaw in the spring of 1923 and then the major surgery the following fall designed to stem what had been diagnosed as cancer. She announced that she would never leave her father, and that she was quite satisfied to stay at home with him as his nurse, secretary, helper, companion. She displaced her mother and her aunt from these roles, and the new configuration in the household was apparently not pleasing to either of the sisters.

Anna Freud's analysis was renewed in the spring of 1924, when her father had recovered sufficiently to work with patients again, and it went on for at least a year, up to the time when Freud began to write "Some Psychical Consequences of the Anatomical Distinction between the Sexes." When Freud had drafted his paper, he presented it to an audience of two on his summer vacation: Anna Freud and Lou Andreas-Salomé. Anna Freud had just joined her family on vacation after attending in Vienna the funeral of her *Kinderfrau* Josefine, who had died in a hospital on the outskirts of the city where the Freuds had provided for her financially. Anna Freud told several of her correspondents about the funeral, and affirmed that Josefine was (as she said to Max Eitingon), "the oldest and most real relationship of my childhood." Whether memories of her infancy were stirred by this funeral, she does not say.

Both Anna Freud and Lou Andreas-Salomé reacted to Freud's paper with enthusiasm—Anna Freud suggested that she read the paper to the September meeting of the International Psychoanalytic Association—and also with their own work. Lou wrote a short story (unpublished and unavailable), and Anna Freud prepared a brief report for a December 1925 meeting of the Vienna Psychoanalytic Society called "Jealousy and the Desire for Masculinity" and based on her first analytic cases—two females, one child and one adult, whom she had often discussed with her father while he was formulating his ideas.

That Freud's paper depended upon the second phase of his analytic work with his daughter and also on her first cases, which she reported to him, seems clear. In Anna Freud's early life, the hostility she felt toward her mother, and her own jealousy of her sister and of others, were related to her penis envy, her "masculinity complex." But what does not emerge from Freud's paper or any of Anna Freud's correspondences is the still elusive topic of daughterly mother love or anything about the complexities of having more than one mother figure.

II

It is at this point that certain passages in Freud's next essay on female psychology loom up. In early 1931, he drafted the paper called "Female Sexuality," which responded to the continuing debates led by Horney and Klein over his views—although he wrote without mentioning his 1925 paper, and treated the debates as though they had arisen spontaneously, not in relation to his own work. By this time, Anna Freud had entered into a kind of partnership or "Boston marriage" with Dorothy Burlingham, an American woman, separated from her husband, with four children, all of whom had been treated analytically by Anna Freud. The two friends shared the upbringing of the children, traveled together, and had just bought a country house together, a place where they and the children and friends could retreat from Vienna on the weekends. Also a recent development in their lives was Dorothy Burlingham's termination of an analysis she had undertaken with Theodor Reik and her transfer to a new analyst, Sigmund Freud.

Freud reminded his readers at the beginning of "Female Sexuality" that it had long been a psychoanalytic tenet that females must negotiate a change in genital zone, from clitoris to vagina. That they also had to negotiate a change from their original love object, the mother, to the father was something that had become apparent more slowly. "The way in which the two tasks are connected with each other is not yet clear to us" (p. 225), Freud notes, and then turns to his clinical context with this passage:

It is well known that there are many women who have a strong attachment to their father; nor need they be in any way neurotic. It is upon such women that I have made the observations which I propose to report here and which have led me to adopt a particular view of female sexuality. I was struck, above all, by two facts. The first was that where the woman's attachment to her father was particularly intense, analysis showed that it had been preceded by a phase of exclusive attachment to her mother which had been equally intense and passionate. Except for a change in her love-object, the new phase had scarcely added any new feature to her erotic life. Her primary relation to her mother had been built up in a very rich and many-sided manner. The second fact taught me that the *duration* of this attachment had also been greatly underestimated. In several cases it lasted until well into the fourth year—in one case into the fifth year—so that it covered by far the longer part of the period of early sexual efflorescence. Indeed, we had to reckon with the possibility that a number of women remain arrested in their original attachment to their mother and never achieve a true change-over towards men. This being so, the pre-Oedipus phase in women gains an importance which we have not attributed to it hitherto [p. 225f.].

To square this claim with his earlier notion that the oedipus complex is the nucleus of the neuroses, Freud proposed to call the girl's mother attachment the "negative oedipus complex," and he stressed that in this stage she is active toward her mother as a little boy is. Then he went on to wonder why this preoedipal or negative oedipal stage had not appeared to him, and speculated that it might have undergone an especially inexorable repression, or else that he had "gained this impression because the women who were in analysis with me were able to cling to the very attachment to the father in which they had taken refuge from the early phase" (p. 226).

These passages might fit Anna Freud, whose attachment to her father was certainly strong—to say the least—and whose tie had certainly not been dissolved by her analysis, conducted as it was *by her father*. And, if Freud was making statements about his daughter, the implications were tremendous: he would, then, be seeing her attachment to him as a secondary formation, something she clung to strongly as an escape from the earlier attachment, not for its own sake; and he would be seeing her attachment to women, her reluctance to take up with any man other than himself, as also a function of her mother love, not of her father love. And Anna Freud herself would, as an analysand, have come to the same conclusions—insofar as the therapeutic situation allowed.

These seemed to me fascinating possibilities. But how would one go about testing whether the description really does fit Anna Freud? Or to specify in exactly what way it might fit Anna Freud? This is the point where information fails, where the documents run out. Anna Freud wrote poems, prose pieces, and letters about her two periods of analysis, and thus made it possible to link her case to her father's work intricately; but in the early 1930s she had no intimate correspondents. Lou Andreas-Salomé was aging, ill, unable to visit; Max Eitingon had disappointed Anna Freud and removed himself from her confidence. In her later correspondences and in a series of dreams she wrote out and interpreted after her father's death, there is not one indication that she understood herself as crucially determined by her early mother love. On the contrary, she continued to interpret herself in terms of the classic oedipal configuration, and she continued to express a great deal of ancient grievance against her mother and her aunt Minna Bernays, both of whom she portrayed as too strict, too controlling, too rigid—that is, as interferers with pleasures, forbidders, and, I think it is safe to infer, toilet trainers and masturbation punishers. Quite specifically, Anna Freud held her mother responsible for not telling her, when she was about 13, that a doctor had prescribed an appendectomy for her: Anna Freud went to the hospital under false pretenses and was taken by surprise to find that surgery was planned. Both in and of itself and insofar as it may have echoed earlier prohibitions and punishments—specifically "castration" threats—this incident helped seal Anna Freud's hostility toward her mother.

The most common form that Anna Freud's ancient grievance took was complaint that Martha Freud, who gave a good deal of concern to makeup and wardrobe, criticized her plain face, bottom-heavy figure, and doughty, sexless clothing. (Anna Freud's one concession to elegance was to wear with pride the necklaces her father gave her on her birthdays.) The seriousness of her complaint, in which appearance certainly stood for reality, presentation for essence, is obvious in the letters to Lou Andreas-Salomé, in which Anna Freud often thanks her older friend for accepting her and loving her just as she is, without demanding any changes or hoping for any improvement. The second most common form the grievance took was complaint that the Bernays sisters were too military about mealtimes, stipulating the exact moment at which meals were to begin and the exact menu, which was to be

consumed down to the last morsel. Anna Freud's revenge on this regime was to conduct a series of experiments in her first nursery, the
Jackson Nursery, that showed toddlers to be quite capable of feeding
themselves a nutritionally balanced diet if they were presented with a
smorgasbord of possibilities and left to eat at their own pace.

These are very suggestive details, but because, as I noted, there is
also little direct documentation to illuminate Anna Freud's early childhood or to bring into focus the three maternal figures, separately or in
relation to each other, there was no choice for me but to test Freud's
theory on Anna Freud's later childhood and adulthood—using
Freud's own terms, which would have been the terms familiar to Anna
Freud. For example, in "Female Sexuality," Freud offers one such way
of testing in relation to later childhood. He notes that in their play
children convert passive experiences into active ones: "When a doctor
has opened a child's mouth, in spite of his resistance, to look down his
throat, the same child, after the doctor has gone, will play at being the
doctor himself, and will repeat the assault upon some small brother or
sister who is as helpless in his hands as he was in the doctor's" (p. 236).
This triumph of activity is something that obviously caught Anna
Freud's attention, for she studied it in detail in *The Ego and the Mechanisms of Defense* (1936), under the title "identification with the aggressor" or the aggressor's aggression. (Interestingly, she cites the example from a similar passage in her father's *Beyond the Pleasure Principle*
[1920b], not from "Female Sexuality," and there is no evidence that
this essay was particularly significant for her.)

But there is also, of course, the libidinal identification Freud had
first studied as part of the process of superego formation; we might call
"identification with the caretaker's care" the mechanism that is apparent when a girl feeds and cleans her doll or takes care of her animals. As
Freud put it: "the little girl's preference for dolls is probably evidence
of the exclusiveness of her attachment to her mother, with complete
neglect of her father-object" (p. 237). In Anna Freud's case, though, it
does seem that it was the *Kinderfrau's* ministrations, not the mother's,
which were reproduced. Martha Freud did not, for example, nurse her
youngest; the baby was bottle-fed by the *Kinderfrau*, while her mother
took a long time to recuperate from a strenuous pregnancy—her sixth
pregnancy in eight years, and not a very desired pregnancy at that.
Later, it was the *Kinderfrau* Josefine who taught Anna Freud to knit
and launched her lifelong habit of knitting little clothes for dolls and
for other people's babies. And this habit was a facet of Anna Freud's
lifework: she was herself always a *Kinderfrau*, a person who took care of
other people's children—as an elementary school teacher, as a child

analyst, as surrogate mother to her nephews and the Burlingham children, as a director of nurseries and a clinic. It should be noted, however, that it is identification which is apparent here, not active taking of the mother figure as a love object, the "negative oedipus complex."

There may be some confirmation for this conjecture about identification with the *Kinderfrau* in the fact that Freud carefully noted in 1931 that "someone such as a nurse" can take the mother's place as chief feeder and washer. Similarly, in his 1933 essay, he speaks of the mother "and the figures of wet-nurses and foster-mothers that merge into her" (p. 118). But Freud does not comment on how multiple mothering can effect a little girl. On this count, it seems to me feasible to conjecture that Anna Freud's identification with the *Kinderfrau's* child care sustained a split: the *Kinderfrau* was the good mother, while Martha Freud, who was the mother of six children, not the caretaker for one, who was the disciplinarian, and who was later the rival for the father's attention, was the troublesome mother, the object of hostility. Of course, such a split could not have been total, and the love Anna Freud felt for her mother was obvious at the time of Martha Freud's death, when the intensely private Anna Freud mourned her openly—to the surprise of people familiar with their tensions. But even such mourning may have been tinged with regret that her mother was not the one with whom she could comfortably be a crying, needy child, be passive and taken care of. At least I suspect this to be the case from the fact that it was in the year of her mother's death that Anna Freud prepared for delivery (but never prepared for publication) a justly famous lecture called "Fear of Passivity."

My conjecture about this splitting or dividing of ambivalence seems to me to be supported very graphically by a similar split that was evident in the last year of Anna Freud's life, when she, the last living member of her immediate family, was reduced to a state of childlike dependency after a stroke. Then she had a stubborn, controlling, rigid caretaker to be angry with, to hate—her maid, Paula Fichtl—and a good one, a *Kinderfrau,* the former nursery school teacher Manna Friedmann, who kept her company, shared her knitting projects with her, enjoyed German songs and stories with her. Anna Freud, citing her loyalty to the maid, who had been with the family for half a century, refused to place her in a home; she kept Paula in the house and made herself and her good *Kinderfrau* miserable by doing so.

When Freud turned in "Female Sexuality" and the later essay "Femininity" to manifestations of intense and long mother love in adult female life, he offered an example that had been part of psychoanalytic observation for many years and that he had earlier written about in

"The Taboo of Virginity" (1918). Women often behave in their first marriages in a complex or layered way. They take a husband who is modeled on their fathers, but they replay with the husband the drama of their mother love, with all its passion and hostility, all its ambivalence. This is a particular instance of a general claim that the girl's mother love will be, in some form, carried into her adult object choices: she may vacillate between currents running from her mother love and currents running from her father love; she may return to her mother love after the disappointment of her father love (as Freud had suggested was the case with the female homosexual), and so forth.

In Anna Freud's case, there was no heterosexual later love. There was also no diminution of her father attachment—thus no return to a mother love current in a homosexual mode. It seems to me that what appeared was an equipoise reflected in the choice of a female companion, Dorothy Burlingham, a mother with four children, and the maintenance of the father attachment. As neither relationship was sexual, they did not conflict on that plane; this was, as it were, psychological bisexuality without physical sexuality. Such an arrangement, of course, would presuppose a great capacity for sublimation—but no one who knew Anna Freud had any question about her accomplishments as far as this psychic function was concerned, and her lifework stands as a monument to her capacities.

This conjecture, however, leaves many unanswered questions. Was there a period of active mother-figure love, a "negative oedipus complex," prior to the *Kinderfrau* identification? What became of the hostility directed toward her mother? Were there female objects of hostility other than Martha Freud (and perhaps Minna Bernays, as her mother's ally) and Paula Fichtl? Did the split between good and bad mother figures I have proposed have other manifestations, for example, in Anna Freud's work and in her work settings, her nurseries and clinics, where so many women joined her enterprises? How did the intellectual mother figures like Lou Andreas-Salomé fit into this scheme? Did Anna Freud mother her surrogate children in the *Kinderfrau* way or the mother way or some mixture of the two split-off ways or some reaction to the splitting off of ways?

These questions are hard enough, and they are not illuminated by any mention in Freud's texts on female psychology of friendships or animosities among adult females or of adult females' choices of profession or types of work—his texts are exclusively concerned with how heterosexual love and marriage are related to early childhood events. It is tempting, nonetheless, to read general passages of his essays with these questions in mind. For example: "A woman's identification with her mother allows us to distinguish two strata: the pre-Oedipus one which rests on her affectionate attachment to her mother and takes her as a model, and the later one from the Oedipus complex which seeks to get rid of her mother and take her place with her father" (1933, p. 134). In Anna Freud's case, as I am developing it, the difference is that the two strata seem to have been predominantly tied to two different mother figures.

But there are also other, quite specific passages in these late essays that are suggestive about Freud's—and Anna Freud's—view of her early development. For example, considering Anna Freud's long struggle with masturbation and beating fantasies, about which both father and daughter wrote, one can easily imagine her as the subject of his remarks in "Femininity" on a girl trying to free herself from masturbation:

> She does not always succeed in this. If envy for the penis has provoked a powerful impulse against clitoridal masturbation but this nevertheless refuses to give way, a violent struggle for liberation ensues in which the girl, as it were, herself takes over the role of her deposed mother and gives expression to her entire dissatisfaction with her inferior clitoris in her efforts against obtaining satisfaction from it. Many years later, when her masturbatory activity has long since been suppressed, an interest still persists which we must interpret as a defence against a temptation that is still dreaded. It manifests itself in the emergence of sympathy for those to whom similar difficulties are attributed [p. 127f.].

One can hardly imagine anyone in a better position to give sympathy to people struggling with masturbation conflicts than a child psychoanalyst, and one can hardly find a child psychoanalyst in whose work masturbation conflicts receive more attention than they do in Anna Freud's work.

III

I have now advanced a series of conjectures about the first years of Anna Freud's life and about her relations with her mothers. My technique has been to comb through Freud's essays looking for traces of Anna Freud's story and then to test the results against relationships, configurations, in her later life. As I have said repeatedly, the conclusions are only conjectures, and I did not include them in my biography because I really cannot prove—which in biography means document—them. Further, they have not produced what my vision of a neat merger of stories—Anna Freud's, her father's, psychoanalysis's—

promised: that the vague figure of Martha Freud would emerge. On the contrary, my conclusions reduce her to a function: the bad mother, the object of hostility. Similarly, the question I raised and left hanging about what Freud's changing views on female psychology have to say about Freud's own psychology has simply clouded over.

The impasse I have created could also easily be made more complicated by another standard psychobiographical strategy: a turn to the current literature. For example, with Anna Freud's case in mind, it is very instructive to look at the work of contemporary child analysts—heirs to Anna Freud's theory and practice of child analysis—on children with beating fantasies. Kerry and Jack Novick, in an article called "The Essence of Masochism" (1987), reported on their observations and analyses of a number of girls and boys with beating fantasies and compared their material, arranged along a developmental line, with adult cases. Being contemporaries, they, of course, give a good deal of attention to preoedipal mother-child relations, and they conclude, not surprisingly, that "descriptions of a mutual lack of pleasure on the part of mother and baby were universal in the fixed beating fantasy sample and have recurred in all our subsequent cases of masochistic pathology where social history data have been available" (p. 355). (But there is no mention of a case of multiple mothering.)

The Novicks note as common a great deal of aggressive behavior in their beating fantasy patients' toddler years—and this, too, is in line with Anna Freud's reputation in her family as a naughty child (her father's affectionate nickname for her was "Black Devil"), although she seems to have been really more saucy and impish than truly violent. The mothers of the Novicks' patients were generally unable to contain their children's aggression or to tolerate their messiness and anal play. This, too, accords with the impression one gets of Martha Freud and Minna Bernays, if not of Josefine. The episode of Anna Freud's appendectomy could very well be described with this observation from the Novicks' paper: "parents of patients with masochistic pathology seem unable to protect them from repeated exposure to overwhelming experiences." But the "repeated exposure" is a bit strong for the case, and the following claim about puberty and adolescence does not fit the case well at all, even though the result is similar: "The fathers of the girls continued and intensified their denigration of the mothers and actively involved themselves in overstimulating relationships with their daughters from the oedipal phase on, with the result that a component in the masochistic pathology of the females was intense bisexual conflict and severe penis envy" (p. 377).

Anna Freud, a child with a troika of mothers, fits some but certainly not all of the Novicks' mother-child generalizations. She was not the child, on the other hand, of either a remote, disinvolved father or an overstimulating one; she was the child of a loving, observant, concerned, but passionately preoccupied one. And, so, this route, too, of comparing child analytic clinical results with what little can be seen of Anna Freud's childhood leaves the biographer with more opportunities for "wild analysis" than sure narrative units.

IV

I have sketched three types of biographical bad lands: (1) the subject's writings run out and cease to give confirmation for hypotheses; (2) the contemporary documentation—in this case, Freud's essays—becomes teasing, suggestive, rather than sure; and (3) independent clinical generalizations, not concerned with the particular case, give a bit of confirmation mingled with a great number of mirages. In effect, I have just shown the essential difference between psychobiography and psychoanalysis. To put the matter very simply: in psychobiography there is no next session; one cannot wait for further associations, transference manifestations, or acting-out episodes to lead beyond an interpretative impasse—to show that at this point in the work I am right, wrong, or some mixture of right and wrong.

On the other hand, the matter can be put less despairingly: psychobiography is designed neither for therapy nor for theory (or metapsychology); these are not its purposes. A psychobiographical narrative unit is another sort of thing than an analytic reconstruction. In addition to the general outlines of a life, what we learn, I think, from psychobiography is something about the features of a life that are never clearly documented, which do not leave clear traces, which are not simply evidentiary. For female biographical subjects born before or near the turn of the century, these features have to do primarily, it seems to me, with the complexity of mothering—even though so many famous women have been very obviously deeply father-directed, in the mode of love, or of identification, or both.

In Anna Freud's case, the complexity is mysterious, but not, on the other hand, unusual in what might be called an extended-mothering bourgeois family. We might call to mind contemporaries of hers with similarly strong male identifications in relation to a single father figure who were similarly mothered by many women: Willa Cather, for example, or Gertrude Stein for another. Sorting out what contributions to the subject's psychology are made by each or any of the mothering figures is nearly impossible. Mothers and grandmothers and nurses merge; sisters and aunts slip generations; "role models" and ego ideals are indistinguishable. Speaking sociologically, one of the main reasons why Martha Freud is so vague a character in Freud biographies is that both before and after her marriage she was a woman embedded in an extended female domestic world, and such a world is very difficult to reconstruct beyond the level of social roles. At the level of who meant what to whom, there is mostly silence. Sigmund Freud's family was also, of course, a predominantly female, multigenerational one (with nurses) organized around a single father figure—and compounded by a complex mixture of Jewish traditions and freethinking elements. It was a family—like the one Martha and Sigmund Freud raised—in which it would not be difficult to name the boys' rival or the little girls' male love, but in which it would be much more difficult to sort out the mothers.

Methodologically, psychobiography has a great deal to learn from intrapsychically focused studies of families. And this learning needs to be added to what two decades of fine feminist scholarship has already revealed about how historical an institution motherhood is and how intricately patriarchal cultures shape both that institution and children's identities developing within it. But even feminist scholars have a tendency, when they turn to biography, to focus in on the mother-child dyad, and to isolate it from anything but the near-by oedipal triangle. Sibling groups, extended and multigenerational families fade away. The rest of childhood, the latency and preadolescent and adolescent years, with all their added complexity of new venues and new relationships, also tend to fade away in explanatory terms if not in narrative terms. Psychoanalytic family study is a book of reminders, a technique of question-posing. But from within the ranks of child psychoanalysts there are also, of course, people who pay particular attention to larger family contexts and full developmental lines—and Anna Freud was certainly foremost among these, and the one singly most influential on several generations of others.

What I learned from my interpretative impasse, the collapse of my dream of perfect biographical and historical order, was to pay more attention to my subject's range of vision: her ability to survey a full family network and to range over the whole of an individual's developmental course. My project became consistently to place the mystery of Anna Freud's mothering in that range. What I came to was a less spectacular but nonetheless satisfying sense of biographical and theoretical orderliness: the notion that the range in Anna Freud's thought had its debt precisely to her plural mothering.

BIBLIOGRAPHY

ABRAHAM, K. (1920). Manifestations of the female castration complex. *Selected Papers on Psycho-Analysis*. London: Hogarth Press, 1949, pp. 338–369.

CHODOROW, N. (1978). *The Reproduction of Mothering*. Berkeley: Univ. California Press.

FREUD, A. (1922). Beating fantasies and daydreams. *W.*, 1:137–157.

———(1936). The ego and the mechanisms of defense. *W.*, 2.

FREUD, S. (1900). The interpretation of dreams. *S.E.*, 4 & 5.

———(1905). Three essays on the theory of sexuality. *S.E.*, 7:125–243.

———(1918). The taboo of virginity. *S.E.*, 11: 191--208.

———(1919). 'A child is being beaten.' *S.E.*, 17:175–204.

———(1920a). The psychogenesis of a case of homosexuality in a woman. *S.E.*, 18:145–172.

———(1920b). Beyond the pleasure principle. *S.E.*, 18:3–64.

———(1923). The infantile genital organization. *S.E.*, 19:141–145.

———(1924). The dissolution of the oedipus complex. *S.E.*, 19:173–179.

———(1925). Some psychical consequences of the anatomical distinction between the sexes. *S.E.*, 19:243–258.

———(1931). Female sexuality. *S.E.*, 21:223–243.

———(1933). Femininity. *S.E.*, 22:112–135.

GAY, P. (1988). *Freud*. New York: Norton.

HORNEY, K. (1923). On the genesis of the castration complex in women. *Int. J. Psychoanal.*, 5:50–65, 1924.

JONES, E. (1953–57). *The Life and Work of Sigmund Freud*, 3 vols. New York: Basic Books.

KLEIN, M. (1948). *Contributions to Psycho-Analysis, 1921–1945*. London: Hogarth Press.

NOVICK, K. K. & NOVICK, J. (1987). The essence of masochism. *Psychoanal. Study Child*, 42:353–384.

Index